# FUNDAMENTALS OF HEALTHCARE MANAGEMENT

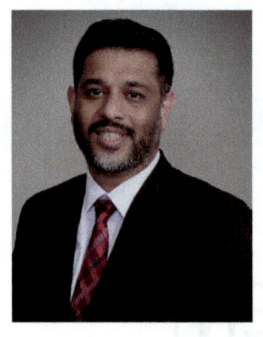

**Soumitra S. Bhuyan, PhD, MPH,** is the Executive Director of Health Administration Programs at the Edward J. Bloustein School of Planning and Public Policy at Rutgers—The State University of New Jersey in New Brunswick, New Jersey, United States. He has also held positions as a visiting research scholar at the Center for Health and Wellbeing, School of International and Public Affairs at Princeton University and at Deloitte's Center for Healthcare Solutions.

Dr. Bhuyan has authored over 50 publications in leading academic peer-reviewed journals and his commentary has been featured in national media outlets such as The Hill, ABC News, and Becker's Hospital Review. He is an Associate Editor of the *British Medical Journal Global Health* and serves on the editorial boards of the *Journal of Health Administration Education*, the flagship journal of the Association of University Programs in Health Administration and *Hospital Topics*. His work on women's health earned him the 2017 Charles E. Gibbs Leadership Prize, and he is also a recipient of the "Rising Star" award from the American Public Health Association's Health Administration Section. Additionally, Dr. Bhuyan is an accreditation fellow with the Commission on Accreditation of Healthcare Management Education (CAHME) and serves on its Standards Council. In 2025, Dr. Bhuyan was the recipient of the CAHME/Baldridge Foundation Award for Leadership Excellence for advancing the quality of healthcare management education.

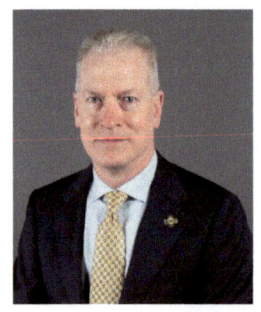

**Kevin D. Broom, PhD, MBA,** is the Vice Chair for Education and Director of the Master of Health Administration (MHA) Program in the Department of Health Policy and Management at the University of Pittsburgh, Pennsylvania, United States. He previously served as the Associate Director for graduate programs at Saint Louis University and the Army-Baylor University Graduate Program in Health and Business Administration.

Dr. Broom has published over 25 papers in prestigious academic journals and contributed to peer-reviewed textbook chapters. He has received accolades for his teaching and research excellence. Before embarking on his academic career, Dr. Broom completed a 23-year tenure in the Army Medical Department where he held roles including Professor, Financial Manager, Health Administrator, and Paramedic. His military service spanned various tactical healthcare delivery organizations and traditional hospitals within the Army's network. Dr. Broom is a Master Fellow at the Commission on Accreditation of Healthcare Management Education (CAHME), having previously served on its Accreditation Council and Candidacy Committee, and has instructed accreditation boot camps and master classes.

# FUNDAMENTALS OF HEALTHCARE MANAGEMENT

## Theory and Practice

*Soumitra S. Bhuyan,* PhD, MPH
*Kevin D. Broom,* PhD, MBA
Editors

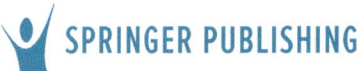

Copyright © 2026 Springer Publishing Company, LLC
All rights reserved.

No part of this publication may be reproduced, stored in a retrieval system, used for text and data mining, machine learning, artificial intelligence model training, or any other automated processing or analysis, or transmitted in any form or by any means, electronic, mechanical, photocopying, recording, or otherwise, without the prior permission of Springer Publishing Company, LLC, via our website at https://www.springerpub.com/permission-requests, or authorization through payment of the appropriate fees to the Copyright Clearance Center, Inc., 222 Rosewood Drive, Danvers, MA 01923, 978-750-8400, fax 978-646-8600, info@copyright.com or at www.copyright.com.

Springer Publishing Company, LLC
902 Carnegie Center/Suite 140, Princeton, NJ 08540
www.springerpub.com
connect.springerpub.com

*Acquisitions Editor*: David D'Addona
*Content Development Manager*: Lucia Gunzel
*Director, Production Project Manager*: Kris Parrish
*Compositor*: S4Carlisle Publishing Services

ISBN: 978-0-8261-4541-3
e-book ISBN: 978-0-8261-4542-0
DOI: 10.1891/9780826145420

**SUPPLEMENTS:**

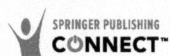 A robust set of instructor resources designed to supplement this text is located at http://connect.springerpub.com/content/book/978-0-8261-4542-0. Qualifying instructors may request access by emailing textbook@springerpub.com.

**Instructor Materials:**
*LMS Common Cartridge With All Instructor Resources ISBN*: 978-0-8261-5469-9
*Instructor's Manual ISBN*: 978-0-8261-4543-7
*Instructor Test Bank ISBN*: 978-0-8261-4546-8
*Instructor Chapter PowerPoints ISBN*: 978-0-8261-4544-4
*Instructor Sample Syllabus ISBN*: 978-0-8261-4539-0

25 26 27 28 / 5 4 3 2 1

Medicine is an ever-changing science. Research and clinical experience are continually expanding our knowledge, in particular our understanding of proper treatment and drug therapy. The authors, editors, and publisher have made every effort to ensure that all information in this book is in accordance with the state of knowledge at the time of production of the book. Nevertheless, the authors, editors, and publisher are not responsible for any errors or omissions or for any consequence from application of the information in this book and make no warranty, expressed or implied, with respect to the content of this publication. Every reader should examine carefully the package inserts accompanying each drug and should carefully check whether the dosage schedules therein or the contraindications stated by the manufacturer differ from the statements made in this book. Such examination is particularly important with drugs that are either rarely used or have been newly released on the market.

The work is provided, "as is," and the publisher disclaims any and all warranties, express or implied, including any warranties as to accuracy, comprehensiveness, or currency of the content of this work or any information that can be accessed through the work via a hyperlink or otherwise, the persistence and accuracy of which is hereby disclaimed. Neither the publisher nor its licensors shall be liable to you or anyone else for any inaccuracy, error or omission, regardless of cause, in the work or for any damages resulting therefrom.

Library of Congress Cataloging-in-Publication Data

Names: Bhuyan, Soumitra S. editor | Broom, Kevin D. editor
Title: Fundamentals of healthcare management : theory and practice /
  [edited by] Soumitra S. Bhuyan, PhD, MPH, Kevin D. Broom, PhD, MBA.
Description: Princeton, New Jersey : Springer Publishing Company, [2026] |
  Includes bibliographical references and index. |
Identifiers: LCCN 2025019614 (print) | LCCN 2025019615 (ebook) | ISBN
  9780826145413 paperback | ISBN 9780826145420 ebook
Subjects: LCSH: Health services administration—Textbooks
Classification: LCC RA394 .F86 2025 (print) | LCC RA394 (ebook)
LC record available at https://lccn.loc.gov/2025019614
LC ebook record available at https://lccn.loc.gov/2025019615

Contact sales@springerpub.com to receive discount rates on bulk purchases.

*Publisher's Note*: New and used products purchased from third-party sellers are not guaranteed for quality, authenticity, or access to any included digital components.

Printed in the United States of America by Gasch Printing.

*I dedicate this book to my mother, Swarnalata Bhuyan; my wife, Urmi Basu; and our two beloved furbabies, Lucy and Phisku. Without their unconditional love, patience, and support, this journey would not have been possible.*
—*Soumitra S. Bhuyan*

*First and foremost, I dedicate this book to my loving wife, Polly, whose love, support and encouragement have sustained me, both personally and professionally. I also dedicate this book to all my mentors, professional colleagues, and students who continually inspire me.*
—*Kevin D. Broom*

# CONTENTS

*Contributors  xi*
*Preface  xv*
*Acknowledgments  xix*
*Instructor Resources  xxi*

## SECTION I. SYSTEMS THINKING IN HEALTHCARE MANAGEMENT

1. **Systems Thinking in Healthcare**  3
   *Soumitra S. Bhuyan, Akash Rai, and Kevin D. Broom*

2. **Overview of Healthcare Organizations**  19
   *Patrick D. Shay and Anupam Lahiri*

3. **Managing the Healthcare Workforce**  29
   *Katherine A. Meese and Anthony Patterson*

4. **Health Economics**  43
   *Mark Bonica and Stephen Mihalacki*

5. **Organizational Design**  63
   *Soham Sengupta and Prabhat Singh*

6. **Public Health System in the United States**  73
   *Nizar K. Wehbi and Koshy Koshy*

7. **Introduction to Health Policy and Healthcare Reform**  85
   *Mark Bonica and Peter Wright*

8. **Community and Population Health Management**  99
   *Christopher E. Johnson, Thomas Walton, and Mary Curnutte*

9. **Case: Population/Community Health Improvement: Improving Maternal and Child Health in Rural America**  115
   *Rocco Gonzalez, Nathalie Occean, and Kashif Khan*

## SECTION II. HEALTHCARE MANAGEMENT: THEORIES AND APPLICATIONS

10. Strategic Planning    123
    *Nalin Johri and Kenneth M. Morris, Jr.*

11. Healthcare Financial Management    143
    *Kevin D. Broom and Joseph C. (Chris) Rheney*

12. Health Insurance and Reimbursement    157
    *Jason S. Turner and Angela L. Perri*

13. Human Resources Management    173
    *Dae Hyun "Daniel" Kim and William "Marty" M. Keith*

14. Quality and Performance Improvement in Healthcare    189
    *Jill Suzanne Fennimore and Diane Denny*

15. Project Management in Healthcare    215
    *Allen K. Solenberg, Jr. and Roie S. Rennert*

16. Healthcare Marketing    231
    *Steven W. Howard and Jacob S. Collins*

17. Healthcare Information Technology    241
    *Suzanne J. Paone and Ann Marie Evans*

18. Data Management and Analytics in Healthcare Management    255
    *Elizabeth K. McNutt and Bankole Olatosi*

19. Introduction to Healthcare Compliance    271
    *Tina Batra Hershey and Natalie C. Bulger*

20. Case: Healthcare Finance, Service Line Development, Health Outcome, and Quality Initiative    283
    *Laura Griffin, MariaRita Genovese, and Shashank Rao*

## SECTION III. LEADERSHIP THEORIES, APPLICATION, AND ACTIONS IN HEALTHCARE MANAGEMENT

21. Journey of a Healthcare Leader    291
    *William Tuttle and Patrick Grusenmeyer*

22. Leadership Theories and Applications in Healthcare Management    301
    *Lee Bewley and Matthew P. Ayers*

23. Healthcare Law and Ethics    317
    *Elizabeth Van Nostrand and Nicholas J. Barcellona*

24. **Crisis Management in Healthcare**   *329*
    *Aram Dobalian and Pete Brewster*

25. **Diversity, Equity, and Inclusion in Healthcare Management**   *343*
    *Ebbin Dotson, Darren Brownlee, and James E. Taylor*

26. **Leadership and Professional Performance**   *359*
    *Laurie Baedke and Natalie Lamberton*

27. **Case: A Leadership Dilemma: Navigating Culture Change in a Surgical Department**   *373*
    *Tiara Walz, Tiara Owens, and Lina Maria Alfonso*

*Glossary*   *379*
*Index*   *391*

# CONTRIBUTORS

**Lina Maria Alfonso, MHA**  Business Process/Quality Improvement Specialist, Columbia University Irving Medical Center, Vagelos College of Physicians and Surgeons, New York, New York

**Matthew P. Ayers, MBA**  Chief Administrative Officer, Norton Hospital at Norton Healthcare, Louisville, Kentucky

**Laurie Baedke, MHA, FACHE, FACMPE**  President and CEO, Growth Edge Leadership, Omaha, Nebraska

**Nicholas J. Barcellona, MBA**  Chief Financial Officer, WVU Medicine, Morgantown, West Virginia

**Lee Bewley, PhD, FACHE**  Associate Professor, Director, Health Management Programs, University of Louisville School of Public Health and Information Sciences, Louisville, Kentucky

**Soumitra S. Bhuyan, PhD, MPH**  Associate Professor, Edward J. Bloustein School of Planning & Public Policy, Rutgers, The State University of New Jersey, New Brunswick, New Jersey

**Mark Bonica, PhD, MBA**  Associate Professor, Health Management and Policy, University of New Hampshire, Durham, New Hampshire

**Pete Brewster, BS**  Program Manager for Strategic Planning and Quality, Office of Emergency Management, Veterans Health Administration, U.S. Department of Veterans Affairs, Martinsburg, West Virginia

**Kevin D. Broom, PhD, MBA**  Associate Professor, Health Policy and Management, School of Public Health, University of Pittsburgh, Pittsburgh, Pennsylvania

**Darren Brownlee, DrPH, MHA**  Senior Division Chair, Education at Mayo Clinic, Jacksonville, Florida

**Natalie C. Bulger, FACHE, CHC, MHA**  Former Director, VHA Risk Management, Office of Integrity and Compliance, Veterans Health Administration, Washington, DC; Former Director of Compliance, Risk, and Regulatory, The Children's Institute of Pittsburgh, Pittsburgh, Pennsylvania

**Jacob S. Collins, MS**  Associate Vice President for Enterprise Intelligence, Atrium Health, Pittsburgh, Pennsylvania

**Mary Curnutte, PhD, MS, RD, LD**  Department of Health Management and Systems Science, University of Louisville School of Public Health and Information Sciences, Louisville, Kentucky

**Diane Denny, DBA, MHA, CPXP, CPHQ, CPPS, FACHE, CSSGB**  Professor, Health Care Administration, Purdue University Global, West Lafayette, Indiana; Senior Associate Professor, Healthcare and Operations Management Concentrations, Jack Welch Management Institute, Herndon, Virginia

**Aram Dobalian, PhD, JD, MPH**  Associate Dean of Graduate Studies, Professor, and Division Chair of Health Services Management and Policy, The Ohio State University College of Public Health, Columbus, Ohio; Founding Director, Veterans Emergency Management Evaluation Center, Veterans Health Administration, U.S. Department of Veterans Affairs, North Hills, California

**Ebbin Dotson, PhD, MHSA**  Program Director, MPH Program, Department of Health Policy and Management, University of California Los Angeles Fielding School of Public Health, Los Angeles, California

**Ann Marie Evans, MBA**  Assistant Adjunct Faculty, College of Arts and Sciences, Carlow University, Pittsburgh, Pennsylvania

**Jill Suzanne Fennimore, MBA, PMP, MBB**  Lecturer, Master of Health Administration, Edward J. Bloustein School of Planning & Public Policy, Rutgers, The State University of New Jersey, New Brunswick, New Jersey

**MariaRita Genovese, MHA, CPC**  Director of Revenue Cycle and Business Operations, MD Anderson Cancer Center at Cooper University Hospital, Camden, New Jersey

**Rocco Gonzalez, MPH, CPH**  Community Health, Access, and Informatics Director; Mercy, Chesterfield, Missouri

**Laura Griffin, MHA**  Vice President Nursing Operations, ECU Health, Greenville, North Carolina; Adjunct Professor, Department of Health Policy and Management, University of Pittsburgh Graduate School of Public Health, Pittsburgh, Pennsylvania

**Patrick Grusenmeyer, ScD, FACHE**  Associate Professor, Department of Health Services Administration, University of Alabama at Birmingham (UAB), Birmingham, Alabama

**Tina Batra Hershey, JD, MPH**  Associate Professor, Health Policy and Management, University of Pittsburgh School of Public Health, Pittsburgh, Pennsylvania

**Steven W. Howard, PhD, MBA**  Associate Professor, Health Services Administration, The University of Alabama at Birmingham, School of Health Professions, Birmingham, Alabama

**Christopher E. Johnson, PhD**  Director, Institute of Health Administration, Robinson College of Business, Georgia State University, Atlanta, Georgia

**Nalin Johri, PhD, MPH, MA (Social Work)**  Program Director and Associate Professor, Masters of Healthcare Administration Program, School of Health and Medical Sciences, Seton Hall University, Nutleyz, New Jersey

**William "Marty" M. Keith, SPHR, SHRM-SCP**   Market Vice President, Human Resources, CommonSpirit Health, Lexington, Kentucky

**Kashif Khan, MHA**   Senior Consultant, Healthcare Strategy, Alvarez and Marsal, Washington, DC

**Dae Hyun "Daniel" Kim, PhD**   Assistant Professor, Health Management and Policy, Georgetown University School of Health, Washington, DC

**Koshy Koshy, PhD**   Associate Professor, Environmental and Occupational Health & Justice, Rutgers School of Public Health, Piscataway, New Jersey

**Anupam Lahiri, MBA, OTR, FACHE**   CEO, Select Specialty Hospital—West Tennessee, Jackson, Tennessee

**Natalie Lamberton, FACHE**   Chief Executive Officer, NDL Holdings, Denver, Colorado

**Elizabeth K. McNutt, MS, FACHE, PMP**   RWJBarnabas Health, System Strategy, West Orange, New Jersey

**Katherine A. Meese, PhD**   Faculty (Adjunct), Department of Health Services Administration, University of Alabama at Birmingham, Birmingham, Alabama

**Stephen Mihalacki, MBA PMP, FACHE**   Vice President, Network Strategy and Cost of Care, Magellan Health, Cranberry Township, Pennsylvania

**Kenneth M. Morris, Jr., MA, MHA**   Vice President External Affairs, St. Joseph's Health, Paterson, New Jersey

**Nathalie Occean, MHA, CPHQ**   Chief Operating Officer, MedHaul, Memphis, Tennessee

**Bankole Olatosi, PhD, MPH, MS, FACHE**   Associate Professor, Health Services Policy and Management, Arnold School of Public Health at the University of South Carolina, Columbia, South Carolina

**Tiara Owens, MHA**   Practice Administrator, Kids First Pediatric Group, Atlanta, Georgia

**Suzanne J. Paone, MBA, DHA, RHIA**   Associate Adjunct Faculty, School of Public Health, University of Pittsburgh, Pittsburgh, Pennsylvania

**Anthony Patterson, MSHA**   Assistant Professor and Associate Dean for Clinical Affairs and Strategy, University of Alabama at Birmingham, Birmingham, Alabama

**Angela L. Perri, MBA**   President, UPMC Medicare Products, UPMC Insurance Services Division; Adjunct Professor, University of Pittsburgh School of Public Health, Pittsburgh, Pennsylvania

**Akash Rai, MBBS, MHA**   Edward J. Bloustein School of Planning & Public Policy, Rutgers, The State University of New Jersey, New Brunswick, New Jersey

**Shashank Rao**  Senior Director of Healthcare and Life Sciences Strategy, EY-Parthenon, New York, New York

**Roie S. Rennert, MHA, PMP**  Senior Director, Special Projects, PRISM Vision Group, New Providence, New Jersey

**Joseph C. (Chris) Rheney, MHA, MBA, FACHE**  Healthcare Finance and Operations Executive, Federal and For-Profit Institutions, San Antonio, Texas

**Soham Sengupta, PhD, MIB, MS**  Assistant Professor, Jones College of Business, Middle Tennessee State University, Memphis, Tennessee

**Patrick D. Shay, PhD, MS**  Associate Professor, Department of Health Care Administration, Trinity University, San Antonio, Texas

**Prabhat Singh, MHA, MBBS**  Practice Management Consultant / Financial Analyst, InnovateUMD, Cullman, Alabama

**Allen K. Solenberg, Jr., PhD, CHFP**  MHA Program Director and Associate Professor, Health Administration and Health Policy, College of Public Health, UNT Health, Fort Worth, Texas

**James E. Taylor, PhD**  Chief Diversity, Inclusion, and Talent Management Officer, UPMC, Pittsburgh, Pennsylvania

**Jason S. Turner, PhD, MAE**  Professor, Department of Health Systems Management, Rush University, Chicago, Illinois

**William Tuttle, DSc, MHA, LFACHE**  Baptist Health Sciences University; School of Public Health at the University of Memphis; Memphis, Tennessee

**Elizabeth Van Nostrand, JD**  Associate Professor, Health Services Administration and Policy, College of Public Health, Temple University, Philadelphia, Pennsylvania

**Thomas Walton, MDiv, MS**  Executive in Residence, Department of Management and Systems Science, University of Louisville School of Public Health and Information Sciences, Louisville, Kentucky

**Tiara Walz, PhD**  Assistant Professor, Baylor University Graduate Program in Health Care and Business Administration, Baylor University, Waco, Texas

**Nizar K. Wehbi, MD, MPH, MBA**  Senior Health Administration Fellow, Edward J. Bloustein School of Planning & Public Policy, Rutgers University, New Brunswick, New Jersey

**Peter Wright, FACHE**  Chief Executive Officer, Northwestern Medical Center, St. Albans, Vermont

# PREFACE

Healthcare organizations are becoming increasingly complex. To improve operational efficiencies and promote equity in healthcare, healthcare managers must adopt a systems thinking approach to address both micro- and macro-level issues affecting these organizations. *Fundamentals of Healthcare Management: Theory and Practice* is a competency-driven textbook designed to build a solid foundation for acquiring the skills necessary to effectively manage 21st-century healthcare organizations while aligning with professional standards. This book focuses on a systems thinking perspective, emphasizing the interconnected elements that influence healthcare organizations, with the goal of improving both clinical outcomes and operational efficiencies. It integrates key theories of healthcare management with real-world applications, bridging the gap between theoretical understanding and professional practice.

Each chapter is coauthored by an academic and a practitioner, balancing theoretical rigor with practical application. Through this dyad authorship model, chapters introduce critical concepts, explore real-world scenarios, and help develop management competencies to address the challenges of a complex healthcare system. Each chapter also includes learning objectives, reflection questions, vignettes, and learning activities to foster participation and active learning. Additionally, the textbook features chapters on Project Management in Healthcare; Healthcare Compliance; Crisis Management in Healthcare; and Diversity, Equity, and Inclusion. The content is organized into three sections:

- Section I: Systems Thinking in Healthcare Management
- Section II: Healthcare Management: Theories and Applications
- Section III: Leadership Theories, Applications, and Actions in Healthcare Management

This comprehensive structure ensures a well-rounded exploration of the theoretical and practical dimensions of healthcare management, equipping readers with the knowledge and skills to navigate the complexities of modern healthcare organizations effectively.

## SECTION I. SYSTEMS THINKING IN HEALTHCARE MANAGEMENT

The first section establishes the foundation for understanding the complexity of the U.S. healthcare system. It underscores the importance of a systems thinking approach and the adaptive nature of the U.S. healthcare system, linking macro-level issues—such as health policy and reform, the public health system, and community health issues—to healthcare organizations.

- *Chapter 1: Systems Thinking in Healthcare* explores foundational theories of systems thinking, including tools, methodologies, applications, and key challenges to implementation in healthcare settings.
- *Chapter 2: Overview of Healthcare Organizations* provides an overview of the various types of healthcare organizations and their roles within the healthcare ecosystem, including acute care, nursing homes, and long-term care facilities.

- *Chapter 3: Managing the Healthcare Workforce* highlights the importance of a sustainable healthcare workforce in achieving the Quintuple Aim by focusing on recruitment, retention, and professional development.
- *Chapter 4: Health Economics* introduces core health economics concepts, emphasizing supply-demand dynamics and cost analysis in healthcare delivery.
- *Chapter 5: Organizational Design* examines organizational design theories in healthcare, highlighting how structure impacts efficiency and decision-making.
- *Chapter 6: Public Health System in the United States* discusses the core functions of public health, emphasizing disease prevention and health promotion through community-based approaches.
- *Chapter 7: Introduction to Health Policy and Healthcare Reform* reviews the principles of health policy development, the role of the U.S. federal government, and recent healthcare reform initiatives.
- *Chapter 8: Community and Population Health Management* explores health disparities and evolving strategies for population health and community management aimed at improving health outcomes.

## SECTION II. HEALTHCARE MANAGEMENT: THEORIES AND APPLICATIONS

This section focuses on the core management areas and strategies required for successfully operating a healthcare organization. It covers topics such as strategic planning, quality and performance improvement, financial management, healthcare marketing, information technology, compliance, and project management frameworks essential for healthcare operations.

- *Chapter 10: Strategic Planning* introduces strategic planning processes and tools critical for healthcare organizations, illustrating their role in overall organizational success.
- *Chapter 11: Healthcare Financial Management* discusses essential accounting concepts and financial principles needed for managing a healthcare organization.
- *Chapter 12: Health Insurance and Reimbursement* covers health insurance, payment models (from fee-for-service to value-based care), and the alignment of financial incentives to improve patient outcomes.
- *Chapter 13: Human Resources Management* examines workforce issues, employment laws, and the importance of fostering a diverse healthcare workforce.
- *Chapter 14: Quality and Performance Improvement in Healthcare* focuses on quality, patient safety, and performance measurement, introducing improvement tools and frameworks such as plan-do-check-act, Lean, change management, and Six Sigma and their role in enhancing healthcare delivery systems.
- *Chapter 15: Project Management in Healthcare* details the phases of healthcare project management and tools, including regulatory constraints and multidisciplinary coordination, while offering practical strategies.
- *Chapter 16: Healthcare Marketing* analyzes strategies for marketing health services, emphasizing market competition and patient engagement.
- *Chapter 17: Healthcare Information Technology* highlights the critical role of information systems in improving patient outcomes, addressing data interoperability, electronic health records, and telehealth.

- *Chapter 18: Data Management and Analytics in Healthcare Management* examines the significance of data analytics and tools for decision-making and operational management in healthcare.
- *Chapter 19: Introduction to Healthcare Compliance* discusses compliance issues in healthcare, focusing on regulations, ethics, and strategies for reducing fraud, waste, and abuse in healthcare organizations.

## SECTION III. LEADERSHIP THEORIES, APPLICATION, AND ACTIONS IN HEALTHCARE MANAGEMENT

The final section of the textbook highlights the leadership competencies essential for managing healthcare organizations effectively. The COVID-19 pandemic posed significant challenges for many healthcare organizations, and this section includes a chapter on crisis management to introduce students to emergency management, their roles during crises, and strategies for improving preparedness for future emergencies.

- *Chapter 21: Journey of a Healthcare Leader* explores the professional development journey of healthcare leaders, discussing essential attributes and the evolving leadership competencies required for success at different stages of their careers.
- *Chapter 22: Leadership Theories and Applications in Healthcare Management* reviews foundational leadership theories and their practical applications in the healthcare setting.
- *Chapter 23: Healthcare Law and Ethics* provides an overview of healthcare laws and ethical issues in decision-making, emphasizing patient rights, confidentiality, and legal compliance.
- *Chapter 24: Crisis Management in Healthcare* discusses the roles of leadership during a crisis, key strategies for effective communication, resource allocation, and ensuring the continuation of patient care.
- *Chapter 25: Diversity, Equity, and Inclusion in Healthcare Management* emphasizes the importance of building a diverse, equitable, and inclusive workforce and examines their impact on patient experiences and outcomes.
- *Chapter 26: Leadership and Professional Performance* focuses on key leadership principles in healthcare, including ethics, professionalism, and lifelong learning, with a specific focus on self-awareness and emotional intelligence.

The healthcare system is evolving rapidly and there is a growing need for competent and adaptable healthcare leaders who can make data-driven, informed, ethical, and impactful decisions. This book provides the foundation necessary to build out the knowledge base and to develop the skills necessary to become an effective change agent and drive meaningful improvements in the healthcare industry.

*Soumitra S. Bhuyan*
*Kevin D. Broom*

# ACKNOWLEDGMENTS

This first edition of *Fundamentals of Healthcare Management: Theory and Practice* is the result of a meaningful collaboration between academic scholars and health industry professionals, aiming to provide a foundational, engaging, and practical introduction to healthcare management. We are deeply grateful to the many individuals and institutions whose support made this book possible.

We extend our heartfelt gratitude to the contributing authors whose valuable expertise, diverse perspectives, and dedication have significantly enriched this volume. Their insights have ensured that the content remains relevant, insightful, and beneficial for readers. Our sincere appreciation also goes to our colleagues, mentors, and students for their thoughtful input, constructive feedback, and intellectual curiosity. Your contributions have been instrumental in shaping the ideas and approaches presented in this text.

Special thanks are due to our editorial team at Springer Publishing Company, whose guidance, patience, and meticulous oversight were critical to the successful completion of this project. We also thank the administrative staff and technical editors for handling the publication process with exceptional professionalism and attention to detail. We gratefully acknowledge Rutgers University and the University of Pittsburgh for providing stimulating academic environments, supportive resources, and the encouragement necessary to see this book to completion.

Finally, we recognize the broader community of scholars, practitioners, students, and readers whose ongoing pursuit of knowledge inspires continuous growth in the field of healthcare management. We sincerely hope this book serves as a valuable resource and inspires future leaders to achieve success in their careers.

# INSTRUCTOR RESOURCES

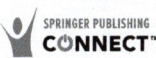 A robust set of instructor resources designed to supplement this text is located at http://connect.springerpub.com/content/book/978-0-8261-4542-0. Qualifying instructors may request access by emailing **textbook@springerpub.com**.

Available resources include:

- LMS Common Cartridge With All Instructor Resources and Instructions for Use
- Instructor's Manual
- Instructor Test Bank
- Instructor Chapter PowerPoints
- Instructor Sample Syllabus

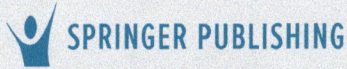

Visit https://connect.springerpub.com and look for the **"Show Supplementary"** button on the book homepage.

# SECTION I: SYSTEMS THINKING IN HEALTHCARE MANAGEMENT

# CHAPTER 1

# SYSTEMS THINKING IN HEALTHCARE

Soumitra S. Bhuyan, Akash Rai, and Kevin D. Broom

## LEARNING OBJECTIVES

- Define and apply systems thinking in healthcare as a complex adaptive system.
- Explore theoretical foundations of systems thinking and application to healthcare.
- Utilize systems thinking tools to drive improvement in healthcare delivery.
- Identify the challenges related to applying system thinking principles for health systems improvement.
- Understand the role of emerging technologies in system thinking in healthcare.

## KEY TERMS

- Causality
- Causal loop diagram
- Chaos theory
- Complex adaptive system
- Cynefin framework
- Feedback loop
- Healthcare quality
- Interconnectedness
- Network theory
- Systems thinking

## INTRODUCTION

Healthcare is a complex adaptive system characterized by a dynamic network of interdependent components, including hospitals, clinics, providers, patients, and stakeholders. These components interact and connect, adapting to external environmental demands for resources in nonlinear and often unpredictable ways. Due to these inherent complexities, a holistic approach is essential to understanding healthcare systems.

The term **systems thinking** was first introduced in 1987 by Barry Richmond, a pioneer in system dynamics. Richmond defines systems thinking as "the art and science of making reliable inferences about behavior by developing understanding of the underlying structure" (Richmond, 1994). Systems thinking provides a framework for examining interrelationships among components rather than focusing solely on isolated elements. It emphasizes recognizing patterns of change rather than static snapshots (Senge, 1990).

A more contemporary definition by Arnold and Wade (2015) describes systems thinking as "a set of synergistic analytic skills used to improve the capability of identifying and understanding systems, predicting their behaviors, and devising modifications to them in order to produce desired effects." Simply put, systems thinking views problems as interconnected parts of a broader dynamic system. This approach prioritizes understanding the relationships, interactions, and interdependencies among components that contribute to a system's behavior (World Health Organization, n.d.).

Healthcare leaders are increasingly considering factors beyond the individual patient or healthcare system when developing interventions and policies aimed at improving population and community health. Research estimates that hospital care accounts for only 10% to 20% of health outcomes, while the remaining 80% to 90% is influenced by social determinants of health—factors such as socioeconomic conditions, physical environments, and individual behaviors (Tan et al., 2005). Systems thinking helps leaders and clinicians explore the linkages and interactions among individual, community, and systemic factors, facilitating solutions that address the structural dynamics of these challenges (Peters, 2014).

Healthcare leaders must critically examine inefficiencies in existing systems to identify the root causes of organizational problems. Examples of systems thinking in healthcare include (a) Evaluating social, cultural, and emotional factors that influence a patient's health to optimize treatment plans; (b) enhancing healthcare quality by integrating treatment plans across specialties, primary care, and emergency care services; and (c) leveraging demographic, healthcare utilization, and disease data to improve population health and community services (Peters, 2014; Xia et al., 2017).

In recent years, systems thinking has gained widespread recognition in healthcare. A study revealed that 75% of healthcare stakeholders have adopted systems thinking to address organizational challenges, underscoring its growing importance in tackling the complexities of modern healthcare systems (Rocio et al., 2023).

## FOUNDATIONS OF SYSTEMS THINKING

The foundational concepts of interconnectedness, synthesis, emergence, feedback loops, causality, and systems mapping are vital to understanding how independent agents within healthcare organizations interact and influence each other in their environment.

**Interconnectedness** refers to how various elements within a healthcare system are linked and impact one another in the real world. Healthcare leaders must shift from a linear to a circular thinking mindset, acknowledging the interconnected nature of health systems where one action often depends on—or influences—a combination of factors to function effectively. By embracing this principle, leaders can better understand the benefits and pitfalls of decisions within their immediate environment and anticipate the ripple effects of changes throughout the broader system (Segal, 2020).

For example, consider the impact of an ED or hospital closure in a local area. A recent study analyzed how such closures or openings affect nearby hospitals. The findings revealed that ED closures increased driving time to the nearest alternative by at least 30 minutes. Moreover, the 1-year mortality rate and 30-day readmission rates for heart attack patients at crowded hospitals rose significantly due to the closure of a nearby ED (Hsia & Shen, 2019). Similarly, healthcare organizations are adopting a team-based approach that includes clinician and nonclinical caregivers to address unmet nonmedical needs—such as transportation, housing, and food—when caring for individuals without high medical and social needs. This holistic approach recognizes that addressing social determinants of health is as critical as providing medical care.

The growing population of patients with multiple chronic conditions underscores the importance of interconnectedness across medical specialties. Currently, one in three American adults and four in five Medicare beneficiaries live with multiple chronic illnesses (Bierman et al., 2021). Effective management of such patients requires coordinated input from various specialists. For instance, treating a patient with diabetes and hypertension necessitates collaboration among a primary care provider, cardiologist, endocrinologist, nutritionist, and others. This coordinated, interdisciplinary approach ensures holistic and integrated treatment plans, ultimately improving patient outcomes (Zmed Solutions, 2024).

*Synthesis* is the process of combining two or more components to create something new, offering a better understanding of the system compared to its individual parts. Healthcare leaders and clinicians can analyze these components and their interactions to understand how they collectively contribute to the functioning of the system.

For example, healthcare providers use electronic health record (EHR) systems to access patients' clinical and demographic information for treatment. A specialist may review notes from a primary care provider to make recommendations for preventive care, such as screenings and vaccinations. Additionally, an increasing number of hospitals are collecting social determinants of health data during patient admissions, enabling providers to gain a holistic understanding of patients' medical and social needs (Davis et al., 2023).

Another example of synthesis is the use of evidence-based practice guidelines by clinicians to treat patients. These guidelines are developed by synthesizing information from multiple resources. For instance, a surgeon treating a patient with prostate cancer might evaluate various treatment options, including active surveillance, while considering the patient's preferences. By integrating these diverse elements, the clinician can develop a patient-centered care plan tailored to the individual's needs.

*Emergence* describes how complex behaviors or patterns arise from the interactions between different components within a system, resulting in new phenomena that are distinct from the individual components. For example, in recent years, many patients have begun receiving behavioral healthcare in primary care settings. This collaborative care model exemplifies the emergence of a new model of care, as it integrates two distinct specialties—primary care and behavioral health. Since a significant number of patients with chronic health conditions also experience mental health issues, this model has led to improved patient outcomes by addressing both physical and mental health needs in a cohesive manner (Reising et al., 2023). Similarly, during the COVID-19 pandemic, various systems—including hospitals, pharmaceutical companies, emergency services, and public health and government organizations—coordinated efforts to increase vaccination rates and curb the spread of the virus (Filip et al., 2022). These collaborations demonstrated emergence by enabling faster responses, quicker decision-making, efficient resource allocation, and improved information sharing. The interplay between these systems created a collective impact far greater than the sum of their individual efforts.

**Feedback loops** refer to the mechanisms through which a system responds to changes. A key characteristic of feedback loops is that the output of one cycle becomes the input for the next cycle. Healthcare systems routinely use feedback loops to implement quality improvement initiatives.

For instance, healthcare organizations often survey patients to gather feedback after visits. This real-time data is then used to make adjustments and improvements to ensure continuity of care. Similarly, clinical and nonclinical staff regularly provide feedback to enhance the overall patient experience. For example, a hospital aiming to reduce medical errors during surgical procedures might collect information from surgeons about their practice patterns and error rates. This feedback is then analyzed and shared to identify areas for improvement.

There are two major types of feedback loops: reinforcing loops and balancing loops. In a reinforcing loop, elements of the system amplify or strengthen each other. A good example of this is the vaccination drive during the COVID-19 pandemic. As vaccination rates increased, infection and death rates declined, reducing the burden on hospital systems. This, in turn, reinforced public confidence in vaccination programs, leading to further participation and higher vaccination rates.

In contrast, a balancing loop works to bring a system back into equilibrium. For example, when patient loads increase, healthcare systems may hire additional clinical and nonclinical staff or allocate more resources to manage the demand. These actions help restore balance to the system by addressing the increased workload.

*Causality* illustrates how system behaviors may not always follow linear cause-and-effect relationships. It sheds light on how one factor influences another in the context of a complex, dynamic, and constantly evolving healthcare system. In a complex healthcare system where components are interdependent, it can be challenging to identify a single variable responsible for a particular phenomenon. For example, implementing quality improvement projects in healthcare often faces numerous challenges. Variables such as organizational factors, interprofessional frictions, employee training, work experience, workload, teamwork, and motivation can all influence the outcomes. Pinpointing the most significant barrier among these factors can be difficult due to their interconnected nature.

Another example is hospitals working to reduce 30-day readmission rates following patient discharge. Several factors contribute to readmissions, including poor quality of care, inadequate discharge planning, medication nonadherence, and insufficient social or family support to help patients manage their health (Dhaliwal & Dang, 2024). These interconnected variables make it difficult for hospitals to isolate a single cause responsible for readmissions, as the outcome is often influenced by the interaction of multiple factors.

*Systems mapping* is the visual representation of the components within a system and their interrelationships. It is a crucial tool for systems thinkers, enabling them to identify and map the elements of a system to understand how these elements interact, relate, and behave within a complex framework. Systems mapping provides unique insights to inform decision-making and facilitate shifts that can lead to significant changes in the system in an efficient manner.

The systems mapping process involves several steps. The first step is to define the purpose, such as improving quality, enhancing patient engagement, or increasing provider satisfaction. This purpose serves as the foundation for developing the map. The next step is to gain a clear understanding of the current state of the system. This can be achieved through research or by engaging with system experts who possess in-depth knowledge of its components and processes.

Key elements to include in the map are as follows:

- *Providers*: Organizations such as hospitals, clinics, and other facilities that deliver care
- *Key stakeholders:* Entities like government agencies, health insurance providers, advocacy groups, and social support organizations
- *Services:* Different types of services provided, such as treatments, surgeries, and specialized programs
- *Patient pathways:* Entry points into the system and the flow of patients through various services
- *Policies and regulations:* Frameworks and locations associated with processes like medication-assisted treatments

- *Service interventions:* Locations where changes are tested, or new capacities are introduced
- *Gaps:* Unaddressed or undefined areas identified by stakeholders that need attention

This structured approach enables a comprehensive understanding of the system as it currently exists, which in turn supports targeted improvements and effective planning (Healthcare Improvement Scotland, 2023).

## THEORIES OF SYSTEMS THINKING

Systems thinking relies on several theories to understand and manage complex systems, each offering unique perspectives. Chaos theory, network theory, and adaptive systems theory are particularly valuable for analyzing the dynamics of complex systems. These theories provide frameworks to interpret intricate interactions, emergent behaviors, and unpredictable patterns within such systems.

### CHAOS THEORY

Proposed by Edward Lorenz, a meteorologist at Massachusetts Institute of Technology in the 1960s, *chaos theory* emerged from his work with equations predicting weather patterns (Oestreicher, 2007). This theory helps explain feedback loops in nonlinear systems, where events or processes appear random due to the lack of clear underlying causes. Key principles include the butterfly effect, which illustrates how small changes in initial conditions can lead to significant and unpredictable outcomes. For example, a butterfly flapping its wings in one region might trigger a hurricane in another (Jesmi et al., 2020).

Accurately predicting chaotic systems requires a complete understanding of initial conditions, which is often unattainable. The COVID-19 pandemic exemplifies chaos theory principles. It displayed sensitivity to initial conditions, with its trajectory varying across regions depending on factors such as the timing of the first case, public health responses, population density, and mobility patterns. The pandemic's spread was nonlinear and unpredictable, characterized by sudden case spikes and varied transmission rates, complicating forecasts. It involved complex system dynamics, influenced by the interplay of biological, behavioral, environmental, and socio-economic factors, creating an unpredictable system. Feedback loops were evident in interventions like lockdowns, social distancing, and mask mandates, where the measures' effectiveness influenced the pandemic's progression and, in turn, public behaviors and policies. Furthermore, the spread reflected fractal patterns—local transmission dynamics mirrored broader regional and global trends. The pandemic operated on the edge of chaos, with sudden shifts, such as the emergence of new variants or outbreak clusters, triggering phase transitions that altered its dynamics unpredictably (Calistri et al., 2024).

### NETWORK THEORY

*Network theory* explores the connections between discrete objects and the nature of their interactions. Widely used in systems thinking, this theory is vital for understanding the complex relationships between agents, particularly when introducing technology-driven innovations in healthcare. The availability of extensive data sources and advancements in data science make it possible to leverage network theory to analyze complex relationships, such as interpreting healthcare big data and assessing the effectiveness of public health interventions.

In healthcare, network theory has diverse applications. It aids in analyzing disease transmission patterns, optimizing resource allocation, and designing care delivery pathways. It also informs decision-making processes, helping to explain the implementation of health policies and the adaptability of health systems in changing environments. Additionally, network theory supports processes such as data sharing, improving treatment protocols, resource sharing, and collaborative research across healthcare participants. By identifying and understanding the relationships between these elements, network theory contributes to more effective healthcare systems and interventions.

## ADAPTIVE SYSTEMS THEORY

Adaptive systems theory, also known as **complex adaptive systems** (CAS) theory, describes systems as complex, self-organizing, and unpredictable, characterized by numerous interactions among individual parts. Drawing on game theory in economics, CAS explores how interactions between these parts can result in cooperation or competition. Healthcare teams are often examples of CAS.

In CAS, the smallest components, known as agents, are individual units capable of producing a response to a given stimulus. These agents interact within homogeneous or heterogeneous groups, engaging in limited interactions that collectively yield outcomes comparable to the sum of all potential interactions. When agents combine to produce emergent behaviors, the process is called aggregation, and the resulting entities are referred to as aggregate agents. These aggregate agents can interact further to form broader systems with richer behaviors and interactions.

CAS theory offers a valuable framework for addressing challenges in healthcare and other fields. For example, its principles can be applied to healthcare research and planning to address chronic diseases and lifestyle-related health issues. By viewing patients and healthcare organizations as CAS, providers can better understand the dynamic interactions between factors influencing disease progression and treatment outcomes. CAS theory thus enables the development of more effective healthcare strategies that account for the intricacies of human systems.

## CYNEFIN FRAMEWORK: DECISION-MAKING IN A COMPLEX SYSTEM

The *Cynefin framework*, developed by David J. Snowden in 1999, helps leaders recognize that every situation is unique and requires a tailored approach for effective decision-making. This tool enables more accurate assessment of situations and appropriate responses by categorizing scenarios into five domains based on cause-and-effect relationships: simple, complicated, complex, chaotic, and disorder.

*Simple:* Also referred to as "clear" or "obvious," the simple domain involves situations where cause-and-effect relationships are stable, evident, and predictable. Solutions are straightforward, and standard operating procedures are typically sufficient. In healthcare, tasks such as routine patient check-ins, administering vaccinations, or following established infection control protocols fall within this domain.

*Complicated:* In the complicated domain, problems have multiple possible solutions, and while cause-and-effect relationships exist, they may not be immediately obvious and require expert analysis. This domain often requires specialized knowledge or consultation with experts to determine the best approach. For instance, developing a treatment plan for a patient with multiple chronic conditions may fall into this category. These situations demand critical thinking and expertise to navigate effectively.

*Complex:* The complex domain deals with "unknowns," where there is insufficient data or evidence to determine cause-and-effect relationships. Solutions emerge through experimentation, observation, and adaptability rather than predefined procedures, for example, responding to a novel infectious disease outbreak, like the early stages of the COVID-19 pandemic, where the virus' characteristics, transmission methods, and effective treatments were initially unclear. In these scenarios, healthcare teams must experiment and adapt to evolving information.

*Chaotic:* Chaotic situations occur when there is no clear cause-and-effect relationship, and events are out of control. The primary goal in this domain is to stabilize the situation and restore order before transitioning to the complex domain for further assessment and resolution. Crisis management in healthcare, such as responding to a mass casualty event or handling an acute outbreak of a highly contagious disease, will fall into this domain.

*Disorder:* The disorder domain applies when it is unclear which of the other four domains the situation belongs to. This occurs when there is confusion about how to interpret a situation or which approach to use. In a healthcare organization, disorder may arise when conflicting information from different departments or experts delays decision-making. The goal in this domain is to understand the problem better and break it down into smaller components that can be categorized into the appropriate domains for resolution.

## SYSTEMS THINKING TOOLS

Systems thinkers employ a variety of tools to analyze and improve the performance of complex systems (Table 1.1). The following are three key tools widely used in this approach:

**TABLE 1.1. SYSTEMS THINKING TOOLS AND APPLICATION IN HEALTHCARE**

| TOOL | DEFINITION/USE | APPLICATION IN HEALTHCARE |
| --- | --- | --- |
| Causal loop diagrams | Visual representation of cause-and-effect relationships | Understanding complex interactions in healthcare systems |
| Stock and flow diagrams | Illustrates the flow of resources within a system | Modeling resource allocation in healthcare facilities |
| Process mapping | Visual representation of workflow processes | Identifying inefficiencies in healthcare workflows |

*Causal loop diagrams:* **Causal loop diagrams** (CLDs) help in understanding the mechanisms or actions driving system behaviors. They illustrate feedback—interactions between system elements resulting in cause-and-effect behavior cycles—and loops, which are the cyclical patterns of behavior within the system. These diagrams highlight desirable and undesirable behaviors and can identify spillover effects from interventions or actions that lead to unintended outcomes (Sustainability Methods, n.d.).

CLDs have diverse applications in health systems research and policy. They can inform the design of health interventions or policies and guide the development of a theory of change for evaluation. They are also valuable for identifying risks to future programs, enabling course corrections during implementation. CLDs help in understanding the underlying mechanisms of health system behavior and identifying leverage points to optimize system performance. Additionally, they can be used to study how policy implementation evolves over time and why certain health policies succeed or fail. CLDs have also proven useful in analyzing health systems' responses to shocks or disruptions and identifying factors that foster system resilience, specifically in terms of absorptive, adaptive, and transformative capabilities (Baugh Littlejohns et al., 2018).

*Stock and flow diagrams:* Stock and flow diagrams visualize the interconnectedness of various elements within a system, such as customer interactions, service delivery processes, or data flows. These diagrams include two main components:

- *Stocks:* Quantities or collections within the system, such as population, inventory, or money.
- *Flows:* Rates of change affecting the stocks, like income, births, or sales.

These components are connected through valves or converters, representing the variables that influence flows. For example, the amount of water in a bathtub (stock) is affected by the flow of water from the faucet and the drain, which are controlled by valves.

Stock and flow diagrams are widely used across disciplines such as economics, environmental sciences, and social systems analysis. In healthcare, they are instrumental in modeling patient flows through healthcare facilities, tracking medical supply distribution, and assessing policy impacts on population health outcomes. These diagrams help stakeholders visualize complex systems with feedback loops, providing insights into how stocks and flows interact and affect overall system behavior.

*Process mapping:* Process mapping is a systems thinking tool designed to understand, evaluate, and optimize processes within complex systems. It promotes collective thinking, improves communication among stakeholders, and visualizes system inefficiencies or design flaws that hinder performance. Process mapping tools include flow diagrams, closed-loop diagrams, and others.

This tool has numerous applications in healthcare and other fields. For instance, process mapping can be used to visualize the patient journey, redesign healthcare procedures to enhance efficiency, and improve service delivery. It has also been used to assess how point-of-care testing for diseases such as tuberculosis and HIV affects care delivery in large urban healthcare clinics (Durski et al., 2020). By clarifying stakeholder relationships and identifying bottlenecks, process mapping supports the optimization of healthcare systems and processes.

## METHODS/MODELS OF SYSTEMS THINKING

Systems thinking employs various methods and models to analyze and understand complex systems (Table 1.2). The following are key approaches that provide valuable insights and strategies:

**TABLE 1.2. METHODS/MODELS OF SYSTEMS THINKING**

| METHOD | DEFINITION/USE | APPLICATION IN HEALTHCARE |
| --- | --- | --- |
| Systems dynamics modeling | Analyzing the dynamic behavior of complex systems | Understanding healthcare system responses to changes |
| Agent-based modeling | Simulation modeling of interactions between agents | Studying patient flows and disease spread in populations |
| Scenario planning | Anticipating future scenarios and planning | Planning for healthcare resource allocation and demand |
| Collaborative decision-making processes | Collective problem-solving and decision-making | Enhancing interdisciplinary collaboration in healthcare |

*Systems dynamics modeling:* Systems dynamics modeling (SDM) utilizes tools to identify and analyze the behavior of complex systems over time (Azar, 2012). This approach focuses on concepts like stocks, flows, and feedback loops. It addresses the challenge of simultaneity by adjusting variables over small time increments, while allowing for feedback, interactions, and delays. Common tools used in SDM include CLD and stock and flow diagrams.

SDM is widely applied across various fields, including healthcare. For instance, it is used to simulate patient flow in hospitals, predict the outcomes of different treatment strategies, and evaluate healthcare policies. Specifically, SDM can model disease spread, assess the effectiveness of vaccination programs, and optimize resource allocation in healthcare facilities (Rwashana & Williams, 2008).

*Agent-based modeling:* Agent-based modeling (ABM) is a method for studying interactions among individuals, entities, environments, and time. In ABM, a system is modeled as a collection of autonomous decision-making units called agents. Each agent operates based on a set of programmed rules, analyzing its situation and making decisions accordingly. Agents may simulate behaviors such as producing, consuming, or selling.

ABM differs from SDM in that it explores systems where individual agents are interdependent, with feedback loops in causal mechanisms. It also allows for modeling hypothetical scenarios that might be impractical or unethical to conduct in real life (Bonabeau, 2002). ABM has been applied in areas such as studying the interactions between fly populations, climate, and the environment. In healthcare, ABM can model dynamic patient or healthcare worker activities that other simulation tools may not accommodate effectively.

*Scenario planning:* Scenario planning is a strategic method that uses tools to identify and evaluate potential future events and their alternative outcomes. It involves both quantitative projections and qualitative assessments. The primary value lies in learning from the planning process rather than solely focusing on the final scenarios. Scenario planning organizes perceptions of how future events might unfold and guides strategic decision-making to ensure success in uncertain contexts.

Applications of scenario planning include developing sustainable long-term strategies, making informed decisions under uncertainty, fostering flexible and creative thinking within organizations, and aligning stakeholders toward a shared vision. In healthcare, scenario planning can assist organizations in strategizing responses to complex challenges like resource allocation, patient care delivery, healthcare innovation, and policy development (Rawson et al., 2023).

*Collaborative decision-making processes:* Collaborative decision-making is a systematic approach in which multiple stakeholders work together to make decisions. This process seeks to find optimal solutions for the group while valuing the contributions of each participant. Collaborative decision-making builds trust, improves team dynamics, enhances communication, and ensures transparency in decision-making.

In healthcare, where decisions directly affect patient outcomes, collaborative approaches among providers, patients, caregivers, and other stakeholders lead to more effective care plans, increased patient satisfaction, and improved health outcomes. From selecting treatment options to designing care management strategies, collaborative decision-making incorporates the expertise, preferences, and concerns of all entities, resulting in more informed and integrated decisions (Bendowska & Baum, 2023).

## CHALLENGES AND LIMITATIONS OF ADOPTING SYSTEMS THINKING IN HEALTHCARE

Systems thinking is a powerful approach that acknowledges organizational and societal capacities while emphasizing multidisciplinary collaboration and teamwork. However, its implementation in healthcare faces several challenges.

*Resistance to change:* Resistance to change is a significant obstacle when introducing systems thinking in healthcare. This resistance arises from individual, interpersonal, and organizational factors.

At the individual level, healthcare professionals may resist due to negative attitudes, fear, uncertainty, or reluctance to abandon established habits. At the interpersonal level, communication challenges, cultural differences, and peer influence can deter change acceptance. At the organizational level, structural barriers like insufficient resources, lack of participatory management, and inadequate support impede progress (Cheraghi et al., 2023).

In healthcare education, resistance to enhancing traditional models hinders the adoption of systems thinking. Strategies like fostering inclusive, forward-thinking environments and showcasing tangible benefits can mitigate these barriers (Jones & Bartlett Learning, 2024).

*Data complexity and availability:* The healthcare sector generates nearly 30% of the world's data (RBC Capital Markets, n.d.), encompassing diverse formats like electronic records, medical imaging, and visual content. Managing this vast volume presents storage challenges and security risks. Complex data relationships hinder understanding of true cause-effect dynamics within systems, limiting the effectiveness of systems thinking models and resulting in inefficiencies in mapping system behaviors.

*Stakeholder engagement:* Effective stakeholder engagement is critical yet challenging in healthcare systems thinking. Fragmented health systems often force stakeholders to operate in silos, limiting collaboration and integration across healthcare components. The lack of participatory management and insufficient involvement of key stakeholders can result in implementation failures and reduce the impact of systems-thinking initiatives.

*Ethical considerations:* Ethical considerations in systems thinking involve navigating interconnected relationships while ensuring equitable access and resource distribution. Healthcare organizations must balance operational needs with moral obligations to patients and providers, addressing equity, fairness, and inclusivity in their systems-thinking approaches.

# FUTURE DIRECTIONS

## INTEGRATION OF ARTIFICIAL INTELLIGENCE AND MACHINE LEARNING

Artificial intelligence (AI) and machine learning are transforming healthcare systems by enhancing decision-making processes. AI can simulate individual agent behaviors and model collective emergent properties, providing insights into complex systems. In healthcare education, AI tools help students anticipate system behaviors and conduct scenario analysis using complex data sets (Jones & Bartlett Learning, 2024). A Canadian study on AI integration in healthcare highlights the importance of supportive organizational culture, transparent leadership, and bridging technical and clinical domains. However, barriers such as insufficient real-world evidence, misaligned processes, and a lack of governance frameworks persist (Alami et al., 2024).

## BIG DATA ANALYTICS AND PREDICTIVE MODELING

Predictive analytics is enabling healthcare organizations to transition from reactive to proactive care. By analyzing patterns in patient data, predictive models can identify individuals at risk of adverse outcomes, optimize treatment plans, and anticipate disease progression (Alowais et al. 2023). In medical education, data analytics equips students to interpret complex healthcare patterns and correlations (Jones & Bartlett Learning, 2024).

## EXPANSION OF SYSTEMS THINKING IN HEALTHCARE EDUCATION

As healthcare evolves, education systems must adapt to teach systems-thinking competencies. Accrediting bodies like the Quality and Safety Education for Nurses (QSEN) and public health institutions have integrated systems thinking into core curricula (Dolansky & Moore, 2013). Modern healthcare demands graduates who understand collaborative care, informatics, and group dynamics (Clark & Hoffman, 2019). Educational strategies such as case studies, interactive simulations, systems mapping workshops, and interdisciplinary collaboration are effective in developing systems-thinking skills (Jones & Bartlett Learning, 2024).

## EMERGING RESEARCH AREAS

Research is increasingly focused on integrating AI and machine learning to model complex systems. Immersive simulations are emerging as a critical trend, allowing learners to navigate real-time healthcare scenarios and apply systems-thinking principles effectively (Yahya et al., 2024).

## CASE STUDY 1.1: TRANSFORMING HEALTHCARE DELIVERY THROUGH SYSTEMS THINKING

### BACKGROUND

Good Health Community Hospital (GHCH), a 250-bed hospital located on the East Coast of the United States, has been experiencing increasing challenges in recent years. The ED was facing numerous issues, including overcrowding, poor resource allocation, and declining patient satisfaction ratings. Following the COVID-19 pandemic, staff burnout and turnover rates, especially among nurses and doctors, reached record levels. A recent outbreak of a new infectious disease further exacerbated these problems, pushing the system to its breaking point. To tackle these challenges, GHCH leadership embraced a systems-thinking approach to identify and address the underlying causes of these issues.

### APPLYING SYSTEMS THINKING

#### NETWORK THEORY: STRENGTHENING CONNECTIONS

The GHCH team utilized network theory to visualize the relationships within the hospital and with external partners. This analysis uncovered significant fragmentation among departments, such as inadequate coordination between ED, diagnostic labs, and outpatient clinics. By reconfiguring workflows and enhancing communication pathways, the hospital was able to optimize patient transfers and diagnostic procedures. For example, the implementation of a centralized referral system boosted efficiency and minimized delays in care delivery. These modifications also enabled stronger collaboration with local health agencies during the infectious disease outbreak.

#### CHAOS THEORY: ADDRESSING UNCERTAINTY

By applying chaos theory, GHCH management investigated how minor issues could escalate into widespread disruptions across the system. For instance, delays in patient diagnosis triggered a chain reaction that resulted in overcrowding and extended hospital stays. Leaders acknowledged that although chaos is an inherent feature of complex systems, stabilizing critical components can help alleviate its effects. Consequently, the team implemented point-of-care diagnostics to fast-track diagnoses, thereby reducing bottlenecks and enhancing patient flow.

### CYNEFIN FRAMEWORK: CATEGORIZING PROBLEMS

The **Cynefin framework** assisted GHCH management in classifying challenges into various domains to tailor their interventions:

- *Simple:* Routine tasks such as patient intakes were standardized via streamlined protocols.
- *Complicated:* Diagnostic issues needing expert input were managed through collaborative consultations.
- *Complex:* The outbreak enforced iterative problem-solving and scenario planning to foresee potential rises.
- *Chaotic:* The initial chaos during the outbreak was handled through urgent crisis management, such as establishing triage systems to prioritize critical cases.

### OVERCOMING CHALLENGES

*Resistance to change:* Healthcare providers were reluctant to adopt new processes due to concerns about increased workloads. To tackle this issue, the management emphasized transparent communication, offered targeted training, and showcased early successes to boost confidence.

*Data complexity:* GHCH faced difficulties in utilizing the extensive data from EHRs and diagnostic tools to manage patient care effectively. The implementation of a centralized data platform allowed for predictive modeling, which identified high-risk patients and improved resource allocation.

*Stakeholder engagement:* The lack of collaboration among stakeholders impeded progress. By involving all key players, including hospital administrators, frontline staff, and community partners, GHCH built trust and aligned efforts toward common goals.

### RESULTS AND IMPACT

Within a year, GHCH achieved substantial improvements:

- Reduced hospital readmission rates by 25%, thereby enhancing patient satisfaction
- Improved diagnostic efficiency, resulting in faster turnaround times for patients
- Enhanced collaboration, leading to stronger and integrated healthcare delivery systems
- Increased patient satisfaction scores by 10%, reflecting improved care and efficiency

GHCH's use of systems thinking reshaped its healthcare delivery model. By applying network theory, chaos theory, and the Cynefin framework, the hospital developed a more resilient and efficient system. This case demonstrates the potential of systems thinking in addressing complex challenges and enhancing outcomes in global healthcare systems.

## CONCLUSION

Systems thinking represents a transformative approach to understanding and improving healthcare delivery systems. By analyzing interconnected relationships, dependencies, feedback loops, and system dynamics, healthcare leaders can address systemic challenges comprehensively. Tools like CLD, stock and flow diagrams, and process mapping empower leaders to visualize the problems and optimize solutions. Theoretical foundations, including chaos theory, network theory, and CAS theory, provide robust frameworks for understanding interconnected healthcare complexities. With increasing number of stakeholders employing systems-thinking methods and tools to improve efficiency, its importance in healthcare management is evident. Successful implementation requires strategic integration of systems-thinking principles, fostering interdisciplinary collaboration, and comprehensive training programs. Looking forward, emerging technologies like AI and big data analytics will be essential in building resilient healthcare systems and improving patient outcomes. By addressing challenges and embracing innovation, systems thinking will remain pivotal in shaping the future of healthcare.

## END-OF-CHAPTER RESOURCES

### CRITICAL THINKING QUESTIONS

- How does the interconnected nature of healthcare systems both facilitate and complicate efforts to improve patient outcomes? Provide specific examples from your experience where this interconnectedness was pivotal.
- What potential ripple effects could you anticipate if a major hospital in your area closed, and how would systems thinking help address these challenges?
- Consider the role of feedback loops in healthcare quality improvement. How might reinforcing and balancing loops interact when implementing a new patient safety initiative in a hospital setting?
- Compare and contrast how chaos theory and network theory could be applied to manage a hospital ED during a crisis situation.
- Using the Cynefin framework, analyze a recent healthcare challenge you have encountered and explain how understanding its domain could have led to better decision-making.
- How might process mapping and CLD be used to improve patient flow in an ED? What key variables and relationships would you include in your analysis?
- How can healthcare organizations better integrate data analytics and predictive modeling while ensuring ethical considerations and patient privacy? What potential system-wide impacts should be considered?
- Discuss how collaborative decision-making processes could be improved in healthcare settings using systems-thinking principles. What role do different stakeholders play?
- Consider the GHCH case study. What lessons can healthcare organizations in other countries learn from their experience?
- Reflecting on the data complexity challenges mentioned in the chapter, how can healthcare organizations better manage and utilize vast amounts of data while maintaining security and privacy?

### LEARNING ACTIVITIES

**CourseConnect ▸**

To access self-assessment questions and interactive, competency-based learning activities for this chapter, visit www.springerpub.com/courseconnect. See inside front cover and tear-out card for CourseConnect details.

### REFERENCES

Alami, H., Lehoux, P., Papoutsi, C., Shaw, S. E., Fleet, R., & Fortin, J. P. (2024). Understanding the integration of artificial intelligence in healthcare organisations and systems through the NASSS framework: A qualitative study in a leading Canadian academic centre. *BMC Health Services Research*, 24(1), 701. https://doi.org/10.1186/s12913-024-11112-x

Alowais, S. A., Alghamdi, S. S., Alsuhebany, N., Alqahtani, T., Alshaya, A. I., Almohareb, S. N., Aldairem, A., Alrashed, M., Saleh, K. B., Badreldin, H. A., Al Yami, M. S., Al Harbi, S., & Albekairy, A. M. (2023). Revolutionizing healthcare: The role of artificial intelligence in clinical practice. *BMC Medical Education*, 23(1), 689. https://doi.org/10.1186/s12909-023-04698-z

Arnold, R. D., & Wade, J. P. (2015). A definition of systems thinking: A systems approach. *Procedia Computer Science*, 44, 669–678. https://doi.org/10.1016/j.procs.2015.03.050

Azar, A. T. (2012). System dynamics as a useful technique for complex systems. *International Journal of Industrial and Systems Engineering, 10*(4), 377–410. http://doi.org/10.1504/IJISE.2012.046298

Baugh Littlejohns, L., Baum, F., Lawless, A., & Freeman, T. (2018). The value of a causal loop diagram in exploring the complex interplay of factors that influence health promotion in a multisectoral health system in Australia. *Health Research Policy and Systems, 16*(1), 126. https://doi.org/10.1186/s12961-018-0394-x

Bendowska, A., & Baum, E. (2023). The significance of cooperation in interdisciplinary health care teams as perceived by Polish medical students. *International Journal of Environmental Research and Public Health, 20*(2), 954. https://doi.org/10.3390/ijerph20020954

Bierman, A. S., Wang, J., O'Malley, P. G., & Moss, D. K. (2021). Transforming care for people with multiple chronic conditions: Agency for Healthcare Research and Quality's research agenda. *Health Services Research, 56*(Suppl. 1), 973. https://doi.org/10.1111/1475-6773.13863

Bonabeau, E. (2002). Agent-based modeling: Methods and techniques for simulating human systems. *Proceedings of the National Academy of Sciences, 99*(Suppl. 3), 7280–7287. https://doi.org/10.1073/pnas.082080899

Calistri, A., Roggero, P. F., & Palù, G. (2024). Chaos theory in the understanding of COVID-19 pandemic dynamics. *Gene, 912*, 148334. https://doi.org/10.1016/j.gene.2024.148334

Cheraghi, R., Ebrahimi, H., Kheibar, N., & Sahebihagh, M. H. (2023). Reasons for resistance to change in nursing: An integrative review. *BMC Nursing, 22*(1), 310. https://doi.org/10.1186/s12912-023-01460-0

Clark, K., & Hoffman, A. (2019). Educating healthcare students: Strategies to teach systems thinking to prepare new healthcare graduates. *Journal of Professional Nursing, 35*(3), 195–200. https://doi.org/10.1016/j.profnurs.2018.12.006

Davis, V. H., Rodger, L., & Pinto, A. D. (2023). Collection and use of social determinants of health data in inpatient general internal medicine wards: A scoping review. *Journal of General Internal Medicine, 38*(2), 480–489. https://doi.org/10.1007/s11606-022-07937-z

Dhaliwal, J. S., & Dang, A. K. (2024). Reducing hospital readmissions. In StatPearls [Internet]. StatPearls Publishing.

Dolansky, M. A., & Moore, S. M. (2013). Quality and safety education for nurses (QSEN): The key is systems thinking. *Online Journal of Issues in Nursing, 18*(3). https://doi.org/10.3912/OJIN.Vol18No03Man01

Durski, K. N., Naidoo, D., Singaravelu, S., Shah, A. A., Djingarey, M. H., Formenty, P., Ihekweazu, C., Banjura, J., Kebela, B., Yinka-Ogunleye, A., Fall, I.-S., Eteng, W., Vandi, M., Keimbe, C., Abubakar, A., Mohammed, A., Williams, D. E., Lamunu, M., Briand, S., ... Osterholm, M. (2020). Systems thinking for health emergencies: Use of process mapping during outbreak response. *BMJ Global Health, 5*(10), e003901. https://doi.org/10.1136/bmjgh-2020-003901

Filip, R., Gheorghita Puscaselu, R., Anchidin-Norocel, L., Dimian, M., & Savage, W. K. (2022). Global challenges to public health care systems during the COVID-19 pandemic: A review of pandemic measures and problems. *Journal of Personalized Medicine, 12*(8), 1295. https://doi.org/10.3390/jpm12081295

Healthcare Improvement Scotland. (2023). *Systems mapping: Tool directory*. Retrieved from https://www.hisengage.scot/equipping-professionals/designing-person-centred-services/tool-directory/systems-mapping/

Hsia, R. Y., & Shen, Y. C. (2019). Emergency department closures and openings: Spillover effects on patient outcomes in bystander hospitals. *Health Affairs, 38*(9), 1496–1504. https://doi.org/10.1377/hlthaff.2019.00125

Jesmi, A. A., Jouybari, L. M., & Sanago, A. (2020). Application of chaos theory in the patient's safety. *Journal of Nursing and Midwifery Sciences, 7*(2), 131–133. https://doi.org/10.4103/JNMS.JNMS_34_19

Jones & Bartlett Learning. (2024, January 3). *What is system thinking in health care? Strategies for educators to encourage holistic thinking*. https://www.jblearning.com/blog/jbl/2024/01/03/health-systems-thinking

Oestreicher, C. (2007). A history of chaos theory. *Dialogues in Clinical Neuroscience, 9*(3), 279–289. https://doi.org/10.31887/DCNS.2007.9.3/coestreicher

Peters, D. H. (2014). The application of systems thinking in health: Why use systems thinking? *Health Research Policy and Systems, 12*(51), 1–6. https://doi.org/10.1186/1478-4505-12-51

Rawson, J. V., & Stevens, J. P. (2023). Scenario planning approach to adapting in the COVID era. *Academic Radiology, 30*(4), 572–578. https://doi.org/10.1016/j.acra.2022.11.032

RBC Capital Markets. (n.d.). *The healthcare data explosion*. Retrieved from https://www.rbccm.com/en/gib/healthcare/episode/the_healthcare_data_explosion

Reising, V., Diegel-Vacek, L., Dadabo, L., & Corbridge, S. (2023). Collaborative care: Integrating behavioral health into the primary care setting. *Journal of the American Psychiatric Nurses Association, 29*(4), 344–351. https://doi.org/10.1177/10783903211041653

Richmond, B. (1994). Systems thinking/system dynamics: Let's just get on with it. *System Dynamics Review, 10*(2–3), 135–157. https://doi.org/10.1002/sdr.4260100204

Rocio, S., María Paulina, E., Karol, R., Luis Fernando, S., & Ingrid, G. (2023). Accelerating systems thinking in health: Perspectives from the region of the Americas. *Frontiers in Public Health, 11*, 968357. https://doi.org/10.3389/fpubh.2023.968357

Rwashana, A. S., & Williams, D. W. (2008). System dynamics modeling in healthcare: The Ugandan immunisation system. *International Journal of Computing and ICT Research, 1*(1), 85–98.

Segal, E. (2020, October 26). Systems thinking 101: Making positive systems change. The Unschool. https://www.unschools.co/journal-blog/2019/8/11/week-14-systems-thinking-101

Senge, P. (1990). *The fifth discipline: The art and practice of the learning organization*. Doubleday/Currency.

Sustainability Methods. (n.d.). *System thinking & causal loop diagrams*. https://sustainabilitymethods.org/index.php/System_Thinking_%26_Causal_Loop_Diagrams

Tan, J., Wen, H. J., & Awad, N. (2005). Health care and services delivery systems as complex adaptive systems. *Communications of the ACM, 48*(5), 36–44. https://doi.org/10.1145/1060710.1060737

World Health Organization. (n.d.). *Systems thinking*. https://ahpsr.who.int/what-we-do/thematic-areas-of-focus/systems-thinking

Xia, S., Zhou, X.-N., & Liu, J. (2017). Systems thinking in combating infectious diseases. *Infectious Diseases of Poverty, 6*(1), 144. https://doi.org/10.1186/s40249-017-0339-6

Yahya, L. B., Naciri, A., Radid, M., & Chemsi, G. (2024). Immersive simulation in nursing and midwifery education: A systematic review. *Journal of Educational Evaluation for Health Professions, 21*. https://doi.org/10.3352/jeehp.2024.21.19

Zmed Solutions. (2024, January 30). *Innovating together: Interdisciplinary healthcare for a better future*. Retrieved from https://www.zmedsolutions.net/innovating-together-interdisciplinary-healthcare-for-a-better-future/

# CHAPTER 2

# OVERVIEW OF HEALTHCARE ORGANIZATIONS

Patrick D. Shay and Anupam Lahiri

## LEARNING OBJECTIVES

- Describe the variety of types of healthcare organizations within the U.S. healthcare system across the continuum of care.
- Identify and discuss key preventive and primary care settings and their role in promoting patient health.
- Identify and discuss key acute care settings, including hospitals and hospital systems as well as nonhospital-based acute care sites.
- Identify and discuss healthcare organizations comprising the post-acute care sector, including their relation to other sectors across the continuum of care.
- Identify and discuss long-term care settings and healthcare organizations providing end-of-life care.

## KEY TERMS

- Acute care
- Continuum of care
- End-of-life services
- Healthcare organizations
- Long-term care
- Post-acute care
- Preventive care
- Primary care

## INTRODUCTION TO HEALTHCARE ORGANIZATIONS

In this chapter, we examine the landscape of healthcare organizations that comprise a critical part of the U.S. healthcare system, considering organizations according to where they are situated along the **continuum of care**, which is "the spectrum of personal and population healthcare needed throughout all stages of a condition, injury, or even throughout a lifetime" (World Health Organization, & United Nations Children's Fund, 2020, p. viii). Within this approach, **healthcare organizations** are categorized according to the types of services they predominantly provide, spanning from preventive to end-of-life care, with broader categories of services including primary care, acute care, post-acute care, and long-term care. Such categories also commonly align with consideration of where such services tend to be administered, including outpatient, inpatient, or residential settings. Figure 2.1 illustrates this common approach to categorizing healthcare organizations.

**FIGURE 2.1.** The continuum of care.

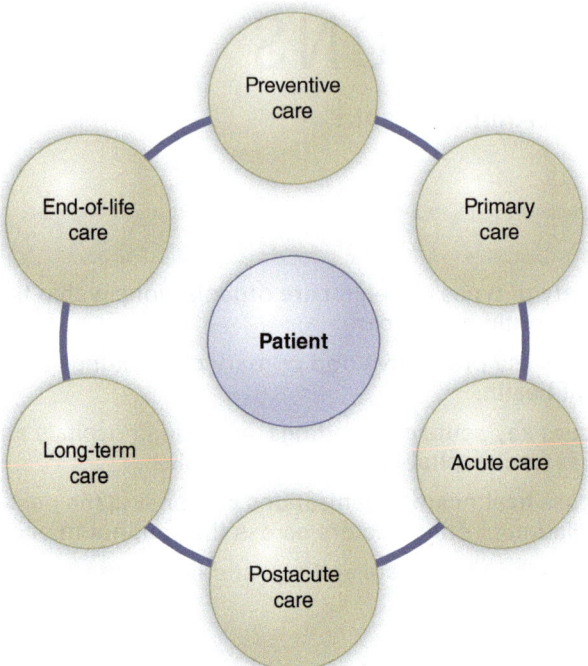

In navigating this continuum, we begin by exploring primary and preventive care organizations. Next, we progress to consider acute care organizations, including hospitals and hospital systems, followed by an evaluation of post-acute care, long-term care, and end-of-life care providers.

## PRIMARY AND PREVENTIVE CARE SERVICES

For many, primary and preventive care represent an initial entry point to medical services, but they also serve a critical role in ensuring coordinated, accessible, integrated, and relational healthcare experiences for patients. Primary and preventive care services go hand-in-hand; **primary care** maintains a focus on addressing and identifying initial healthcare needs, while **preventive care** supports a robust primary care effort to identify, correct, treat, or avoid any problematic health issues. Although primary and preventive care efforts can take place in healthcare organizations across the continuum of care, such as hospitals and nursing homes, some settings are particularly common for such services, including primary care clinics, physicians' offices, community health centers, retail clinics, and fitness and wellness centers, among others.

Throughout the history of the U.S. healthcare delivery system, *medical clinics and physician offices* have served as the foundation for outpatient care, providing the vast majority of primary care and preventive services, including education, examination, testing, screenings, immunizations, and chronic disease management. In such settings, physicians and their staff—including physician assistants, nurse practitioners, nurses, or nursing aides, among other medical professionals—provide routine primary care, basic diagnostic services, and minor treatments for an array of patient needs and a broad range of health conditions. They also serve as connection points to other healthcare providers and provider organizations across the continuum of care, referring patients to specialists or hospital-based services when needed.

During the 21st century, *retail clinics* have grown substantially as a healthcare setting in which patients can seek care without an appointment on a nonroutine, episodic basis to address minor and nonemergent medical issues as well as receive basic diagnostic and preventive care services. These clinics are characterized as retail due to both their typical locations in retail settings—including supermarkets, drugstores, and similar conveniently accessible retail spaces—and their retail-based approach to providing services, offering walk-in availability on a daily basis across extended hours of operation with affordable pricing for basic services that do not require insurance coverage.

Along with retail clinics, *urgent care facilities* are commonly referred to as a "convenient care" setting, characterized by their offering of walk-in medical services at convenient times and locations for patients. However, in contrast to retail clinics, urgent care facilities provide services for medical needs that are more complicated or immediate in nature. At the same time, they are not intended to address complex health conditions or critical medical needs that are more appropriately provided in emergency departments, instead serving a vital role in the healthcare landscape by offering convenient and accessible services for needs that require prompt care but do not justify the use and cost of emergency settings.

In underserved communities, *community health centers* serve as a critical source of primary care and preventive services, providing care regardless of an individual's ability to pay for the services they receive. These facilities work to increase access to needed care for patients who experience varied obstacles, and they offer comprehensive medical and supportive services that are tailored to meet the unique needs of the diverse populations they serve, such as dental care, laboratory testing, pharmacy services, radiology services, therapy services, transportation, language translation, mental and behavioral health support, and health education. *Federally qualified health centers* are a specific type of community health center that receive enhanced funding from the U.S. Department of Health and Human Services' Health Resources and Services Administration in order to comprehensively care for underserved and vulnerable populations such as minorities, women of childbearing age, infants, persons with HIV/AIDS, patients struggling with substance abuse, persons living below the poverty line, and individuals and families experiencing health service access barriers for any reason.

In addition, a variety of other settings also offer primary and preventive care services to meet the needs of the populations they serve. For example, *school-based health centers* provide services to school-age children and adolescents in clinics physically located on or adjacent to a school campus. *Mobile clinics*, which are health clinics built into customized motor vehicles such as vans, buses, or recreational vehicles, are transportable healthcare settings that bring a variety of services to patients at varied locations. They offer an efficient and convenient means for patients to receive primary and preventive care, playing a critical role in enhancing patients' access to care and delivering needed services to difficult-to-reach populations (Leibowitz et al., 2021; Malone et al., 2020). *Diagnostic imaging centers* serve as key providers of secondary and tertiary preventive services, employing trained specialists and utilizing advanced technological equipment to perform noninvasive diagnostic services such as x-ray, mammography, ultrasound, MRI, CT scans, PET scans, bone density scans, or fluoroscopy. *Medically based fitness and wellness centers* promote care in settings that, in addition to standard exercise equipment, often include cardiovascular equipment, personal training, fitness professionals, nutrition systems, sports performance, health and fitness education, massage therapy, fitness assessments, outpatient rehabilitation services, and the ability to connect continued fitness and exercise as part of an individual's broader plan of care. Finally, *complementary and alternative medicine* facilities represent a growing element of the healthcare delivery system that offer different services, including homeopathy, herbal remedies, acupuncture, meditation, yoga, exercises, chiropractic care, and more, to either complement or substitute traditional preventive or primary care approaches.

## ACUTE CARE SERVICES

When compared to preventive and primary care, **acute care** refers to short-term medical services that intervene in the event of an acute illness or injury. Acute care services are required for serious or sudden health needs that demand prompt medical attention, including emergency medicine, surgery, trauma care, critical care, and intensive care. When people think about acute care organizations, perhaps general acute care hospitals are what most commonly come to mind. However, it is important to recognize the variety of acute care settings that are a part of the U.S. healthcare delivery system, including specialty hospitals, freestanding emergency departments, and ambulatory surgery centers, among others.

*General acute care hospitals* are widely recognized as inpatient institutions that operate at least six inpatient beds; maintain physician staffing; provide around-the-clock nursing care; and primarily diagnose, treat, and offer a variety of surgical and therapeutic services for a broad range of patient medical conditions (Centers for Disease Control and Prevention, 2024). In contrast, *specialty hospitals* admit only certain types of patients, focusing on providing a narrower range of services for the specific conditions, health needs, or patients they specialize in. Examples, among others, include heart hospitals that provide comprehensive cardiac care; orthopedic hospitals that focus on care across the orthopedic service line; or women's hospitals that specialize in women's health services, including breast health, gynecology, obstetrics, and care for newborns. Similarly, *children's hospitals* are specialized facilities with staff trained to deal with children's unique medical needs on both an inpatient and outpatient basis. These settings provide the vast majority of highly specialized care for children, including organ transplants, cancer care, advanced tertiary care, and care for rare diseases and disorders (Casimir, 2019). Additionally, *behavioral health hospitals* play a particularly important but often overlooked role as a type of specialty hospital within the U.S. healthcare delivery system, providing diagnostic services and treatment on an inpatient and outpatient basis in a safe and therapeutic environment for patients who have mental and behavioral health diagnoses or psychiatric illnesses.

Another important category of hospitals includes *public hospitals*, which represent roughly 19% of U.S. hospitals including federal government hospitals as well as community hospitals owned by state and local government entities (American Hospital Association, 2025). Although these hospitals are referred to as "public," it is essential to consider that not all public hospitals are open to the general public; rather, they are simply owned by public governmental entities. For instance, Veterans Affairs (VA) hospitals—owned by the U.S. Department of Veterans Affairs—solely operate to treat and care for veterans of the U.S. armed forces, including war veterans and retired military personnel. Similarly, the U.S. Department of Defense operates 45 military hospitals across the Military Health

System (MHS) and Defense Health Agency to provide inpatient acute care specifically for active duty and reserve-component members of the U.S. armed forces and their families (MHS, 2024). Moreover, for the medical and health needs of more than 2.8 million Indigenous peoples and 574 federally recognized tribes across the country, the Indian Health Service (IHS)—a part of the U.S. Department of Health and Human Services—maintains 21 hospitals as well as an array of health centers, health stations (IHS, 2024).

General acute care hospitals situated in nonmetropolitan counties are known as *rural hospitals*. To help ensure these hospitals can viably provide needed care to their rural communities, many rural hospitals—over 1,350 of them as of 2023 (Rural Health Information Hub, 2023)—have obtained designation as *critical access hospitals*, enabling them to receive more comprehensive reimbursement for the essential services they provide that would otherwise be unavailable. These facilities typically operate more than 35 miles from any other hospital, maintain fewer than 25 acute care inpatient beds, and care for patients with an average length of stay of 4 days or less.

*Teaching hospitals* play a key role in the U.S. healthcare system, operating as acute care facilities that care for patients while also serving as the primary site for educating residents; medical students; and other healthcare professionals completing their education in clinical settings, such as nurses, therapists, and medical assistants. Similar to teaching hospitals, *academic medical centers* maintain a focus on medical education in addition to providing patient care, yet the settings are distinct; academic medical centers, which are affiliated with a medical school, are distinguished in their ability to confer medical degrees as well as their commitment to conducting clinical and biomedical research, recognized as part of their "tripartite mission" of education, research, and patient care.

Beyond inpatient acute care facilities, a variety of acute care organizations provide services to patients on an outpatient basis, meaning they treat patients without requiring an inpatient stay or overnight hospitalization. *Ambulatory surgery centers* (ASCs), which are sometimes referred to as "surgicenters" or outpatient surgery centers, provide surgical services on an outpatient basis in high-quality, low-cost settings. They often tend to focus on a specific specialty or type of surgical procedure, and after their procedures and some brief observation, patients are dismissed on the same day to recover in their place of residence. *Freestanding emergency departments* (FSEDs), also referred to as "freestanding ERs," provide emergency care to patients, including those who arrive by ambulance and those seeking care on a walk-in basis. Unlike emergency departments within acute care hospital facilities, FSEDs are separate from a hospital campus and are equipped to specifically provide emergency care services on an outpatient basis. Because they do not provide inpatient care and do not utilize operating rooms, any patients requiring inpatient services are transported to hospital facilities for inpatient admission following their stabilization at the FSED. *Multiservice outpatient centers* are facilities in which a variety of outpatient settings are located in the same facility to meet varied patient needs. These settings can often be referred to by a wide variety of terms—including health hubs, outpatient centers, multipurpose ambulatory care centers, health parks, or health malls, among others—and they also can widely vary in terms of their combinations of different types of services. For example, one outpatient center may combine an FSED with an imaging center, an urgent care center, and a retail clinic; another may combine an outpatient rehabilitation clinic, a fitness and wellness center, and a sports medicine practice; and another may combine an ASC, a specialty physician practice, and a diagnostic services facility. In the 21st century, as hospital systems have worked to expand their geographic presence across their local markets, many systems across the country have pursued the development of multiservice outpatient centers in varied parts of their surrounding communities (Shay & Mick, 2017).

Acute care services can also be provided on an outpatient basis in settings devoted to specialty care. For example, in some instances, specialty physicians provide acute care services in their practice or clinic settings. Similarly, at *vision centers*, optometrists can provide medical treatments or minor procedures for eye conditions, and ophthalmologists can perform medical and surgical interventions on patients' eyes, in addition to routine eye exams and basic optometry services. *Dental clinics*, besides providing routine dental care, preventive treatments, or cosmetic dental services, can often offer advanced dental and oral procedures, including endodontic, periodontal, orthodontic, prosthodontic, or oral and maxillofacial services and surgeries. At *birth centers*, nurses and midwives assist mothers in prenatal care and childbirth, specifically in low-risk pregnancies, in settings that are often homelike and holistic in nature. *Cancer centers* are a crucial acute care setting, specializing in the research, diagnosis, and treatment of cancer, including on an inpatient and outpatient basis. *Wound care centers* specialize in clinical care and treatments for complex, difficult-to-heal wounds, offering comprehensive services such as surgical wound debridement, antibiotic therapies, skin grafts, negative pressure-assisted wound closures, and hyperbaric oxygen therapy. Finally, *dialysis centers* provide lifesaving dialysis services for patients suffering from chronic kidney disease or end-stage renal disease, offering in-center dialysis treatments on an outpatient basis as well as training and support for at-home dialysis.

## POST-ACUTE CARE, LONG-TERM CARE, AND END-OF-LIFE CARE SERVICES

A critical component of the continuum of care involves the healthcare services focused on "downstream" health needs such as post-acute care, long-term care, and end-of-life services. Settings relating to these needs can easily be overlooked in our healthcare delivery system, but they represent essential sectors that are important to know in understanding the broader healthcare landscape.

The **post-acute care** sector provides medical services—including inpatient and outpatient services—to patients following an acute care stay or episode. The primary goal and philosophy of post-acute care providers is to aid and expedite the recovery process, helping to restore the patient to their maximum possible level of functioning and easing their transition back into the community. Similar but distinct from post-acute care facilities, **long-term care** settings provide services to patients navigating the aging process who may suffer from chronic, degenerative conditions and need health support. Long-term care facilities offer a variety of individualized and coordinated services—including medical care and therapy, social support, recreation, and case management—across an extended period of time, with the aim of maximizing the individual's functional independence and quality of life. In that sense, long-term care services contrast with short-term or post-acute care settings in that they are administered across broader (and sometimes indefinite) periods of time without specifically defined conclusions for treatments to a particular disease or injury. Long-term care services can also be provided in community-based settings, including patients' homes, and many long-term care patients face numerous health services needs due to chronic conditions and aging. Across both the post-acute and long-term care sectors, there is a wide variety of settings.

*Inpatient rehabilitation facilities* (or IRFs) provide intensive therapeutic and rehabilitative services to care for patients recovering from recent disability due to illness, injury, or accident. Patients receiving care in these inpatient facilities will generally have a length of stay spanning between 1 and 2 weeks, although some may stay for a longer duration of time depending upon their medical needs. IRFs can include freestanding rehabilitation hospitals and inpatient rehabilitation units in acute care hospitals, and patients commonly receive 3 or more hours of therapy—including physical and occupational therapy, as well as speech therapy if needed—on a daily basis during their stay.

IRFs will often provide outpatient services within their facilities, but in other instances, *outpatient rehabilitation clinics* or *outpatient rehabilitation centers* exist as freestanding facilities beyond an IRF or hospital campus. Sharing an emphasis on rehabilitative care, these settings enable patients to receive needed therapy services on an outpatient basis. This can include continued rehabilitative care for patients after they have been discharged from an inpatient setting—whether that is a stay at an inpatient acute care hospital or care in an inpatient post-acute facility such as an IRF—or it can involve outpatient care for patients who never needed an inpatient stay but have been prescribed rehabilitative therapy services such as physical therapy, occupational therapy, speech therapy, or cardiac rehabilitation, among others.

For patients needing advanced post-acute services over an extended inpatient stay, *long-term acute care hospitals* (LTACs) operate as certified hospitals that provide concentrated care to patients suffering from complex comorbidities and chronic conditions. Also referred to as "LTACHs" or "LTCHs," these facilities maintain an average length of stay greater than 25 days, with many patients requiring significant respiratory care.

*Skilled nursing facilities* (SNFs) are settings that provide high levels of individualized medical care from licensed health professionals—including nurses and therapists—for short-term rehabilitation from illness or injury and long-term care for patients with frequent or high levels of care needs due to chronic medical conditions. Skilled nursing care involves various services that support patients' needs around the clock and aim to maximize patients' functional independence, including nursing services as well as speech, occupational, and physical therapy, among others. Due to their provision of services for both rehabilitation patients and long-term care patients, SNFs are considered part of both the post-acute care and long-term care sectors.

*Home health* includes a wide variety of services that are provided by healthcare professionals in a patient's personal residence. These services—potentially including intermittent or part-time skilled nursing care, therapy services (physical, occupational, or speech), medical supplies, and durable medical equipment, among others—provide patients with a meaningful alternative to institutionalization, catering to patients' preferences for independence, comfort, and convenience. Similar to SNFs, home health plays an integral role in both post-acute and long-term care sectors; it is not uncommon for patients to receive care from home health agencies after discharge from an acute care hospital, a long-term care facility, or an inpatient rehabilitation hospital, while in other instances, patients may be prescribed home health services for long-term care and maintenance without having been admitted for inpatient services previously in their episode of care.

*Assisted living facilities* (ALFs) are long-term care settings providing personal care support and round-the-clock assistance for residents who have difficulty independently caring for themselves or are unable to live safely in an independent setting, including individuals who cannot access needed support from informal caregivers but who also do not require 24-hour medical supervision that is provided in long-term care settings such as SNFs. When ALF residents periodically require rehabilitative services or advanced nursing care, the facilities will commonly make arrangements for such services to be provided through home health care, as needed. Related to ALFs, *continuing care retirement communities* (CCRCs) provide a progressive spectrum of long-term care services and settings on the same campus. By including different facilities separately dedicated to independent living, personal care (i.e., nonmedical custodial care), assisted living, skilled nursing, and—in some instances—specialized care such as Alzheimer care or intensive rehabilitation, CCRCs allow residents to "age in place" on the same campus. CCRCs appeal to seniors who desire living situations that can be flexible and adapt to their evolving needs for domestic services and medical care, all within an environment that embraces comfortable amenities, maintenance-free living, personal convenience, and social engagement.

At the furthest end of the continuum of care are **end-of-life services**, which include hospice and palliative care. *Hospice* involves an approach to care for patients in the final stages of their terminal illness—with a prognosis anticipating less than 6 months to live—who have elected to discontinue curative treatments. Hospice care prioritizes patient comfort and quality of life by providing noncurative medical services; pain management; and emotional, psychosocial, and spiritual support while respecting patient dignity. Although hospice services can be provided at freestanding hospice facilities, they are not limited to a specific setting; the majority of hospice services are provided at patients' places of residence, and hospice care can also be provided in hospitals or long-term care settings such as SNFs or CCRCs. Similar to hospice, *palliative care* (alternatively referred to as supportive care) is provided to individuals with a chronic incurable or terminal illness, focusing on relieving symptoms of the disease to promote dignity, comfort, and quality of life. Like hospice, palliative care focuses on comprehensive comfort care rather than curative orientations, supporting the best possible quality of life for patients. However, in contrast to hospice, palliative care can be offered regardless of the stage of the disease or the provision of other interventions or therapies, and it can be paired in a supplementary fashion with curative treatments.

## CONCLUSION

As the U.S. healthcare delivery system has progressed, healthcare organizations have served as key settings in the story of patient care, representing where much of the "action" takes place among patients and healthcare professionals. However, these settings also function as key characters in that story, serving as critical stakeholders across the broader healthcare delivery system and involving a wide array of resources. Over time, healthcare organizations have evolved to meet a variety of changing forces, including economic, social, and demographic factors, among others. As a result, today's healthcare organizations are complex entities employing myriad healthcare professionals who provide services throughout the continuum of care at varied settings and locations throughout their local markets. This complexity is further intensified by the many trends and pressures observed both across the healthcare industry and within its varied organizations, particularly as healthcare leaders pursue aims such as increased service coordination, community engagement, and alignment across providers and payers. Looking ahead, we can anticipate that healthcare's evolution will continue, hopefully leading to a future in which healthcare organizations progressively realize gains in lowering costs, improving quality, expanding access, and enhancing the care experiences for patients and providers alike.

# END-OF-CHAPTER RESOURCES

## CRITICAL THINKING QUESTIONS

- The U.S. healthcare system is vast and complex. How can understanding the different types of healthcare organizations help us navigate the system more effectively?
- The concept of the continuum of care emphasizes the need for a coordinated approach to healthcare delivery across different settings. However, there are several potential challenges that patients may face while navigating the continuum of care. These challenges can make it difficult for patients to transition smoothly between different healthcare providers. Adopting the perspective of the patient, discuss some of these challenges in navigating the continuum of care to receive needed health services, and propose strategies that can improve communication and coordination between different healthcare providers involved.
- Discuss the different roles that each of the following continuum of care sectors play in the healthcare delivery system: preventive care, primary care, acute care, post-acute care, long-term care, and end-of-life care. What values do you see are reflected in each of these sectors? In what ways do these sectors compete, and why? How do you see each of these sectors either aligning with or conflicting with other values in the healthcare delivery system and across society?
- The U.S. healthcare system is known for its fragmentation. Discuss how this fragmentation creates challenges for patients, and evaluate the pros and cons of some potential solutions, including the standardization of healthcare procedures and the introduction of a single-payer system.
- What are the differences in healthcare organizations available to those living in rural areas versus major cities, and what are the implications of these differences?
- Weigh the pros and cons of choosing an ASC versus a hospital for a surgical procedure, and determine when each option may be more appropriate.
- With the rise of telehealth services, which types of healthcare organizations in the United States might benefit most from this service and why?
- Please discuss the specific advantages that post-acute care services can offer to patients after a hospitalization or acute illness, considering their potential to improve patient outcomes and reduce healthcare costs. In what conditions should these services be a mandatory part of the healthcare journey for certain patient populations?
- In numerous long-term care settings, organizations have the added responsibility to care for patients as residents. What challenges may that entail, and what unique dynamics must be taken into consideration of caring for patients who are at the same time residents?
- How do healthcare organizations' financing structures in the United States, such as Medicare, Medicaid, and private insurance, impact the services provided and patients served?

## LEARNING ACTIVITIES

**CourseConnect**

To access self-assessment questions and interactive, competency-based learning activities for this chapter, visit www.springerpub.com/courseconnect. See inside front cover and tear-out card for CourseConnect details.

## REFERENCES

American Hospital Association. (2025). *Fast Facts on U.S. Hospitals, 2025*. https://www.aha.org/statistics/fast-facts-us-hospitals

Casimir, G. (2019). Why children's hospitals are unique and so essential. *Frontiers in Pediatrics*, 7, 305. https://doi.org/10.3389/fped.2019.00305

Centers for Disease Control and Prevention. (2024). Health, United States. https://www.cdc.gov/nchs/hus/sources-definitions/hospital.htm

Indian Health Service. (2024). *Quick Look*. https://www.ihs.gov/newsroom/factsheets/quicklook

Leibowitz, A., Livaditis, L., Daftary, G., Pelton-Cairns, L., Regis, C., & Taveras, E. (2021). Using mobile clinics to deliver care to difficult-to-reach populations: A COVID-19 practice we should keep. *Preventive Medicine Reports*, 24, 101551. https://doi.org/10.1016/j.pmedr.2021.101551

Malone, N. C., Williams, M. M., Smith Fawzi, M. C., Bennet, J., Hill, C., Katz, J. N., & Oriol, N. E. (2020). Mobile health clinics in the United States. *International Journal for Equity in Health*, 19, 40. https://doi.org/10.1186/s12939-020-1135-7

Military Health System. (2024). *MHS health facilities*. https://www.health.mil/News/Media-Resources/Media-Center/MHS-Health-Facilities

Rural Health Information Hub. (2023). *Critical Access Hospitals (CAHs)*. https://www.ruralhealthinfo.org/topics/critical-access-hospitals

Shay, P. D., & Mick, S. S. F. (2017). Clustered and distinct: A taxonomy of local multihospital systems. *Health Care Management Science*, 20(3), 303–315. https://doi.org/10.1007/s10729-016-9353-7

World Health Organization, & United Nations Children's Fund. (2020). *Operational framework for primary health care: Transforming vision into action*. World Health Organization. https://www.who.int/publications/i/item/9789240017832

# CHAPTER 3

# MANAGING THE HEALTHCARE WORKFORCE

Katherine A. Meese and Anthony Patterson

## LEARNING OBJECTIVES

- Understand the importance of maintaining the healthcare workforce in achieving the Quintuple Aim.
- Identify environmental and industry factors that threaten the healthcare workforce.
- Describe risks to the healthcare organization when the workforce is not adequately maintained.
- Identify organizational causes of burnout and opportunities to increase resources and reduce work demands.
- Describe the role of communication and perceptions in shaping the employee experience.
- Explore team-level considerations for improving employee engagement and experience.

## KEY TERMS

- Belonging
- Burnout
- Conflict
- Job demands-resources theory
- Psychological safety
- Turnover

## INTRODUCTION

Healthcare is a human-centric industry. Relative to other industries like manufacturing or oil and gas, the main product is not produced by heavy machinery and equipment but by people. As a result, understanding how to create a healthy and engaged workforce is central to providing high-quality care for patients. Financial challenges have long been a concern of healthcare executives, topping the list of leader concerns on the American College of Healthcare Executives' annual survey for years. However, in the wake of the COVID-19 pandemic, workforce challenges rank first (American College of Healthcare Executives, 2023). This chapter provides an overview of the overarching goals for the healthcare workforce, a review of the current state of the workforce and external challenges, and solutions that can help maintain a healthy and sustainable workforce within an organization and team.

## THE QUINTUPLE AIM

Defining the goals for the healthcare workforce is important before exploring the barriers to progress and solutions. The Institute for Healthcare Improvement proposed the Quintuple Aim, an extension of the widely recognized Triple Aim (Nundy et al., 2022). The Quintuple Aim seeks to achieve five interconnected goals within healthcare to create a high-functioning and sustainable system:

- Aim 1: Improving population health
- Aim 2: Enhancing patient experiences
- Aim 3: Reducing costs
- Aim 4: Improving workforce well-being and safety
- Aim 5: Advancing health equity

Many of these aims are interrelated, though some will be difficult to achieve simultaneously. For example, hiring more staff to reduce workload and help with burnout may lead to increased costs in the short term. The Quintuple Aim reflects a holistic approach to healthcare improvement that recognizes the interdependence of these five dimensions. By striving to achieve all five goals simultaneously, healthcare organizations aim to create a more balanced, effective, and sustainable healthcare system.

## FINANCIAL, REGULATORY, AND LEGAL RISKS ASSOCIATED WITH THE HEALTHCARE WORKFORCE

The fourth aim of the Quadruple Aim framework focuses on improving the well-being and safety of the healthcare workforce. Organizations that do not prioritize this aim may face significant financial, regulatory, legal, and reputational risks. Many of these risks are exacerbated when employees leave the organization.

### FINANCIAL COST OF TURNOVER

While percentages vary among organizations, the largest expense in delivering care is typically wages and benefits, which on average account for more than 50% of the hospital's total expense (Statista, 2019). Healthcare has always been subject to over- and undersupply of various health professionals. Turnover costs include the expense of recruiting, hiring, and training new employees, as well as the cost of temporary staffing required to cover any shortfalls. Healthcare organizations and, by extension, patient care can suffer when costs exceed reimbursement from services delivered. Hospital expense increases between 2019 and 2022 are more than double the increases in Medicare reimbursement for inpatient care during that same time, resulting in tremendous financial strain (American Hospital Association, 2024).

While some turnover is inevitable and can bring new ideas into an organization through new employees, high turnover can be harmful. Employee turnover in healthcare organizations can incur significant costs and negatively impact quality of care and organizational reputation. High turnover rates among nurses, for example, are estimated to cost the average hospital $3.6 to $6.5 million per year (Plescia, 2021). The estimated cost to replace one physician is up to $1.2 million after considering lost productivity, billing, and recruitment costs (Berg, 2018). Other industries estimate that replacing an employee typically costs one half to two times their annual salary (Gandhi & Robison, 2021). However, the nonfinancial costs may be even greater in terms of patient safety, care quality, reputation, and workforce relations and engagement.

## THREAT TO QUALITY AND SAFETY

High turnover threatens patient safety and the delivery of safe care (Aiken et al., 2023). It leads to frequent staff changes, resulting in patients not receiving care from the same team of nurses and physicians over time. Experienced clinicians leave and are frequently replaced with new hires with less experience. The learning curve for new clinical staff increases the risk of medical errors. New staff members need to become more familiar with organizational processes to do things safely and efficiently. This disruption in care teams makes it hard to coordinate complex patient care.

When people leave, the remaining staff can feel overworked when positions remain unfilled. Nurses left caring for too many patients have less time to spend with each one. Staff can become overwhelmed and are more likely to make mistakes or experience burnout. They also have less ability or incentive to adopt and follow time-intensive safety practices or require additional training, such as checklists and time-outs in surgery. Health organizations struggle to make care better and safer with a constantly changing workforce that is systemically underresourced.

## HARM TO REPUTATION

High turnover also hurts the organization's reputation and brand, both as an employer and healthcare provider. When staff turnover is high, it can make the workplace seem unappealing for clinicians and nonclinical workforce. It also gets harder to recruit and retain top talent. The organization must spend more effort and money trying to recruit new hires. Losing staff with long-term experience can also directly worsen patients' experiences. Staff friendliness, promptness, communication, and preparation for discharge often suffer. This results in lower scores on patient surveys and rating sites, which can affect the hospital's reputation (Pappas et al., 2022).

## COLLECTIVE ACTION AND UNIONIZATION

Healthcare leaders need to improve the work environment, workforce relations, and engagement to address turnover. When staff feel heard and valued, they are more likely to stay. On the other hand, poor management-staff relations can lead to unionization campaigns when employees feel that they are not able to accomplish their goals in direct discussions with management (National Labor Relations Board, 2022; Nelson, 2023). Unions try to give healthcare professionals more bargaining power over wages, work rules, and policies that affect their jobs (Lin et al., 2022). The main benefits of unions are that they can result in higher pay and better worker benefits. However, union contracts also reduce managers' flexibility in assigning staff efficiently. Healthcare leaders aim to build positive relationships that avoid the need for unionization and potential labor strikes down the road (Hut, 2023).

## ENVIRONMENTAL AND INDUSTRY FACTORS

Despite the risk to the organization of workforce shortages and high turnover, there are many environmental and industry-level factors that pose challenges to maintaining adequate staffing and a healthy and engaged workforce. Environmental level factors such as economic conditions, demographic shifts, and regulatory changes can significantly impact the supply and demand for healthcare workers. For example, an economic downturn may lead to layoffs and reduced hiring, while an aging population increases the need for healthcare services and puts strain on the existing workforce.

### AGING POPULATION

A substantial challenge facing the healthcare sector is the aging population. As individuals age, their healthcare needs increase, necessitating a sufficient workforce to meet the increased need for care. However, the sizeable baby boomer generation in the United States coexists with a relatively smaller proportion of younger individuals. This demographic imbalance strains the availability of the healthcare workforce, particularly given the departure of older but experienced clinicians. The retirement of aging clinicians not only means they are not available to deliver care but also that they cannot provide mentorship and training to newer clinicians, resulting in a loss of institutional and technical knowledge and experience. According to projections from the Association of American Medical Colleges (2021), the United States could face a shortage of between 37,800 and 124,000 physicians by 2034, further exacerbating the impact of retiring clinicians. While there is some debate about overall nursing shortages, recent reports have found that nurses are increasingly choosing ambulatory settings, which leaves a shortage of nurses to handle complex patients in inpatient and hospital settings (Auerbach et al., 2024).

### THE EFFECTS OF THE COVID-19 PANDEMIC AND GREAT RESIGNATION

The effects of the COVID-19 pandemic, coupled with broader socioeconomic dynamics, have led to significant shifts in how we view work broadly, specifically within the healthcare workforce. The "great resignation," characterized by an unprecedented number of employees leaving their jobs, swept across various industries, including healthcare (Parker & Menasce Horowitz, 2022). The healthcare sector offers meaningful and purposeful work and presents substantial demands and risks, such as exposure to diseases and violence, regulatory constraints, and inflexible schedules. Consequently, many healthcare workers chose to exit the field, seeking improved work-life balance, appreciation, and recognition. Between 2020 and 2022, 54% of healthcare and pharmaceutical industry workers who switched jobs did not return to the same industry (De Smet et al., 2022). In 2021, 117,000 physicians left the workforce, which accounts for over 10% of the total number of active physicians in the United States (Popowitz et al., 2022; Young et al., 2023).

### BURNOUT AND PSYCHOLOGICAL STRAIN

Burnout among the healthcare workforce was a challenge before the pandemic and remains a pressing issue. **Burnout** is when people experience a sense of detachment or cynicism, ineffectiveness or diminished personal accomplishment, and emotional exhaustion

(Maslach & Leiter, 2006). Healthcare workers are highly resilient, but the challenging work environment and strenuous demands of the job have resulted in persistent burnout. This phenomenon extends beyond clinicians, affecting nonclinical healthcare workers and executives as well (Mensik, 2022). The psychological toll is evident in alarming rates of depression, anxiety, and even suicide among physicians.

Sadly, 55% of physicians know a physician who considered, attempted, or died by suicide (The Physicians Foundation, 2021). The suicide rates for female physicians are 46% higher than other professional women of similar age (Duarte et al., 2020). Research early in the COVID-19 pandemic found that healthcare employees were at risk of high distress, with 75% of administrative and nonclinical employees, 90% of advanced practice providers, 92% of clinical support staff, and 90% of nurses reporting high distress (Meese et al., 2021). Beyond the impact on the individual, these dynamics can affect the entire healthcare team. Emotional contagion research has shown that positive and negative emotions can spread among others, which means that an individual's burnout and distress are likely to have wider reaching effects (Herrando & Constantinides, 2021).

## ECONOMIC FACTORS AND LABOR SHORTAGES

In parallel, broader economic factors have compounded the challenges faced by the healthcare sector. Escalating inflation rates and decreasing unemployment complicated the financial landscape (Mondragon & Wieland, 2022). These macroeconomic shifts bore a two-fold impact on healthcare organizations. On the one hand, they grappled with higher supply costs and reduced revenue due to canceled elective procedures and short staffing (Weise et al., 2020). On the other hand, employees, confronted with mounting inflation and heightened job risks, demanded higher compensation. This surge in labor costs strained healthcare organizations, particularly those with narrower financial margins. Furthermore, other industries' labor shortages enticed workers with offers of higher salaries, flexibility, and enhanced benefits, further intensifying the competition for healthcare talent (De Smet et al., 2022; Liu, 2022). While the most recent labor reports show that the national healthcare workforce appears to be growing beyond prepandemic levels, merely having enough people does not mean we have the right employees in the right places with the necessary skills and experiences to meet the growing demand for care (Meese, 2024).

### DECLINING REIMBURSEMENT

Hospital reimbursement from government payors like Medicare and Medicaid has generally been declining over time. Both payors reimburse hospitals at rates that are often below the actual costs of care, with 67% of hospitals reporting negative Medicare margins in 2022 (American Hospital Association, 2024). Rising healthcare costs have also pressured private insurer reimbursement to maintain an acceptable margin, thus putting more pressure on healthcare organizations to contain the costs of delivering care. Hospital operating costs continue to increase, driven by new medical technology, drug costs, medical supplies and equipment, nonlabor expenses such as information technology, facility maintenance, food and nutrition, regulatory compliance, staffing shortages, and more. Driven by workforce shortages, labor costs have been increasing faster than inflation (International Federation of Employee Benefit Plans, 2023).

As a result of declining reimbursement and rising costs, hospital profit margins have been declining over the past several decades (Trends Affecting Hospitals and

Health Systems, 2015). Many hospitals now operate on very low margins. Rural and public hospitals tend to have even lower margins than the industry average. Declining reimbursement and rising costs have forced hospitals to find ways to operate more efficiently (Jamalabadi et al.,2020). This has included strategies such as supply chain management, clinical standardization, and efforts to improve care coordination and outcomes. However, the trends have also led to hospital closures, especially in rural areas (Kaufman et al., 2015). Financial pressures on hospitals are expected to continue.

## CHANGING WORK EXPECTATIONS AND PRIORITIES

As new generations enter the workforce, they bring shifting expectations and priorities. Flexibility is a core desire, especially among women and those with caregiving responsibilities (De Smet et al., 2022). This distinction is especially important in healthcare, where females comprise 70% of the healthcare workforce globally (Boniol et al., 2019). Flexibility is not always a feature of clinical work, where an individual must work set shifts at the patient's location. Across industries, employees increasingly prioritize workplaces that value their well-being and offer improved conditions, leading to better pay, advancement opportunities, and a healthier work-life balance (Parker & Menasce Horowitz, 2022).

The combination of pandemic-era effects, economic shifts, burnout, an aging population, and evolving work expectations has reshaped the healthcare workforce. Organizations must grapple with various challenges, including retaining skilled professionals, addressing burnout and psychological distress, adapting to changing demographics, and meeting the evolving needs of a new generation of caregivers. Navigating these complexities will require innovative strategies and increasing focus on creating desirable work environments to facilitate retention of the healthcare workforce.

## ORGANIZATIONAL FACTORS INFLUENCING THE WORKFORCE

While industry-level changes have shaped how people generally relate to work, many factors contribute to burnout, disengagement, and ultimately, turnover, which are work-related factors within an organization. Some of these occur at the organizational level, while others may occur at the team or individual levels.

### WORK-RELATED CAUSES OF BURNOUT

Burnout is considered an occupational phenomenon, meaning it is a specific work-related condition that differentiates it from other types of personal life stress. The six causes of burnout are described in Table 3.1 (Maslach & Leiter, 2006), along with examples in the healthcare context. Any steps organizations and leaders can take to address these six domains will likely help alleviate the growing problem of burnout within the healthcare workforce.

## TABLE 3.1. SIX CAUSES OF BURNOUT IN HEALTHCARE

| CAUSE OF BURNOUT | DESCRIPTION | HEALTHCARE EXAMPLE |
|---|---|---|
| Work overload | The duration or difficulty of the work exceeds human limits. This can refer to long hours or the difficulty of the work. | Physicians work 16 hours per week longer than the average U.S. employee, and in some specialties, 24-hour shifts are routine. |
| Lack of control or autonomy | When a person feels they do not have control over how their work is carried out | Intense regulation and the transition from private practice to employed physician models with additional policies and procedures can reduce feelings of autonomy. |
| Lack of reward | Feelings of inadequate pay, recognition, or appreciation or feeling devalued. | Many healthcare workers had paycuts or salary reductions during the COVID-19 pandemic while also working longer hours and facing increased exposure to an infectious virus. |
| Lack of fairness | Actual or perceived inequity in treatment, compensation, promotions, shift assignments, or other allocation of resources. | Employees with a longer tenure in an organization feel it is unfair when contract labor or travel nurses are paid more to do similar work. |
| Low sense of community | A sense of community at work is created through positive social interactions with colleagues but can be damaged by gossip, hostility, incivility, or isolation. | Long hours, heavy patient loads, and a demanding pace of work can make it difficult to make time for friendships or relationships at work and at home. |
| Conflict in values | Feeling that your personal values are out of alignment with the organization's values or activities. | The personal value of wanting to help others who are suffering may conflict with an organizational policy of not performing certain procedures if a patient is unable to pay. |

*Source:* Adapted from Maslach, C., & Leiter, M. (2006). Burnout. *Stress and Quality of Working Life: Current Perspectives in Occupational Health, 37*, 42–49 Statista. (2023). *Average hours per week physicians worked in the United States in 2023, by specialty*. Retrieved May 16, 2025, from https://www.statista.com/statistics/1534917/us-physician-working-hours-by-specialty/

# JOB DEMANDS-RESOURCES THEORY

The **job demands-resources theory** provides a framework for understanding how leaders and organizations can support a thriving healthcare workforce. The theory posits that motivation, well-being, and engagement thrive when individuals possess the necessary resources to meet the demands of the job. This balance can be achieved by enhancing resources or reducing demands (Bakker & Demerouti, 2007).

## ADDING RESOURCES

Leaders and organizations may add resources at the organizational, team, and individual levels to help employees meet the work demands. The three categories of resources are physical, structural, and social (Bakker & Demerouti, 2007).

### PHYSICAL RESOURCES

Physical resources include ensuring enough supplies and equipment to do the job well. Supply chain disruptions and global drug shortages can pose challenges to this goal. Lack of appropriate physical resources can often result in workarounds where employees expend time and energy (and often experience increased stress) trying to devise backup solutions.

## STRUCTURAL RESOURCES

Structural resources are individual attributes or organizational aspects of the job that may help achieve work goals or support personal growth. These can include a well-designed organizational structure, clear reporting structures, straightforward policies and procedures, leadership development programs, and autonomy. Structural resources may include mental health and well-being programs, on-site childcare, paid time off, and tuition benefits.

## SOCIAL RESOURCES

These are resources that an employee gets from those they interact with at work. These include mentorship, good collegial relationships, and a sense of belonging. These resources can be enhanced through mentorship programs, team-building activities, and clarifying team norms and expectations of behavior so that leaders create conditions that support the development of good coworker relationships.

The absence of these resources strains employees, potentially leading to disengagement and burnout. While some resources are costly, many social and structural resources are developed through time and intentionality but do not require a heavy financial investment.

## REDUCING DEMANDS

Solely adding resources without also addressing the work's demands is not sufficient to support a flourishing workforce. If a unit is shortstaffed and the manager is not able to hire more employees, they can still help reduce the workload by removing inefficiencies and unnecessary or redundant tasks. Clinicians have cited heavy administrative burdens as a leading cause of burnout, particularly around duplicative documentation, inefficiencies in the electronic medical record, or activities and data collection that multiple groups within the organization request. Many physicians spend more time charting than interacting with patients (Stein, 2015).

### CASE STUDY 3.1: SOLICITING EMPLOYEE FEEDBACKS

Programs that solicit employee feedback on which processes can be refined or eliminated can yield positive results for the organization. Melinda Ashton, MD, executive vice president and chief quality officer at Hawaii Pacific Health, launched an initiative called "Getting Rid of Stupid Stuff" at her health system (Ashton, 2018, 2019). The program involved the following:

- Seeking feedback
- Including compliance and legal
- Developing a partnership with IT
- Creating a leadership group to address concerns

The program produced promising initial results. Just eliminating a single component of nursing documentation saved over 1,700 nursing hours per month within the health system. That time can be used to reduce the nursing workload and to invest more in spending time with patients and demonstrating empathy and compassion.

## PERCEPTION AND COMMUNICATION

Perception and communication play an important role in how organizational decisions affect the workforce, including their well-being and motivation. Humans are sense-making beings that connect disconnected bits of information into stories that make sense to them.

People tend to filter out information that does not already align with their values, beliefs, and experiences. Healthcare leaders may make a decision that is in the best interest of the organization and in alignment with the organization's values, but if not communicated well, employees may perceive or interpret the actions differently, which can cause harm. People tend to act on their perceptions of a situation rather than on objective information surrounding an event.

Gallup found that only 7% of workers strongly agree that they get timely, open, and accurate communication at work. Workers who strongly agree that leadership within the organization communicates effectively are 73% less likely to feel burned out (Robison, 2021). Leaders must pay careful attention to how information is communicated within an organization and to how they craft a cohesive story around organizational decisions to prevent any damage that may unintentionally occur from inaccurate perceptions (Case Study 3.2).

## CASE STUDY 3.2: PERCEPTIONS OF NEW BUILDINGS AND STAGNANT WAGES

A large academic medical center was experiencing a financial crisis as the COVID-19 pandemic extended into its second year. They had received a large government stimulus to help offset the increased costs of staffing the hospitals during the pandemic, but the extra funding was expiring. The high cost of hiring traveling nurses, increased supply costs due to global shortages, and paying bonuses to retain employees meant that the health system was expecting to incur a financial loss during the fiscal year. The communication team from the CFO's office managed the messaging to the organization about the dire situation. Leaders, managers, and employees received updates about the "financial crisis" facing the organization. When employees asked for raises to help offset the rising costs from inflation, they were reminded of the financial crisis and raises were denied.

Around the same time, the organization received a very generous gift from the state. The state gave the organization $50 million, specifically to build a state-of-the-art research facility. Even though the organization was in financial crisis, they could only use the money for the stipulated donation's purpose. Executives at the organization were very excited about the new resources, especially during a financially lean year. The public relations team from the marketing department handled the communications about the new building. There were many press releases about the $50 million building, pictures of the architectural renderings on social media, and a highly publicized ribbon cutting ceremony. During these communications, the size and cost of the building were celebrated, but there was less information about the source of funds.

When the organization conducted their annual employee engagement survey, employees expressed anger, frustration, and distrust about the new building. They were angry that the "greedy executives" spent money on new buildings instead of giving raises to the frontline employees. People expressed an intention to leave an organization that valued "buildings over people."

What should have been excitement and celebration over a donated gift did damage to morale and engagement. Why?

### QUESTIONS

1. What misperceptions did employees have about the new building that damaged trust in leadership?
2. How could the leadership of the health system prevent misperceptions about the new building?
3. How could better coordination of the two messages result in a different outcome?

## TEAM-LEVEL FACTORS

In addition to organizational factors, there are experiences that happen within an employees' team or work group that affect their well-being and engagement at work, which in turn influences their likelihood of remaining in the organization.

These include their relationships with their direct supervisor or manager, the ability to feel a sense of psychological safety and belonging, and the ability to navigate conflict.

### THE ROLE OF THE MANAGER

There are many organizational and individual factors that affect a person's motivation, performance, well-being, engagement, and ultimately, intention to remain with the organization. While a person's direct manager or supervisor does not have the power to influence all these factors, they play a major role in shaping the employee's experience. Gallup has found that 70% of the variation in team performance is determined by the manager (Suellentrop & Bauman, 2021). Leaders have a responsibility to select managers that will represent the values of the organization to the employee. Furthermore, organizations must invest in developing managers and supervisors, so they feel equipped to create a positive environment for their teams.

### PSYCHOLOGICAL SAFETY AND BELONGING

People want to feel that they can belong at work, get along well with others, and use their specific skills and strengths to contribute to the team's goals. **Belonging** is a human need to feel connected to others and to feel that one is socially accepted. Feeling a sense of belonging is an important predictor of performance and mental and physical health. Feeling as though one does not belong or is socially rejected is associated with increased risk of mental illness, lower immune function, and even early mortality (Allen et al., 2021). A healthy team culture is one where people of all different backgrounds, beliefs, and characteristics have an opportunity to belong based on a shared set of values and where individual differences are appreciated and respected.

**Psychological safety** is another important element of ensuring that people are able to belong and contribute to a team. Team psychological safety is a shared belief among members of the team that it is acceptable to speak up, voice concerns, express ideas, and admit mistakes without fear of negative consequences (Gallo, 2023). When people feel safe to share their expertise, thoughts, experiences, and knowledge, it is more likely that they will be able to experience a sense of belonging.

### MANAGING CONFLICT

Conflict is an inevitable and even necessary part of work. Ideas are shaped and challenged through productive conflict, and often, a better result emerges. However, some types of conflict can damage employee relationships, morale, and performance. The first step to managing conflict is identifying which type(s) of conflict are involved. There are several types of conflict, each of which requires a different approach to resolve (Table 3.2). By first diagnosing the cause(s) of the conflict, leaders and managers can develop a strategy to address it.

**TABLE 3.2. TYPES OF CONFLICT IN HEALTHCARE**

| TYPE OF CONFLICT | DEFINITION | HEALTHCARE EXAMPLE |
|---|---|---|
| Goal | Two or more outcomes are incompatible with each other. | An operating room nurse is asked to implement a new policy by the nurse manager, and the surgeon is asking the nurse to use a different process. |
| Cognitive | Ideas or thoughts are incompatible. | Two physicians disagree on how to interpret the scientific evidence for prescribing a medication. |
| Relationship | Arises from differences in personality, style, or behaviors between individuals. | One person's direct form of communication is offensive to another person who does not have a blunt communication style. |
| Process | People disagree on how a task or objective should be completed or what process is used to execute. | The organization must cut expenses by 5% but leaders disagree about how they should decide which programs to cut. |
| Values | Arises from differing beliefs, moral, ethical or political views or values. | Employees disagree about whether it is ethical to mandate that healthcare workers get vaccines. |
| Status | Occurs when there is disagreement about who is in charge or which party has the authority to make decisions. | A more experienced employee is not willing to follow the direction or guidance of a younger employee who has been assigned to lead a project. |

*Source:* Adapted from Gallo, A. (2017). *HBR guide to dealing with conflict (HBR Guide Series)*. Harvard Business Review Press; Kolb, D., & Bartunek, J. M. (1992). *Hidden conflict in organizations: Uncovering behind-the-scenes disputes* (Vol. 141). Sage; Vaske, J. J., Donnelly, M. P., Wittmann, K., & Laidlaw, S. (1995). Interpersonal versus social-values conflict. *Leisure Sciences, 17*(3), 205–222. https://doi.org/10.1080/01490409509513257.

## CONCLUSION

The healthcare workforce is rapidly changing, and staffing shortages and workforce concerns rank highly among concerns for healthcare executives. Environmental and industry-level changes are resulting in people leaving the healthcare workforce for a variety of reasons which can pose great risks to an organization in terms of financial performance, quality and safety, and reputational harm. Organizations and managers have a responsibility to address organization-level factors that are negatively impacting the workforce, including addressing the sources of burnout, increasing resources, and reducing work demands. Individual managers have an important role in maintaining a positive work culture that promotes psychological safety and belonging while navigating various forms of conflict to a successful resolution. Creating a positive work experience and environment for healthcare workers is critical to maintaining the workforce and reducing organizational risk.

## END-OF-CHAPTER RESOURCES

### CRITICAL THINKING QUESTIONS

- What can organizations do to reduce turnover of the healthcare workforce?
- What policy-level changes may reduce stress among healthcare workers?
- How can individual managers and leaders improve the retention of their employees?
- How does poor workforce management harm the healthcare organization?

### LEARNING ACTIVITIES

**CourseConnect ▸**

To access self-assessment questions and interactive, competency-based learning activities for this chapter, visit www.springerpub.com/courseconnect. See inside front cover and tear-out card for CourseConnect details.

### REFERENCES

Aiken, L. H., Lasater, K. B., Sloane, D. M., Pogue, C. A., Rosenbaum, K. E. F., Muir, K. J., McHugh, M. D., & US Clinician Wellbeing Study Consortium. (2023). Physician and nurse well-being and preferred interventions to address burnout in hospital practice: factors associated with turnover, outcomes, and patient safety. *JAMA Health Forum*, 4(7), e231809. https://doi.org/10.1001/jamahealthforum.2023.1809

Allen, K.-A., Kern, M. L., Rozek, C. S., McInerney, D. M., & Slavich, G. M. (2021). Belonging: A review of conceptual issues, an integrative framework, and directions for future research. *Australian Journal of Psychology*, 73(1), 87–102. https://doi.org/10.1080/00049530.2021.1883409

American College of Healthcare Executives. (2023, February 13). *Survey: Workforce challenges cited by CEOs as top issue confronting hospitals in 2022*. Retrieved 2025, July 29, from https://www.ache.org/about-ache/news-and-awards/news-releases/survey-workforce-challenges-cited-by-ceos-as-top-issue-confronting-hospitals-in-2022

American Hospital Association. (2024). *Medicare significantly underpays hospitals for cost of patient care*. www.aha.org/2024-01-10-infographic-medicare-significantly-underpays-hospitals-cost-patient-care

Ashton, M. (2018). Getting rid of stupid stuff. *New England Journal of Medicine*, 379(19), 1789–1791. https://doi.org/10.1056/NEJMp1809698

Ashton, M. (2019). *Getting rid of stupid stuff: Reduce the unnecessary daily burdens for clinicians*. AMA STEPS Forward. https://edhub.ama-assn.org/steps-forward/module/2757858

Association of American Medical Colleges. (2021). *AAMC report reinforces mounting physician shortages*. www.aamc.org/news/press-releases/aamc-report-reinforces-mounting-physician-shortage

Auerbach, D. I., Buerhaus, P. I., Donelan, K., & Staiger, D. O. (2024). Projecting the future Registered nurse workforce after the COVID-19 pandemic. *JAMA Health Forum*, 5(2), e235389. https://doi.org/10.1001/jamahealthforum.2023.5389

Bakker, A. B., & Demerouti, E. (2007). The job demands-resources model: State of the art. *Journal of Managerial Psychology*, 22, 309–328. https://doi.org/10.1108/02683940710733115

Berg, S. (2018). How much physician burnout is costing your organization. *American Medical Association*. https://www.ama-assn.org/practice-management/physician-health/how-much-physician-burnout-costing-your-organization

Boniol, M., McIsaac, M., Xu, L., Wuliji, T., Diallo, K., & Campbell, J. (2019). *Gender equity in the health workforce: analysis of 104 countries*. https://iris.who.int/handle/10665/311314

De Smet, A., Dowling, B., Hancock, B., & Schaninger, B. (2022). The Great Attrition is making hiring harder. Are you searching the right talent pools? *McKinsey Quarterly*, 1–13. https://www.mckinsey.com/capabilities/people-and-organizational-performance/our-insights/the-great-attrition-is-making-hiring-harder-are-you-searching-the-right-talent-pools

Duarte, D., El-Hagrassy, M. M., Couto, T. C. E., Gurgel, W., Fregni, F., & Correa, H. (2020). Male and female physician suicidality: A systematic review and meta-analysis. *JAMA Psychiatry*, 77(6), 587–597. https://doi.org/10.1001/jamapsychiatry.2020.0011

Gallo, A. (2023). *What Is psychological safety?* https://hbr.org/2023/02/what-is-psychological-safety

Gandhi, V., & Robison, J. (2021). The 'great resignation' is really the 'great discontent'. Gallup. https://www.gallup.com/workplace/351545/great-resignation-really-great-discontent.aspx

Herrando, C., & Constantinides, E. (2021). Emotional contagion: a brief overview and future directions. *Frontiers in Psychology*, 12, 712606. https://doi.org/10.3389/fpsyg.2021.712606

Hut, N. (2023, October 10). Healthcare labor union activity gains steam: The consequences for hospitals and health systems. *Healthcare Financial Management Association*. https://www.hfma.org/finance-and-business-strategy/healthcare-business-trends/healthcare-labor-union-activity-gains-steam-the-consequences-for-hospitals-and-health-systems/

International Foundation of Employee Benefit Plans. (n.d.). *Health care costs pulse survey: 2024 cost trend*. Retrieved September 3, 2023, from https://www.ifebp.org/store/Pages/health-care-costs-report-2024.aspx

Jamalabadi, S., Winter, V., & Schreyögg, J. A. (2020). Systematic review of the association between hospital cost/price and the quality of care. *Applied Health Economics and Health Policy*, 18, 625–639. https://doi.org/10.1007/s40258-020-00577-6

Kaufman, B. G., Thomas, S. R., Randolph, R., Perry, J. R., Thompson, K. W., Holmes, G. M., & Pink, G. H. (2015). The rising rate of rural hospital closures. *Journal of Rural Health*, 32(1), 35–43. https://doi.org/10.1111/jrh.12128

Lin, G. L., Ge, T. J. & Pal, R. (2022). Resident and fellow unions: Collective activism to promote well-being for physicians in training. *JAMA*, 328(7), 619–620. https://doi.org/10.1001/jama.2022.12838

Liu, J. (2022). *There are more than 11 million open jobs in America right now—and workers have the upper hand*. https://www.cnbc.com/2022/03/10/there-are-more-than-11-million-open-jobs-in-america-right-now.html

Maslach, C., & Leiter, M. (2006). Burnout. *Stress and Quality of Working Life: Current Perspectives in Occupational Health*, 37, 42–49.

Meese, K. A. (2024). *Is the healthcare workforce a problem or not? Backer's Hospital Review*. www.beckershospitalreview.com/workforce/is-the-healthcare-workforce-a-problem-or-not.html

Meese, K. A., Colón-López, A., Singh, J. A., Burkholder, G. A., Rogers, D. A. (2021). Healthcare is a team sport: Stress, resilience, and correlates of well-being among health system employees in a crisis. *Journal of Healthcare Management*, 66(4), 304–322. https://doi.org/10.1097/JHM-D-20-00288

Mensik, H. (2022). *Healthcare executives also experiencing burnout: survey*. https://www.healthcaredive.com/news/healthcare-executive-CEO-burnout-COVID-pandemic/638195/

Mondragon, J. A., & Wieland, J. (2022). Housing demand and remote work. (NBER Working Paper No. 30041). *National Bureau of Economic Research*. https://www.nber.org/system/files/working_papers/w30041/w30041.pdf

National Labor Relations Board. (2022). *Union election petitions increase 57% in first half of fiscal year 2022*. www.nlrb.gov/news-outreach/news-story/union-election-petitions-increase-57-in-first-half-of-fiscal-year-2022

Nelson, L. (2023). *University of Utah Health workers unionize due to low wages, staffing issues*. www.fox13now.com/news/local-news/university-of-utah-health-workers-unionize-due-to-low-wages-staffing-issues

Nundy, S., Cooper, L. A., & Mate, K. S. (2022). The quintuple aim for health care improvement: A new imperative to advance health equity. *JAMA*, 327(6), 521–522. https://doi.org/10.1001/jama.2021.25181

Pappas, M. A., Stoller, J. K., Shaker, V., Houser, J., Misra-Hebert, A. D. & Rothberg, M. B. (2022). Estimating the costs of physician turnover in hospital medicine. *Journal of Hospital Medicine*, 17(10), 803–808. https://doi.org/10.1002/jhm.12942

Parker, K., & Menasce Horowitz, J. (2022). Majority of workers who quit a job in 2021 cite low pay, no opportunities for advancement, feeling disrespected. *Pew Research Center*. https://www.pewresearch.org/short-reads/2022/03/09/majority-of-workers-who-quit-a-job-in-2021-cite-low-pay-no-opportunities-for-advancement-feeling-disrespected/

Plescia, M. (2021, October 14). *The cost of nurse turnover by the numbers*. Becker's Hospital CFO Report. Retrieved September 3, 2023, from https://www.beckershospitalreview.com/finance/the-cost-of-nurse-turnover-by-the-numbers.html

Popowitz, E., Bellemare, T., & Tieche, M. (2022, October). Addressing the healthcare staffing shortage. *Definitive Healthcare*. https://www.definitivehc.com/resources/research/healthcare-staffing-shortage

Robison, J. (2021). Communicate better with employees, regardless of where they work. *Gallup*. 1, 11. https://www.gallup.com/workplace/354289/communicate-better-employees-regardless-work.aspx

Statista. (2019, December 4). *Hospital costs distribution by type of expense U.S. 2016 Statista*. Retrieved September 3, 2023, from https://www.statista.com/statistics/204985/percent-of-hospital-costs-by-type-of-expense/

Stein, C. M. (2015). Academic clinical research: Death by a thousand clicks. *Science Translational Medicine*, 7(318), 318fs349. https://doi.org/10.1126/scitranslmed.aab3490

Suellentrop, A., & Bauman, E. (2021). How influential is a good manager? *Gallup*. https://www.gallup.com/cliftonstrengths/en/350423/influential-good-manager.aspx

The Physicians Foundation. (2021). *New survey reveals 55% of physicians know a physician who considered, attempted or died by suicide*. https://physiciansfoundation.org/new-survey-reveals-55-of-physicians-know-a-physician-who-considered-attempted-or-died-by-suicide/

Weise, K., Baker, M., & Bogel-Burroughs, N. (2020). *The coronavirus is forcing hospitals to cancel surgeries*. https://www.nytimes.com/2020/03/14/us/coronavirus-covid-surgeries-canceled.html

Young, A., Pei, X., Arnhart, K., Carter, J. D., & Chaudhry, H. J. (2023). FSMB census of licensed physicians in the United States, 2022. *Journal of Medical Regulation*, 109(2), 13–20. https://doi.org/10.30770/2572-1852-109.2.13

# CHAPTER 4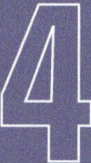

# HEALTH ECONOMICS

Mark Bonica and Stephen Mihalacki

## LEARNING OBJECTIVES

- Identify core economic assumptions in health economics. List and describe key economic assumptions such as individual decision-making, bounded rationality, scarce resources, and the role of institutions.
- Describe supply and demand dynamics in healthcare. Explain how **supply** and **demand** influence prices and quantities of healthcare services and identify factors that cause shifts in these curves.
- Recognize market failures in healthcare. identify examples of market failures in healthcare, including **asymmetric information** and **externalities**, and describe their basic implications.
- Explain the impact of health insurance on consumer behavior. State how health insurance influences consumer demand for healthcare services and define key terms like moral hazard.
- Compare different healthcare payment models. Identify and distinguish between fee-for-service and value-based payment models, such as **case rates**, and recognize their general advantages and challenges.

## KEY TERMS

- Asymmetric information
- Case rate
- Demand
- Equilibrium
- Externalities
- Moral hazard
- Scarce resources
- Supply
- Technological progress

# INTRODUCTION

Health economics emerged as a subfield of economics in the 1960s when economists began to apply the assumptions and tools of economics to questions of health and healthcare. In economics, an assumption is a foundational idea or condition that is accepted as true for the purpose of analysis or discussion. Assumptions simplify complex real-world situations, allowing economists to create models and frameworks that help explain and predict human behavior and market outcomes.

Assumptions are important because they provide a baseline for understanding how individuals and systems operate. By clearly stating assumptions, economists can make logical conclusions, test theories, and explain economic phenomena. While assumptions may not capture every detail of reality, they make it possible to focus on key factors that drive decision-making and market interactions.

The following are core assumptions that underpin economic reasoning and are essential for understanding healthcare markets:

- The individual as the basic unit of analysis: Economists start with individual human beings making choices. Individuals become parts of organizations, such as families, firms, and governments, but understanding organizations requires understanding individuals first. Firms and governments do not make decisions except by metaphor. It is the individual people who are members of the organizations who make decisions on behalf of the organizations.
- Bounded rationality: Individuals make rational choices to improve their happiness (economists call happiness *utility*), but since humans are not omniscient, we are bound by the information and abilities that we have and do the best we can to maximize our happiness.
- Scarce resources. Economics is primarily about choice: Most of the things we want are in limited supply, and we must choose between them. While most of us have our choices limited by our available income and wealth, even the wealthiest people are limited by the number of hours in the day. Because resources are scarce, we must make hard choices between the things we want, choosing some things and not others.
- Institutions matter: Institutions are the rules of society, formal and informal, that help shape the choices we can make as we pursue our happiness goals. The rules range from the formal legal structure that bounds the choices of individuals to informal beliefs, such as religious beliefs, gender roles, and racial/ethnic prejudices that are broadly held in society which also place limits on individual choices. Institutions shape choices by creating incentives, such as punishments and rewards, for particular behaviors.

## MARKETS AND PRICES

With these four assumptions in place, economists imagine people going about working together and trading with each other to improve their happiness. In formal markets, as people seek to trade, prices emerge. Prices provide information about the relative scarcity of any particular good or service and help people who need the good know how much they should buy, and the price also tells the people who make the good how much they should make. A higher price incentivizes a consumer to buy less and a producer to make more, and vice versa.

A basic model of markets involves trade between individuals and/or firms who **supply** a good or service and want to sell it and the individuals, firms, and governments who **demand** the good or service and want to buy it. The price and quantity of the good or service emerges from the interaction between suppliers and demanders. Economists portray this interaction as arriving at an equilibrium when supply matches demand.

## APPLYING MARKETS AND PRICES AT THE MICRO LEVEL: THE LOCAL MARKET FOR PHYSICAL THERAPY

To demonstrate this concept, let us model the supply and demand and physical therapists. Physical therapists (PTs) are allied health providers. They work with patients to improve musculoskeletal function. For example, it is common to work with a PT after a musculoskeletal injury such as a sprain or break to restore mobility.

## SUPPLY OF PHYSICAL THERAPISTS

When people think about a job, they consider a variety of factors such as whether they like the work, what the working conditions are like, and so forth, but one of the most important factors is what wage they will earn. Wages are the price of labor. Let us consider three PTs: Jack, Jill, and Goldy.

Jack is older and has been in practice for many years in Small Town. His children are grown and have moved away to Big City (which is not too far), and he has paid off his mortgage, so his personal expenses are low. Like most providers, he loves his work and loves working with patients. As he thinks about how much he needs to charge in order to keep working as a PT in Small Town, he concludes he needs to charge at least $50 per visit.

Jill also practices in Small Town. She has a young family, a new house, and a lot of expenses. She loves being a PT, but knows she needs to be able to charge at least $75 per visit or she would have to find somewhere else to practice.

Goldy is Jill's college friend. Goldy currently lives in Big City, but Jill talks so fondly about the charms of Small Town that Goldy dreams of moving out of Big City and joining her friend Jill as a PT in Small Town. Goldy currently makes $110 per visit in Big City but would be willing to take $100 per visit if she could work in Small Town.

We now have a sample of the labor market for potential PTs in Small Town. Each of our PTs has revealed their reservation wage, or the minimum amount of money for which they would be willing to work as a PT in Small Town. While each of them will not work for less than their reservation wage, they would happily work for more (Table 4.1).

We can now graph the supply curve for PTs in Small Town (Figure 4.1).

While Jack was willing to work for $50 per visit, he would be very pleased to work for $75 or $100. So if the people of Small Town are willing to pay $75 per visit, both Jack and Jill will continue to practice. If the price per visit rises to $100, Goldy will move to Small Town and provide services there as well. Connecting the dots, we draw the supply curve

### TABLE 4.1. SUPPLY OF PHYSICAL THERAPISTS

| PRICE PER VISIT | QUANTITY OF PTs | PTs |
|---|---|---|
| $50 | 1 | Jack |
| $75 | 2 | Jack and Jill |
| $100 | 3 | Jack, Jill, and Goldy |

PTs, physical therapists.

**FIGURE 4.1.** Supply curve for PTs in small town.

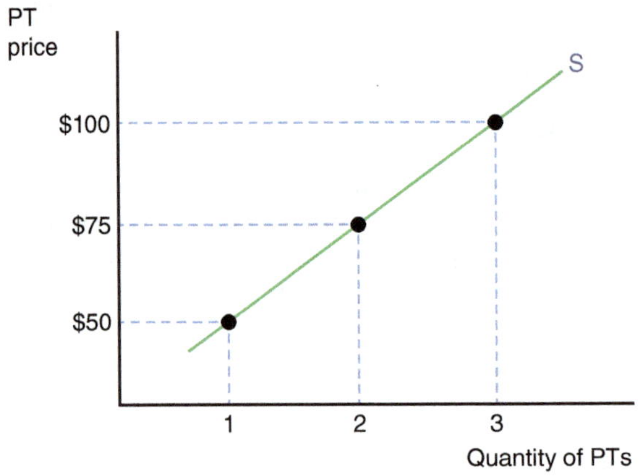

PTs, physical therapists.

for PTs in Small Town. By asking similar questions, we could ascertain the supply curve for any profession, from PTs to nurses to physicians and so forth.

Note that the supply curve slopes up. It slopes up because people have choices about what they do with their time. If the price of a visit falls below $50, Jack would likely retire. If the price falls below $75, Jill will move to Big City where she could earn more money like Goldy. Finally, in order to get Goldy to supply PT visits in Small Town, the price has to rise to at least $100, otherwise Goldy will not move there. Providers of goods and services respond to prices, providing more when the price is high and less when the price is low.

## DEMAND FOR PHYSICAL THERAPISTS

Physical therapy is an essential part of recovering from major surgeries such as knee and hip replacements. As our population ages, we are seeing more of these types of surgeries. This would be a very high-value use of a PT. Let us assume people with those sorts of needs would be willing to pay $100 per visit and there are enough of them to justify one PT in Small Town.

Physical therapy is also useful for less acute conditions such as chronic lower back pain. A PT might educate a patient on exercises, help with soft tissue mobilization, and maybe even perform spinal manipulation. Let us assume people with those sorts of needs would be willing to pay $75 per visit. The need is important but less urgent. Patients with this sort of condition might seek out an alternative to physical therapy, such as massage, if the PT price is too high. At $75 per visit, there would be demand for one PT from the people recovering from surgery, plus demand for an additional PT to address chronic conditions.

Finally, PTs can work with athletes and other active people to improve performance. People who are interested in this sort of support might be willing to pay $50 per visit. The professional guidance is valuable, but if they did not get it, they might be able to find it from a friend or on the internet. At $50, there would be demand from for two PTs from the first two conditions, plus demand for a third to work with people seeking to improve their athletic performance (Table 4.2).

We can now graph the demand curve for PTs in Small Town in Figure 4.2.

Demand curves always slope downward because as the price of a good or service increases, fewer people can afford it, or justify it, and substitutes become more appealing. A person with chronic back pain might be able to justify to themselves spending $75 per

## TABLE 4.2. DEMAND FOR PHYSICAL THERAPISTS

| PRICE PER VISIT | QUANTITY OF PTS DEMANDED |
|---|---|
| $100 | 1 |
| $75 | 2 |
| $50 | 3 |

PTs, physical therapists.

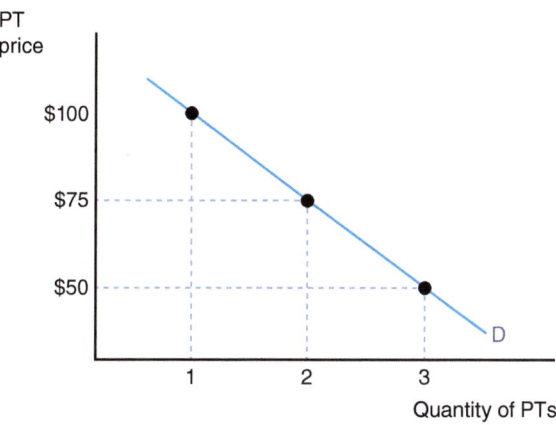

**FIGURE 4.2.** Demand curve for PTs in small town.

PTs, physical therapists.

visit but might decide to try home care or some other means of alleviating the pain if the price is >$75 or might simply go without. This is the reality of healthcare for many people, especially those who do not have health insurance and even for some who do. We could create a similar demand curve for any good or service: physician visits, medicine, exercise classes, and so forth.

## EQUILIBRIUM PRICE FOR PHYSICAL THERAPIST VISITS

How much will a PT visit cost in Small Town? We can figure that out by putting our two curves together. Where the supply and demand curves cross, we have an **equilibrium** (Figure 4.3).

At a price of $75, there is a demand for two providers, and there are two providers who are willing to work for $75. If a provider tries to raise or lower their prices, there will be pressure from the demand side to bring the price back to $75 (Figure 4.4).

In Small Town, we can see from the demand curve that people would like to have three providers who charge $50 per visit. However, only Jack would be willing to work at $50 per visit, so the town would only have one provider. The result would be a shortage of providers. The people who have just had surgery would be desperate to get treatment and would offer more than $50 to be seen, resulting in upward price pressure. The higher price would attract an additional therapist back to Small Town. Higher prices signal to suppliers to switch what they are doing and offer their goods and services—for example, if only Jack were working in Small Town and the price rose to $75 per visit, Jill, or someone like her, would move their practice to Small Town (Figure 4.5).

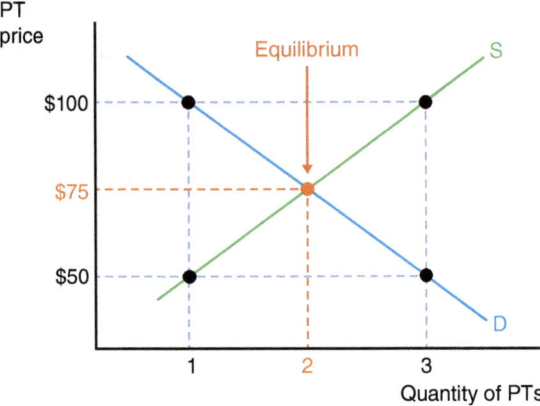

FIGURE 4.3. Example of equilibrium.

PTs, physical therapists.

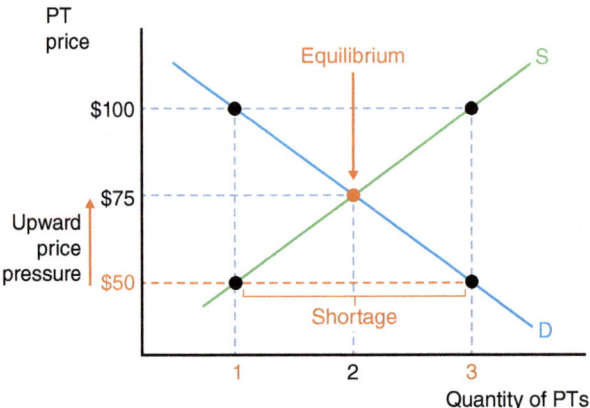

FIGURE 4.4. Results of raising or lowering prices.

PTs, physical therapists.

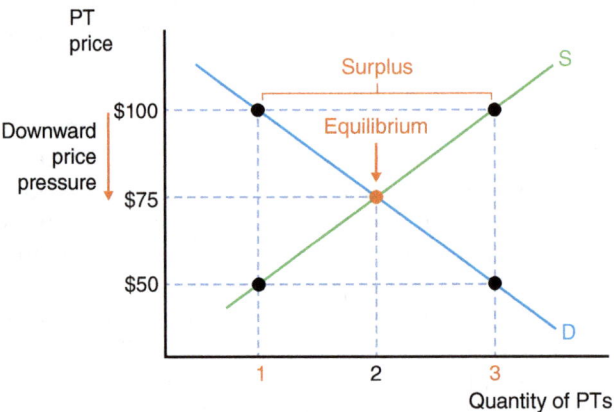

FIGURE 4.5. Shortage of providers results in higher prices.

PTs, physical therapists.

If the PTs try to raise their prices to $100 per visit, Goldy would want to move to Small Town, creating a surplus of two PTs. At $100. there will be only demand for one PT from the people who have just had surgery and were willing to pay that higher price. The people with chronic pain and the athletes would look for other solutions. We could imagine a scenario where Jack and Jill split the demand for one provider, each working part-time, but while that might work for Jack, it would not for work Jill since she needs to work full time. She would cut her price to $75 (her reservation wage) in order to attract more patients, and Jack would have to follow because all of the patients would try to get appointments with Jill, leading us back to the equilibrium.

## APPLYING MARKETS AND PRICES AT THE MACRO LEVEL: THE NATIONAL MARKET FOR HEALTHCARE SERVICES

We can apply this model to the market for healthcare services in the United States (Figure 4.6).

In Figure 4.6, we can see the demand for healthcare services as an aggregate. The curves now represent physical therapy, skilled nursing, surgery, and all the other health services provided in the United States. Demand (D) curves still slope downward because as prices decrease, more consumers are willing or able to purchase more healthcare, making it more attractive and affordable relative to other options. Supply (S) curves still slope upward because higher prices incentivize producers to supply more healthcare as higher revenue can cover increasing costs. As with the PT model, price (P) and quantity (Q) emerge at the intersection of supply and demand curves because this point represents equilibrium: the price where the quantity supplied matches the quantity demanded. At this price, suppliers are willing to produce the exact amount consumers wish to buy, creating a stable balance where no surplus or shortage exists.

## APPLYING ECONOMIC REASONING TO HEALTHCARE: SUPPLY AND DEMAND OF HEALTHCARE SERVICES

This basic model of a market for healthcare services allows us to apply economic reasoning to understand why healthcare services become more or less expensive and more or less scarce. If either the supply or demand for healthcare changes, we can expect a change

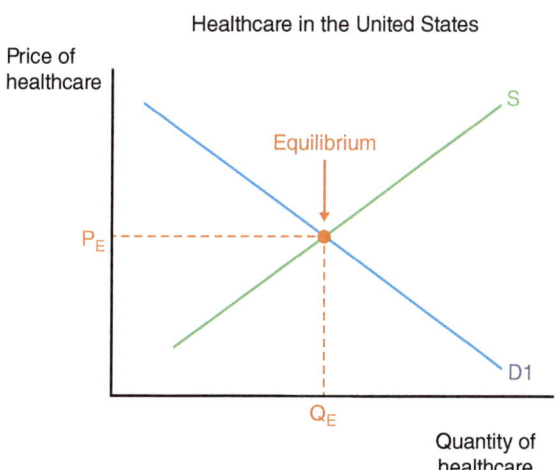

**FIGURE 4.6.** Demand for healthcare services in the United States.

in the overall cost (price) of healthcare and the overall availability of healthcare (quantity). Let us look at things that change supply and demand and see how they interact. Some of these graphs will allow us to discuss why the people in the United States use more healthcare and spend more on it than other countries.

## CHANGES IN DEMAND FOR HEALTHCARE

An increase in the overall demand for healthcare is graphically represented as a rightward shift of the demand curve. Assuming the factors that affect the supply curve remain the same, we can see the effect of an increase in demand in Figure 4.7.

We start at our initial equilibrium (E1) with corresponding price, P1, and the corresponding quantity of care delivered, Q1. Then, the demand curve moves to the right to D2, and pressures on price rise to P2 as people demand more healthcare (Q2). The result of an increase in demand is both higher prices *and* more healthcare delivered at a new equilibrium (E2).

A decrease in demand for healthcare has the opposite effect: a decrease in price and a decrease in the quantity of healthcare delivered (Figure 4.8).

**FIGURE 4.7.** Increase in overall demand for healthcare.

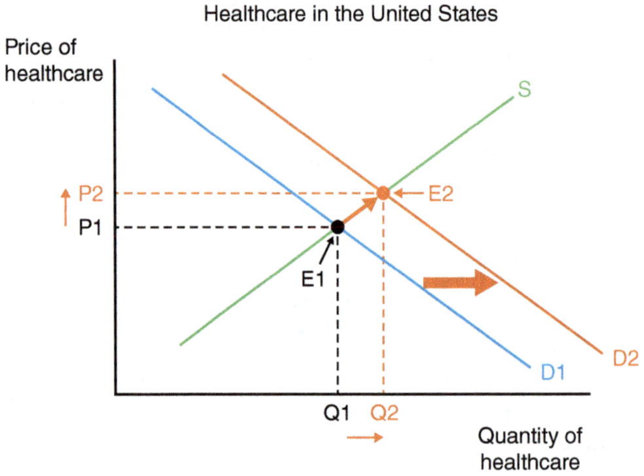

**FIGURE 4.8.** Decrease in demand for healthcare.

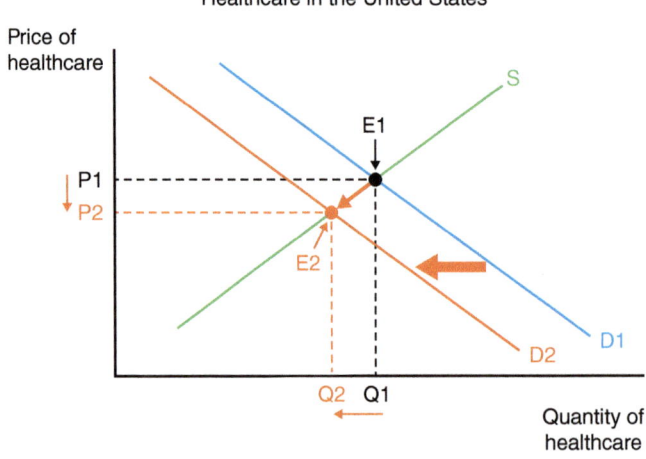

> **BOX 4.1: DEMAND SHIFTERS**
>
> What are some factors that shift the demand for healthcare services?
> - Changes in income
> - Changes in population
> - Technological progress
> - Taxes and subsidies

What are the factors that make demand either increase or decrease? Some typical answers that apply to healthcare are as follows (Box 4.1):

1. *Changes in income:* An increase in income results in a right shift of the demand curve, as portrayed in Figure 4.7. Since World War II, the United States has achieved one of the highest levels of per capita income in the world. If all countries started at the same initial equilibrium (E1), because the incomes of the people of the United States grew more quickly than most other countries, economic theory would help you predict that people in the United States would consume more healthcare and spend more on it, which is true. As people achieve higher levels of income, they want more healthcare. Life-saving care is an example of people wanting more healthcare, such as better access to emergency departments or better oncology care. As income rises, people are also more willing to pay for lifestyle care, such as cosmetic surgery, cosmetic orthodontics, Botox injections, and medically supervised weight loss.

   Economic growth has not happened evenly across the United States. Since the 2000s, many parts of the country began to deindustrialize, and factory jobs that once promised middle-class incomes to workers with little formal education or training disappeared (Green, 2020). In these areas, we have seen an overall decrease in community income, even as the country has continued to become wealthier. So, while on average, Figure 4.7 represents the United States, Figure 4.8 better represents these areas where economic growth has reversed. In these areas, we have seen many hospitals close, and providers leave as the people remaining behind can no longer afford care. Thus, this simple model not only helps us understand factors causing overall prices and consumption of healthcare in the United States to be higher than most other countries, but it also predicts disparities in healthcare services within the United States.

2. *Changes in population:* An increase in population causes the demand curve to shift to the right (Figure 4.7), while a decrease in population causes the demand curve to shift to the left (Figure 4.8). Many rural areas are losing population, and rural hospitals are at a greater risk of closing (Kaufman et al., 2016). Some of the fastest growing areas of the Unites States are in Texas. According to the U.S. Census Bureau, the rural town of Celina, Texas, grew from a population of 17,808 in 2020 to 43,317 in 2023 or approximately 143% in 3 years, making it one of the fastest growing communities in the United States (U.S. Census Bureau, 2024). The increase in population shifted the demand curve for care to the right. This increase in willingness to pay for care attracted healthcare providers, and a new hospital is scheduled to open in 2025 to address the increase in demand (Graham, 2024) and increase the quantity of care provided there.

3. *Technological progress:* Improvements in healthcare technology tend to stimulate demand for healthcare services, resulting in a right shift of the demand curve (Figure 4.7) and both an increase in cost and amount of care demanded. There are

many examples of things that could not be treated historically that now can be treated thanks to technological progress. Antibiotics were not commonly available until the 1930s (Adedeji, 2016). Prior to the discovery of penicillin in 1928, there was little medicine could do for bacterial infections except hope that the body could fight it off. Amputation was commonly used for infections of the extremities (Markatos et al., 2019). Insulin was first used on a human patient in 1922 (American Diabetes Association, 2019). Prior to that, type I diabetes was a death sentence, as children born with it fell into comas and died. These are examples of improvements in technology that generate additional demand, and as a result, higher prices and more healthcare are delivered. The United States leads the world in advances in medical technology, resulting in higher demand. As healthcare technology continues to evolve, healthcare economists are often involved in developing frameworks for measuring healthcare outcomes to ensure progress aligns with patient needs and quality standards (Blumenthal & McGinnis, 2015).

4. *Taxes and subsidies:* The government (at all levels) can affect demand through taxes and subsidies. Health economists study the effects of both. Taxes have the effect of making things more expensive. A tax effectively shifts the consumer's demand to the left, as if their income had been reduced. The result is complicated, but the price to the consumer is raised by the amount of tax charged, reducing the quantity the consumer can afford. Taxes are commonly applied to things the government would like to discourage consumers from consuming, such as cigarettes, alcohol, and sweetened beverages, all of which are bad for individuals' health. These taxes have been shown to effectively reduce the consumption of cigarettes (Bader et al., 2011), alcohol (Gehrsitz et al., 2021), and sweetened beverages (Redondo et al., 2018).

When the government wants to encourage consumers to do something, it can offer subsidies. An example of a subsidy is the Supplemental Nutrition Assistance Program (SNAP), which provides vouchers to low-income families to buy food (formerly the Food Stamp Program). A subsidy like SNAP effectively increases beneficiaries' income with respect to the subsidized product. SNAP increases the amount of money a beneficiary can spend on nutritious food.

## CHANGES IN SUPPLY OF HEALTHCARE

As with demand, a change in the overall supply of healthcare services is represented by a rightward shift of the supply curve (Figure 4.9).

An increase in supply while holding demand constant results in the cost of healthcare decreasing while the quantity supplied increases. This is the ideal outcome for consumers. How we can get to this outcome is an important question.

A decrease in supply while holding demand constant results in the cost of healthcare increasing while we get less of it. Let us look at the factors that make supply shift left or right (Box 4.2).

- *Input prices.* A major factor a firm considers when entering (or leaving) a market (and therefore adding or reducing supply) is the cost of its inputs. The single largest input in healthcare delivery is manpower. Employees represent more than half of the budget for most hospitals and clinics. When wages rise quickly as they have over the last several years, this has a dramatic impact on the cost of delivering healthcare. The result is these organizations are less able to deliver care, and this causes the supply curve to shift left (Figure 4.10), reducing the quantity of care and causing the price to rise. Between February of 2020 and January of 2024, healthcare wages rose more than 20% (Telesford et al., 2024).

**FIGURE 4.9.** Change in overall supply of healthcare services.

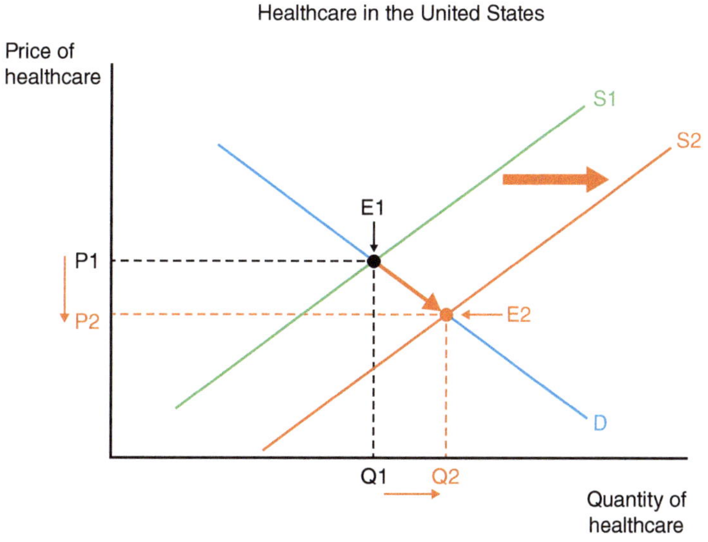

### BOX 4.2: SUPPLY SHIFTERS

What are some factors that shift the supply of healthcare services?
- Input prices
- Number of suppliers
- Technology
- Regulation

In addition to wage inflation, increasing educational requirements are driving up the cost of labor. In 2016, the Commission on Accreditation in Physical Therapy Education (CAPTE) made the Doctor of Physical Therapy (DPT) the minimum level of education for a person to become a PT, extending mandatory training from 4 years to 7 (American Physical Therapy Association, n.d.). The field of pharmacy has similarly adopted the 6-year Doctor of Pharmacy (PharmD) as the entry level of education over the historical 4-year baccalaureate. Other specialties such as physician assistants, nurse practitioners, and occupational therapists are headed in the same direction. Supply constraints in primary care, exacerbated by increasing educational requirements and workload, are well documented by Bodenheimer and Pham (2010). Requiring providers to get additional years of training increases the cost of training medical professionals (a critical input to healthcare delivery) and thus forces the supply curve for health services to the left (Figure 4.10), reducing supply and increasing cost.

- *Number of suppliers:* When the number of suppliers increases in a market, the supply curve shifts right, as in Figure 4.9, resulting in more supply at lower cost to consumers. New providers entering a market will compete with the existing providers to get market share. For example, free-standing imaging centers that enter a market will cut the price of an MRI in order to attract new patients. This forces everyone in the market to cut prices.
- *Technology:* Technological progress on the supplier side can shift the supply curve to the right (see Figure 4.9) if processes can be automated, substituting human

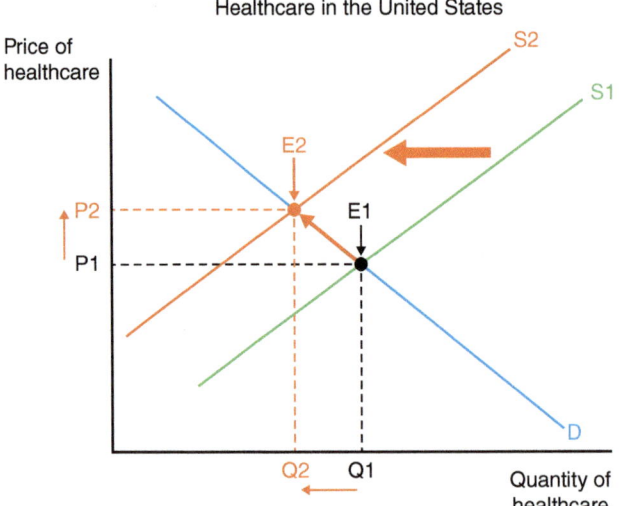

**FIGURE 4.10.** Increase in supply while holding demand constant.

workers with machines. While this has had great success in manufacturing, it has had much less success in healthcare delivery because the process of caring for a patient is stubbornly manpower intensive. One good news story in healthcare delivery has been the advent of telemedicine. Telemedicine allows providers to provide care across broad geographic areas without the cost of travel (Eze et al., 2020). This has been especially valuable in rural areas, resulting in a right shift of supply (see Figure 4.9).

- *Regulation:* The healthcare sector is heavily regulated and with good reason. Most patients lack the ability to determine if their care is being delivered safely and effectively. Regulators such as the Food and Drug Administration (FDA) exist to ensure the safety and efficacy of treatment. The American Hospital Association (AHA) estimated that the average community hospital spends $7.6 million annually to comply with federal regulations, amounting to $1,200 in cost for each patient admission (AHA, 2017). While additional regulations may improve healthcare delivery quality, the increase in cost shifts the supply curve left (see Figure 4.10), reducing the amount of care available and raising prices to consumers who are able to afford the remaining care.

## MARKET FAILURE AND HEALTH

Sometimes, markets do not provide the right incentives to consumers and suppliers. When this happens, the socially optimal amounts of goods and services are not produced. Health economists have made several important observations about health and healthcare delivery using their economic perspectives, particularly by identifying ways that markets for health and healthcare fail. Two sources of market failure in healthcare are asymmetric information and externalities.

### ASYMMETRIC INFORMATION

Most of what health economists study arises out of the problem of **asymmetric information**. Kenneth Arrow's 1963 article, "Uncertainty and the Welfare Economics of Medical Care," is generally regarded as the beginning of the economic study of healthcare markets. Arrow correctly identified that healthcare markets are pervaded by the problem of asymmetric information. Asymmetric information refers to a situation where two parties are negotiating and one party has important information relevant to the outcome of the negotiation and the other does not. This situation is rampant in healthcare because of the imbalance in knowledge between a physician and their patient. If a physician tells a patient they need a procedure or test, even if the patient is presented with the price (which is often not available in advance), the patient rarely has the knowledge to know if the physician is correct or not. This situation becomes particularly challenging if the physician stands to benefit from the patient getting additional procedures or tests.

Asymmetric information can break down the smooth functioning of markets because the buyers (patients) do not have enough information. When markets work properly, they generate prices that accurately reflect the usefulness of the goods and services. When this market process fails, economists call this *market failure*. Asymmetric information is a major cause of market failure.

## EXTERNALITIES

One focus of health economics is understanding market failures associated with **externalities**. Externalities can be positive or negative, both representing cases where the market fails to produce the right quantity at the right price. For instance, when you get an immunization for a contagious disease, such as measles, you reduce your risk of getting sick. Additionally, you also lower the chance of spreading the disease to others. Thus, the immunization benefits you and it also provides a benefit to the people you interact with, many of whom you may not even know, especially in an urban environment. Economists call these added benefits to others a *positive externality*.

In a perfectly efficient market, the price of an immunization would reflect all the value it provides. However, it is impossible for the provider to charge all the people who will benefit, especially since the person receiving the immunization does not know whom they will protect. Because this additional value accrues to someone else, we do not pay for the full social value as individuals. As a result, the market price for immunizations is often too high, leading fewer people to get vaccinated than would be socially optimal.

In contrast, intensive livestock farming (often called *factory farming*) creates conditions that make animals vulnerable to disease. Farmers often use preventive antibiotics to keep animals healthy, lowering production costs and effectively shifting the meat supply curve to the right (see Figure 4.9). However, these antibiotics can lead to the development of antibiotic-resistant bacteria, which may spread to humans and make infections harder to treat (Oliveira et al., 2020). While cheaper meat benefits farmers and consumers, this practice creates a *negative externality* by reducing the effectiveness of antibiotics for society.

Both positive and negative externalities are *market failures*. For negative externalities, the market produces too much of something, while for positive externalities, it produces too little.

## HEALTH INSURANCE—FIXING SOME MARKET FAILURES, INTRODUCING OTHERS

As you will read in Chapter 12, "Health Insurance and Reimbursement," one of the functions of health insurance is to protect individuals from unexpected, high-cost medical expenses that can be difficult to foresee. Consumers pay health insurers to be their financial intermediaries with the consumers' healthcare providers. A consumer pays for a health plan, and a health insurer then pays for the consumer's necessary healthcare.

This arrangement moves the financial risk from the consumer to the insurer. Because the consumer is no longer paying the full price of the healthcare they are receiving, it increases their demand for health services.

Without health insurance, a consumer would demand Q1 amount of healthcare and pay P1 for each unit. The consumer's total cost of care would be P1 × Q1, or the red box (Figure 4.11; e.g., if P1 is $50 and Q1 is five visits, the total cost of care would be $50 × 5 = $250).

Now imagine the consumer purchases a health plan where they pay a co-pay of $10 each time they see their doctor (a co-pay is a fee collected by the provider from the patient for each visit; the provider then bills the patient's insurances for the balance of the negotiated price of the visit). If the patient now faces a price of $10 per visit instead of $50, the patient will visit the doctor more often (Figure 4.12).

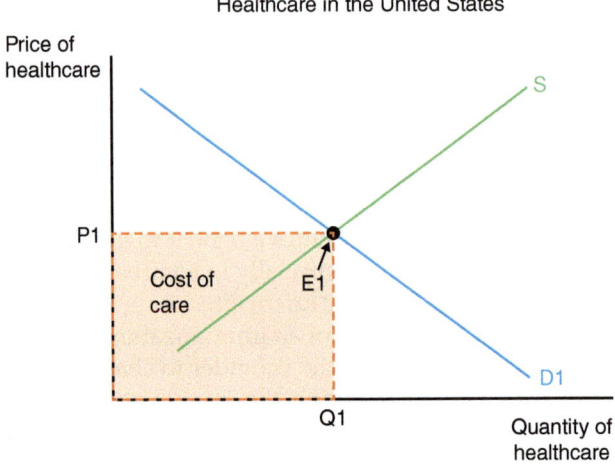

FIGURE 4.11. Total cost of care.

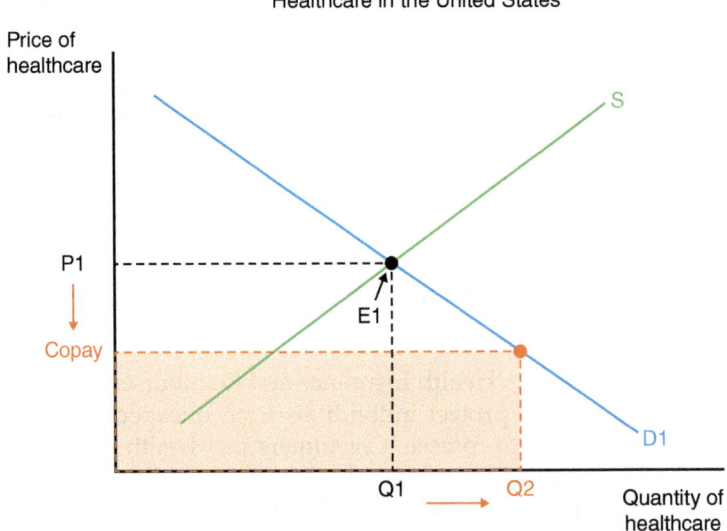

FIGURE 4.12. Price of co-pay.

As long as the co-pay is less than the market price of P1, the consumer will increase their utilization of healthcare services. To find the quantity the consumer will demand, we draw a line from the co-pay price to the right until we hit the consumer's demand curve. At the copay price, the consumer will use Q2 visits. The cost to the patient will be the co-pay × Q2 (Figure 4.13; e.g., if the co-pay is $10 and they now use seven visits, the cost of care to them will be $10 × 7 = $70).

The doctor was willing to provide Q1 visits at P1. To find how much the doctor will require to provide Q2 visits, we draw a line up from Q2 on the quantity axis to the doctor's supply curve. The doctor will want $P_{doc}$, which is >P1. The result is the total cost of care under insurance rises to $P_{doc}$ × Q2 (Figure 4.14; e.g., if we assume $P_{doc}$ is $60, the total cost of care rises to $60 × 7 = $420).

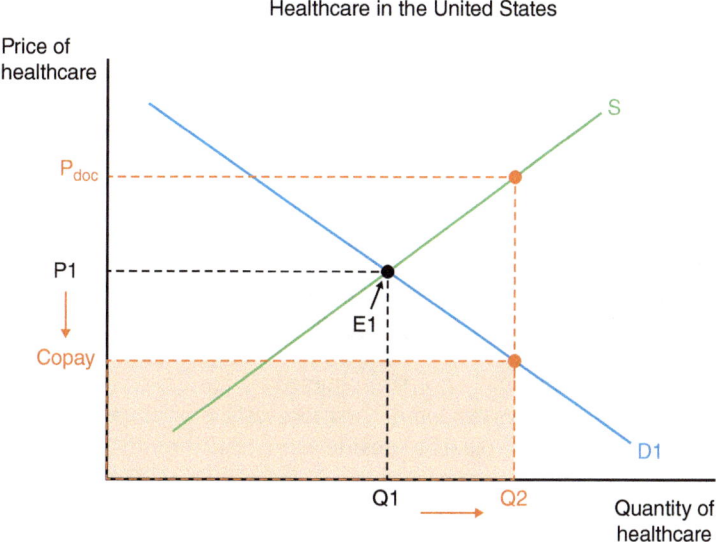

**FIGURE 4.13.** Healthcare quantity consumers will demand.

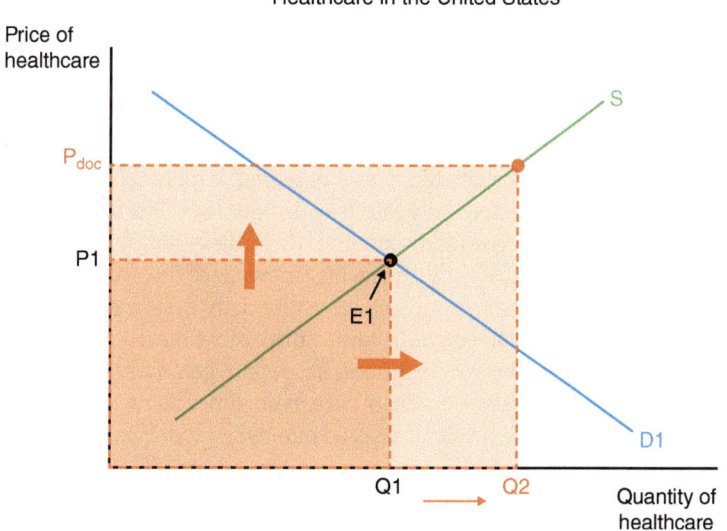

**FIGURE 4.14.** Cost of doctor visit.

Thus, under insurance, the total cost of care expands from P1 × Q1 to $P_{doc}$ × Q2 (from $250 to $420 in this example). When we use more of a resource, like doctor's visits, when someone else (in this case, the insurance company) is paying for them, this is called **moral hazard** (Cutler & Zeckhauser, 2000; Einav & Finkelstein, 2018; Pauly, 1968). Insurance companies are very good at predicting consumer behavior, so the insurance company will set the premium for the consumer to include the $420 in doctor's visits. As a result, the patient pays more for healthcare than they would have under market conditions without insurance, increasing the overall cost of healthcare.

This outcome is not necessarily all bad. Insurance companies use tools like co-pays to manipulate consumer behavior. Because of asymmetric information, consumers often will underutilize services that can keep them healthy and overuse services that they may not need. Unlike consumers, insurance companies employ healthcare professionals (including health economists) to gather information about the best use of healthcare resources. Knowing that prices incentivize consumer behavior, insurance companies will set low co-pays to encourage consumers to use services the insurance company knows are good for consumers and higher co-pays (or refuse to pay for) services the insurance company does not regard as necessary for maintaining good health. The Patient Protection and Affordable Care Act (ACA; discussed further in Chapter 7, "Introduction to Health Policy and Healthcare Reform") requires insurance companies to offer certain services at a co-pay of $0. These services are usually preventive measures, some with positive externalities, such as immunizations.

## CASE STUDY 4.1: INFLUENCING PATIENT CARE AND DECISION-MAKING BY REALIGNING PROVIDER INCENTIVES: A REAL-WORLD EXAMPLE

Healthcare providers have traditionally been reimbursed via fee for service, a method where payment is made for individual services rendered. The more tests, procedures, and services a provider performs, the more they are able to bill. The provider's financial incentive clearly lies in being able to perform more individual services and procedures. This type of incentive is not aligned to the best interest of the patient and often leads to healthcare waste and abuse such as overbilling. Porter and Lee (2013) argue that value-based care models, such as case rates, incentivize providers to focus on patient outcomes rather than service volume, potentially improving efficiency and quality of care.

One technique that insurance providers can implement to control costs and promote efficient care, especially for hospitals and facilities, is called a **case rate**. A case rate is a single or flat reimbursement amount to a provider based on all services rendered as part of one episode of care. This type of arrangement is classified as a "value-based" arrangement because it reimburses the provider for the outcome and care of the patient regardless of the actual costs the provider might have incurred to deliver that care. Value-based contracts will be discussed more in Chapter 12, "Health Insurance and Reimbursement."

Take, for example, an inpatient facility that treats patients for mental health disorders and is reimbursed by an insurer at a negotiated daily rate (say $1,000/day). This facility will be paid $1,000 every day the patient is in their care until discharged. Regardless of how sick a patient is, or how much or little treatment is required, clearly, the facility maximizes their reimbursement the longer a patient stays in their care (and their profit so long as the daily costs are below $1,000 per day).

Under a case rate, the provider can be paid a lump sum every time a patient is admitted, regardless of how little or long a patient stays in treatment. If a patient gets admitted and stays for 1 day or 100 days, the provider receives the same exact amount every time. Using insurance claims data, the provider and insurer can determine the optimal case rate to be paid. Please consider Figure 4.15.

**FIGURE 4.15.** Historical Facility Claims—Provider A.

Cost per day ("per diem") = $1,000

| Avg length of stay (days) | Count of patient admissions | % of cases by length of stay (Admits/Total admits) |
|---|---|---|
| 1 | 5 | 5% |
| 2 | 3 | 3% |
| 3 | 4 | 4% |
| 4 | 2 | 2% |
| 5 | 8 | 8% |
| 6 | 7 | 7% |
| 7 | 6 | 6% |
| 8 | 3 | 3% |
| 9 | 7 | 7% |
| 10 | 10 | 10% |
| 11 | 19 | 19% |
| 12 | 11 | 11% |
| 13 | 9 | 9% |
| 14 | 4 | 4% |
| 15 | 2 | 2% |
| **Total cases** | **100** | **100%** |

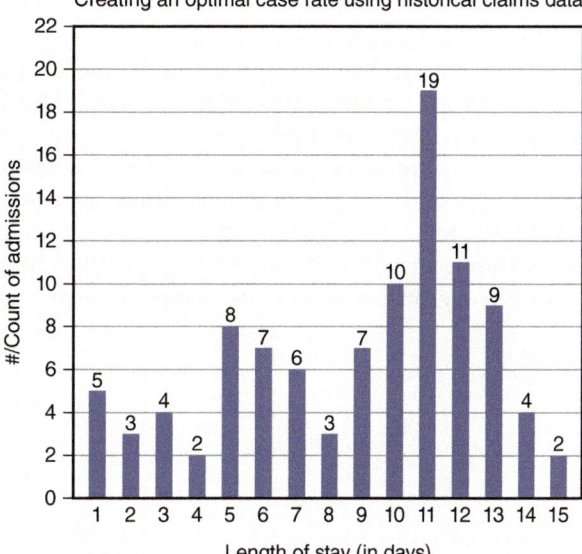

Based on claims that Provider A submitted to their insurer, most admissions cases show a stay of at least 11 days (19% of all cases). Granted some patient admissions are shorter and some are longer, but historically most patients who are treated at this facility stay for 11 days. Under a case rate, the insurer may offer this provider a flat rate of $11,000 for every patient that is admitted ($1,000 per diem × 11 days). The insurer benefits from this arrangement because it will control costs by eliminating spending on outlier cases (those admissions lasting longer than 11 days). They can also budget more appropriately in years to come because this provider's spending is now more predictable. The provider benefits because they can capture more revenue by becoming more efficient and providing better care. For every patient that can be discharged earlier than 11 days, the provider earns an extra $1,000. Finally (and most important), the patient benefits from more streamlined, collaborative, and efficient care by hopefully not having to endure any longer/unnecessary lengths of stay.

Although case rates effectively realign provider incentives for care, this type of arrangement is not without challenges. Without additional controls, a provider might be encouraged to discharge a patient too early in order to maximize profit. Providers might also avoid accepting very sick patients (i.e., adverse selection) knowing that a lengthy stay will be needed, thus incurring more costs than their case rate will cover. Luckily most insurers have ways to protect against this type of "gaming" the case rate. Most insurers will not pay a new case rate if a patient is discharged too early and readmits within a certain time frame, thus protecting the insurer. Additionally, insurers often allow a provision for catastrophic loss cases (patients staying in care past a certain length of stay) where the provider will revert to fee for service once a certain day threshold is met, thus protecting the provider.

## CONCLUSION

Health economics applies the assumptions and tools of economics to questions of health and healthcare delivery. Through basic market models of supply and demand, we can understand why healthcare services become more or less expensive and more or less scarce. The field recognizes that healthcare markets often fail to provide the right incentives to consumers and suppliers, particularly due to asymmetric information between physicians and patients and externalities that affect society. While health insurance helps protect individuals from unexpected, high-cost medical expenses, it can introduce moral hazard when consumers use more healthcare resources because someone else is paying. Modern healthcare systems are exploring payment reforms, such as moving from fee-for-service to case rates, that attempt to realign provider incentives with patient care while controlling costs. These economic perspectives help us understand how to create healthcare delivery systems that work better for both providers and patients.

# END-OF-CHAPTER RESOURCES

## CRITICAL THINKING QUESTIONS

- How does the assumption of the individual as the basic unit of analysis affect the way we understand decision-making in healthcare organizations? Can this perspective be limiting when evaluating collective behaviors?
- In what ways do patients' and providers' limited information impact their healthcare choices? Can you think of examples where this limitation leads to suboptimal outcomes?
- Discuss how formal institutions, such as regulatory bodies, and informal institutions, like cultural beliefs, shape the availability and delivery of healthcare. How do these institutions contribute to disparities in healthcare access?
- Given that scarcity is a fundamental concept in economics, how does it manifest in healthcare, and what are some examples where this scarcity leads to difficult trade-offs?
- How does technological progress influence the demand for healthcare services? Can technological improvements lead to both increased access and higher costs simultaneously?
- Explain the concept of market equilibrium with respect to the supply and demand of healthcare services. What factors might cause this equilibrium to be disrupted, leading to either a surplus or a shortage of services?
- Discuss the implications of positive and negative externalities in the healthcare system. What are some strategies that policymakers could use to address these externalities to optimize health outcomes?
- How does asymmetric information between patients and providers contribute to market failure in healthcare? What measures can be implemented to reduce the impact of this problem?
- How does the existence of health insurance alter consumer demand for healthcare services? What are some potential benefits and drawbacks of this change in consumer behavior?
- Discuss the advantages and challenges associated with value-based payment systems like case rates compared to traditional fee-for-service models. How do these payment systems impact the quality of care provided and the financial incentives for providers?

## LEARNING ACTIVITIES

### CourseConnect ▶

To access self-assessment questions and interactive, competency-based learning activities for this chapter, visit www.springerpub.com/courseconnect. See inside front cover and tear-out card for CourseConnect details.

## REFERENCES

Adedeji, W. A. (2016). The treasure called antibiotics. *Annals of Ibadan Postgraduate Medicine, 14*(2), 56–57.

American Diabetes Association. (2019, July 1). *The history of a wonderful thing we call insulin.* https://diabetes.org/blog/history-wonderful-thing-we-call-insulin

American Hospital Association. (2017, November 3). *Assessing the regulatory burden on health systems, hospitals and post-acute care providers.* https://www.aha.org/guidesreports/2017-11-03-regulatory-overload-report

American Physical Therapy Association. (n.d.). *The clinical doctorate (or "DPT") becomes the only degree conferred by CAPTE-accredited educational institutions*. Retrieved November 11, 2024, from https://timeline.apta.org/timeline/the-clinical-doctorate-or-dpt-becomes-the-only-degree-conferred-by-capte-accredited-educational-institutions/

Bader, P., Boisclair, D., & Ferrence, R. (2011). Effects of tobacco taxation and pricing on smoking behavior in high risk populations: A knowledge synthesis. *International Journal of Environmental Research and Public Health, 8*(11), 4118–4139. https://doi.org/10.3390/ijerph8114118

Blumenthal, D., & McGinnis, J. M. (2015). Measuring vital signs: An IOM report on core metrics for health and health care progress. *Journal of the American Medical Association, 313*(19), 1901–1902. https://doi.org/10.1001/jama.2015.4862

Bodenheimer, T., & Pham, H. H. (2010). Primary care: Current problems and proposed solutions. *Health Affairs, 29*(5), 799–805. https://doi.org/10.1377/hlthaff.2010.0026

Cutler, D. M., & Zeckhauser, R. J. (2000). The anatomy of health insurance. In A. J. Culyer & J. P. Newhouse (Eds.). *Handbook of health economics* (Vol. 1, pp. 563–643). Elsevier.

Einav, L., & Finkelstein, A. (2018). Moral hazard in health insurance: What we know and how we know it. *Journal of the European Economic Association, 16*(4), 957–982. https://doi.org/10.1093/jeea/jvy017

Eze, N. D., Mateus, C., & Cravo Oliveira Hashiguchi, T. (2020). Telemedicine in the OECD: An umbrella review of clinical and cost-effectiveness, patient experience and implementation. *PLoS One, 15*(8), e0237585. https://doi.org/10.1371/journal.pone.0237585

Gehrsitz, M., Saffer, H., & Grossman, M. (2021). The effect of changes in alcohol tax differentials on alcohol consumption. *Journal of Public Economics, 204*, 104520. https://doi.org/10.1016/j.jpubeco.2021.104520

Graham, M. (2024, July 28). New hospital coming to North Texas 'boom town'. *Spectrum News*. https://spectrumlocalnews.com/tx/south-texas-el-paso/news/2024/07/26/new-hospital-coming-to-north-texas--boom-town-?cid=share_clip

Green, G. P. (2020). Deindustrialization of rural America: Economic restructuring and the rural ghetto. *Local Development & Society, 1*(1), 15–25. https://doi.org/10.1080/26883597.2020.1801331

Kaufman, B. G., Thomas, S. R., Randolph, R. K., Perry, J. R., Thompson, K. W., Holmes, G. M., & Pink, G. H. (2016). The rising rate of rural hospital closures. *The Journal of Rural Health, 32*(1), 35–43. https://doi.org/10.1111/jrh.12128

Markatos, K., Karamanou, M., Saranteas, T., & Mavrogenis, A. F. (2019). Hallmarks of amputation surgery. *International Orthopaedics, 43*, 493–499. https://doi.org/10.1007/s00264-018-4024-6

Oliveira, N. A., Gonçalves, B. L., Lee, S. H., Oliveira, C. A. F., & Corassin, C. H. (2020). Use of antibiotics in animal production and its impact on human health. *Journal of Food Chemistry and Nanotechnology, 6*(01), 40–47. https://doi.org/10.17756/jfcn.2020-082

Pauly, M. V. (1968). The economics of moral hazard: Comment. *American Economic Review, 58*(3), 531–537. https://doi.org/10.1016/s0167-6296(99)00015-6

Porter, M. E., & Lee, T. H. (2013). The strategy that will fix health care. *Harvard Business Review, 91*(10), 50–70. https://hbr.org/2013/10/the-strategy-that-will-fix-health-care

Redondo, M., Hernández-Aguado, I., & Lumbreras, B. (2018). The impact of the tax on sweetened beverages: A systematic review. *The American Journal of Clinical Nutrition, 108*(3), 548–563. https://doi.org/10.1093/ajcn/nqy135

Telesford, I., Wager, E., Hughes-Cromwick, P., Amin, K., & Cox, C. (2024, March 27). What are the recent trends in health sector employment? *Peterson-KFF Health System Tracker*. https://www.healthsystemtracker.org/chart-collection/what-are-the-recent-trends-health-sector-employment/

U.S. Census Bureau. (2024, May). *Annual estimates of the resident population for incorporated places of 20,000 or more, ranked by July 1, 2023 population: April 1, 2020 to July 1, 2023 (SUB-IP-EST2023-ANNRNK)*. U.S. Census Bureau, Population Division. https://www.census.gov/data/tables/time-series/demo/popest/2020s-total-cities-and-towns.html

# CHAPTER 5

# ORGANIZATIONAL DESIGN

Soham Sengupta and Prabhat Singh

### LEARNING OBJECTIVES

- Understand the organizational definition and its operational elements.
- Recognize the role of leadership in designing and developing organizational design.
- Explore how leadership influences the antecedents of organizational design.
- Understand the consequences of effective organizational design.
- Understand organizational structure.

### KEY TERMS

- Healthcare
- Hospitals
- Leadership
- Organizational design
- Organizational structure

## DEFINITION OF ORGANIZATIONAL DESIGN

**Organizational design** is how **healthcare** providers (e.g., administrators/managers) design and develop their operational processes to achieve the desired strategic goals, keeping in sync with the organizational structure and culture (Lee & Jang, 2020; Suprapti et al., 2020; Wingfield & Chavez, 2020). For example, healthcare providers design and develop functional ways to address strategies like resource allocation, inventory management, and infrastructure development, to name a few, helping in providing optimal healthcare services. Effective operational design enables healthcare organizations to increase efficiency and performance by bringing time-effective and cost-effective solutions to existing bottlenecks, providing optimum services, and growing **hospital** revenues.

Finetuning different operational aspects or units of healthcare organizations can facilitate compliant and effective organizational design necessary for providing quality care. The operational elements include resource allocation (Turner et al., 2021), inventory management (Ahmadi et al., 2019; Oballah et al., 2015), infrastructure development (Hlavka et al., 2019), patient-centered care (Bokhour et al., 2018), quality and safety

**FIGURE 5.1.** Operational elements of organizational design.

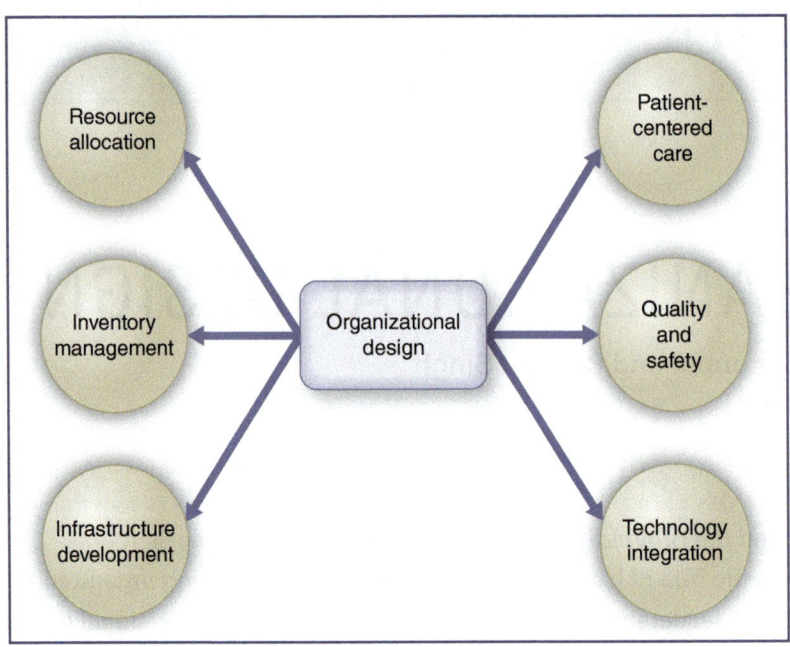

(Lamé & Dixon-Woods, 2020), and technology integration (Satpathy et al., 2024). We discuss the aforementioned operational aspects in detail (Figure 5.1).

## RESOURCE ALLOCATION

Resources enable healthcare organizations to provide timely and effective care, leading to superior organizational performance. An effective organizational design governs the proper utilization and allocation of resources, helping healthcare units to reduce overhead costs while improving service standards. Resource allocation includes human resources like nurses, surgeons, pediatricians, and hospital staff and nonhuman resources like medical equipment (e.g., MRI machines, CAT scan), hospital beds, ventilators, and so forth. All these resources combined contribute toward higher operational efficiency. Proper organizational design is required to synchronize the vital resources to provide quality care.

## INVENTORY MANAGEMENT

Inventory management, guided by an effective organizational design, enables healthcare organizations to address challenges related to inventory control. The inventory control problem is a dilemma organizations face when deciding how much inventory to order or stock to meet demands. For example, **hospitals** with proper inventory management can be better equipped to handle patient demands during flu outbreaks, pandemics, or city-wide emergencies. A robust inventory management system that tracks supplies, such as syringes, vaccines, ventilators, face masks, and so forth, can more effectively handle cyclical variations in patient demands and other healthcare needs.

## INFRASTRUCTURE DEVELOPMENT

The goal is to have a strategic vision that incorporates more beds, opens more specialty units, and so forth. Healthcare organizations must focus on infrastructure development to meet the increasing healthcare needs of an aging population. The upper echelon, likely the board of directors and top management team, should focus on infrastructure development as a strategic priority for sustained competitive advantage. Incorporating infrastructure development within the organizational design framework will enable healthcare units to cater to a larger population with varying healthcare needs.

## PATIENT-CENTERED CARE

The organizational objective is to provide customized patient care tailored to their needs and preferences while maintaining operational efficiency measures like time and cost. It is imperative to have patient-centered care to provide more effective and timely healthcare services to an aging and increasing population. However, delivering such services can lead to increased resource waste and time inefficiencies. Proper organizational design can help manage and neutralize such inefficiencies associated with patient-centered care. For example, scheduling MRIs for patients across different healthcare units within a week requires designing a process that balances the tension between patient needs and the availability of MRI machines. The organizational design should allow nurses and doctors to schedule the appointments so that the availability is more flexible throughout the week instead of all the appointments cramped up in one or a couple of days.

## QUALITY AND SAFETY

The goal is to maintain higher service quality and human safety standards through continuous improvement and compliance with healthcare laws and regulations. Healthcare organizations should provide the highest levels of quality and safety while delivering healthcare services. The organizational design should facilitate organizations' maintenance of standards and compliance with healthcare policies like the Health Insurance Portability and Accountability Act (HIPAA) and the Health Information Technology for Economic and Clinical Health (HITECH) Act. Standard operating procedures (SOPs) adopted by healthcare organizations should be compliant with healthcare security standards (HIPAA security law) and privacy policies like the California Consumer Privacy Act. Organizations should have processes to ensure that organizational policies and SOPs are current and compliant with the updates of the new healthcare privacy and security laws. They should take extra precautions while handling sensitive data like personal health information and other attributes of patient information.

## TECHNOLOGY INTEGRATION

Integrating technological ingenuity into processes to optimize healthcare delivery is the need of the hour. Digital tools like AI-enabled IBM Watson help in faster health diagnosis by evaluating millions of healthcare articles within minutes, helping doctors be more accurate and productive. Automating redundant healthcare processes, such as filing health details of recurring patients, can save time and minimize human error, which will help doctors and nurses have more face time with patients. Integrating telehealth services through the effective and efficient use of Information and Communication Technologies (ICT) will allow the healthcare organization to serve a wide range of patients across the nation, increasing its presence and revenue. To properly utilize the aforementioned digital artifacts and realize the fullest potential of the technology in optimizing healthcare services, digital savviness among healthcare providers is of utmost importance. Lack of digital savviness (Weill et al., 2019; Misron & Hee, 2021) among healthcare workers will be a bottleneck in effectively integrating technology into hospital processes. A well-thought-out operational design will prioritize digital savviness among healthcare workers and technology adoption across the organization to increase operational efficiency and firm performance.

# THEORIES SUPPORTING THE DESIGN AND DEVELOPMENT OF ORGANIZATIONAL DESIGN

## RESOURCE-BASED VIEW

The resource-based view (RBV; Barney, 1991) states that the productive use of firm resources that are valuable, rare, and appropriate leads to short-term competitive advantage, which is sustained over time due to resource imitability, substitutability, and mobility. Low substitutability sustains value, whereas low mobility and imitability sustains rarity (Wade & Hulland, 2004).

## CONTINGENCY THEORY AND STRUCTURAL CONTINGENCY THEORY

Structural contingency theory (SCT; Fiedler, 1964) states that no single organizational structure is optimal for all organizations. The most effective organizational structure necessary for increasing organizational performance is dependent on contingencies like environment, size, and strategy. An effective organizational design (Brown & Bostrom, 1994) will enable a tighter fit between organizational structure and context, increasing performance, long-term growth, and sustainability. The optimal **leadership** style for increasing organizational performance is contingent on the aforementioned factors under SCT. The needs of an organization are better served when it is properly designed and when the management style is appropriate both to the tasks undertaken and the nature of the workgroup.

## CONCEPTUAL FRAMEWORK

Leadership plays a crucial role in shaping and influencing organizational design. The impact of leadership on effective organizational design and its consequences can be seen in Figure 5.2. The antecedents of organizational design are the outcomes of experienced and competent leadership. It is imperative to have an excellent leadership body (board and top management team) that will design and develop effective organizational designs. The desired outcomes of such a process include increased patient care, staff engagement, optimized resource allocation, and a good strategic fit, as seen in Figure 5.2.

*Vision and mission alignment:* Leaders articulate the organization's vision and mission, set the strategic direction, and define the purpose. The organizational design is influenced by the goals and objectives set by leaders. It aligns with the vision to create a structure that supports the overall mission.

*Organizational culture:* Leaders shape the organizational culture by demonstrating and promoting certain values, behaviors, and norms. The cultural aspects fostered by leadership influence how communication flows, how teams collaborate, and how individuals interact. This, in turn, affects the design of the organization.

*Decision-making:* Leaders determine the decision-making processes and the distribution of authority within the organization. Organizational structures, such as hierarchical or decentralized models, are influenced by leadership preferences for decision-making and the level of autonomy granted to different levels within the organization.

The effectiveness of a decision procedure depends on a number of aspects of the situation: the importance of the decision quality and acceptance, the amount of relevant

**FIGURE 5.2.** Antecedents and consequences of effective organizational design.

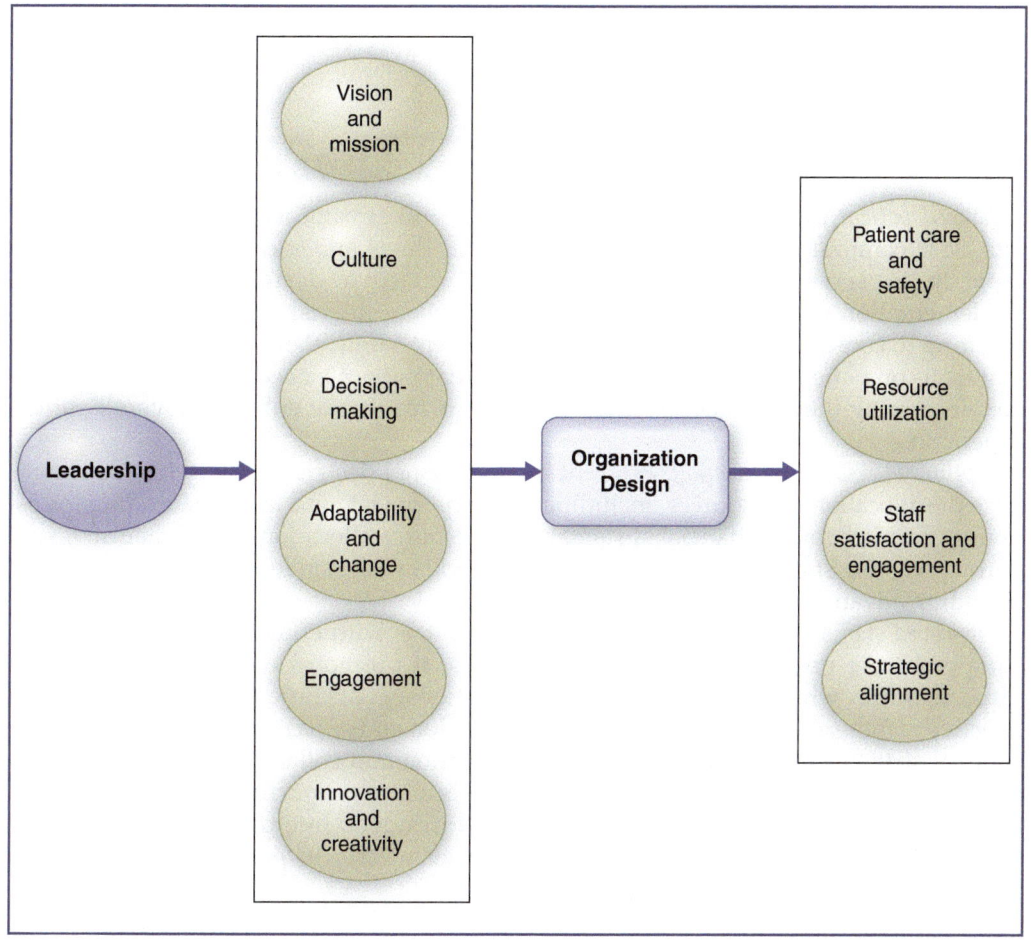

information possessed by the leader and subordinates, the likelihood the subordinates will accept an autocratic decision (centralized) or cooperate in trying to make a good decision if allowed to participate (decentralized) and, the amount of disagreement among subordinates regarding their preferred alternatives.

*Adaptability and change management:* Leaders are responsible for leading organizational change and promoting adaptability. Organizational design must be flexible to accommodate changes in the external environment. Leaders drive the need for adjustments in structure, processes, and systems to respond to market dynamics.

*Employee engagement:* Leaders impact employee engagement, motivation, and job satisfaction through their leadership style and communication. An organization's structure and design can be influenced by the need to create a work environment that aligns with the leadership's approach to employee motivation and engagement.

*Innovation and creativity:* Leaders set the tone for fostering innovation and creativity within the organization. Organizational structures may be designed to encourage cross-functional collaboration, idea-sharing, and experimentation based on the leadership's emphasis on innovation.

Leadership shapes the strategic direction, culture, and overall environment of the organization, which, in turn, influences decisions related to organizational design.

The alignment between leadership philosophy and organizational design is crucial for achieving the organization's goals and sustaining success. Effective leaders continually assess and adapt the organizational design to meet the business' and its stakeholders' evolving needs.

## OUTCOMES OF EFFICIENT ORGANIZATIONAL DESIGN

*Enhanced patient care and safety:* Efficient design will streamline processes and facilitate clear communication, reducing patient wait times and increasing the hospital's capacity to serve more patients efficiently. Effective design will support the implementation of quality improvements by reducing the risk of errors, thereby contributing to consistent, high-quality care and patient safety. Well-organized workflows that focus on patient-centered care help ensure that patient's needs and preferences are met, increasing their satisfaction and engagement, leading to enhanced overall patient experience.

*Optimized resource utilization:* Efficient organizational design will help hospitals optimize the allocation of resources, including staff, equipment, and facilities, leading to cost savings and improved financial sustainability. Resource allocation for mechanisms supporting ongoing staff training and development will build a skilled workforce capable of providing advanced and specialized care.

*Improved staff satisfaction and engagement:* Hospitals with efficient designs are better equipped to respond to emergencies and crises. It promotes well-defined roles and responsibilities which, during emergency situations, contribute to a coordinated and effective response, leading to higher staff satisfaction and engagement. Efficient organizational structures promote effective communication and collaboration among healthcare professionals. Clear communication channels and a supportive work environment foster a positive culture, reducing burnout and turnover. Interdisciplinary collaboration ensures that healthcare teams collaborate seamlessly to provide comprehensive patient care.

*Strategic alignment with healthcare goals:* Organizational design ensures alignment with the hospital's mission, vision, and strategic goals. Clear organizational goals contribute to a shared sense of purpose among staff. For example, staff with a shared sense of purpose will be better able to adapt to emerging healthcare trends and new technologies incorporated by the hospitals. The strategic mindset to quickly adapt to a changing environment is well complemented by the presence of agile structures that facilitate the integration of innovations intended to improve patient care and operational efficiency.

## ORGANIZATIONAL STRUCTURE

Organizational design lays a proper foundation for establishing an excellent **organizational structure** within different divisions and units of a large healthcare organization. A well-oiled organizational structure within a healthcare organization is helpful in facilitating the delivery of high-quality, patient-centered care while ensuring operational efficiency (e.g., resource allocation, inventory management), regulatory compliance, and effective communication and collaboration among healthcare professionals. Organizational structure in a healthcare organization refers to the framework that establishes the hierarchy, roles, relationships, and information-sharing protocols within the healthcare organization. For example, organizational structure will outline how various functional (clinical and nonclinical) departments and their corresponding units and personnel will report to share information with one another on an uninterrupted and need-to-know basis to provide timely and safe healthcare services. The organizational structure of a healthcare organization typically consists of the following elements:

*Hierarchy structure:* Healthcare organizations have an established and well-defined hierarchy, with roles, responsibilities, and level of access assigned to various positions ranging from frontline staff (e.g., doctors, nurses) to top-level executives (e.g., chief financial officer, chief legal officer). An effective organizational design will help develop the standards of communication (e.g., reporting across the hierarchy, sharing sensitive patient information) across the organizational unit or divisions in a timely and secure fashion to ensure patient safety and provide high levels of healthcare service.

*Functional department structure:* Healthcare organizations have both clinical and nonclinical departments where a proper organizational design will help in obtaining the utmost levels of operational efficiency, ensuring competitive advantage and long-term success. Clinical departments are based on medical specialties (e.g., cardiology, pediatrics, oncology) or patient care services (e.g., emergency, medicine, inpatient care, outpatient service). Nonclinical departments, such as finance, human resources, information technology, facilities management, and marketing, play a pivotal role in supporting the smooth operation of healthcare organizations and ensuring compliance with regulatory requirements.

*Interdisciplinary team structure:* Healthcare delivery often requires collaboration across multiple departments and among various healthcare providers (e.g., physicians, nurses, pharmacists, and therapists) based on patient needs. Effective organizational design is the key in enabling effective channels of communication to facilitate collaboration among various disciplines and roles to provide the best possible outcome to medical needs of diverse patient population or a patient with specific health conditions.

*Matrix structure and other departments:* In large healthcare organizations comprising of complex processes, matrix structures are prominent, where research or academic medical centers are operational along with providing hospital services to a large demography. Under such a healthcare setup, employees report to both functional managers (e.g., departmental chairs) and research project managers (e.g., research team leaders). These organizations often have dedicated ancillary departments like quality and safety and regulatory and compliance. The quality and safety department is responsible for monitoring, assessing, and improving the quality and safety of provided healthcare. The regulatory and compliance department overlooks whether the healthcare processes within the organization are compliant with various regulatory and accreditation standards (e.g., HIPAA, HITECH).

The centralized versus decentralized decision-making process is also a significant aspect of organizational structure that determines how operational efficiency is maintained across different levels of the healthcare organization. A centralized decision-making structure concentrates decision-making authority within the top management team, whereas a decentralized structure distributes decision-making authority across various levels or departments.

## CASE STUDY 5.1: ACCOUNTABLE CARE ORGANIZATIONS

The U.S. healthcare system has always been fragmented (lacking a central governing agency, integration, and coordination); highly costly (mainly focusing on acute care); inaccessible (millions with no coverage and millions more with inadequate coverage); and above all, provides average health outcomes (Geller et al., 2023).

The most recent attempt by the Centers for Medicare & Medicaid Services (CMS) to achieve the Triple Aim goal set by the Institute for Healthcare Improvement (IHI) is the implementation of Accountable Care Organizations (ACOs). Launched by CMS in 2012, ACOs are largely based on the Medicare Physician Group Practice (PGP) Demonstration pilot program (CMS, n.d.). The PGP pilot program took place from 2005 to 2010, and it was CMS's first attempt to move risk and profit directly toward providers.

According to CMS, ACOs are groups of doctors, hospitals, and other healthcare providers who come together voluntarily to give coordinated, high-quality care to the Medicare patients they serve. Coordinated care helps ensure that patients, especially the chronically ill, get the right care at the right time, with the goal of avoiding unnecessary duplication of services and preventing medical errors. When an ACO succeeds in both delivering high-quality care and spending healthcare dollars more wisely, it will share in the savings it achieves for the Medicare program (CMS, 2018).

## CASE STUDY 5.2: ELECTRONIC HEALTH RECORDS IMPLEMENTATION

The American Recovery and Reinvestment Act (ARRA) of 2009 was signed into law by President Obama. The use of electronic health records (EHR) was mandated under this law. All eligible professionals were required to adopt and demonstrate the "meaningful use" of EHR by January 1, 2014, so that eligible professionals could maintain their existing Medicare and Medicaid reimbursement levels. Since that day, EHR has been adopted by many professionals and healthcare organizations and has shown its many benefits to all healthcare organizations everywhere. As part of the ARRA, financial incentives were provided to those who were able to adopt and implement EHRs in a timely fashion and show their meaningful use. On the other hand, penalties were also issued for those health organizations/professionals who were noncompliant. HealthIT.gov published a report in 2021 titled "National Trends in Hospital and Physician Adoption of Electronic Health Records," based on data collected from the American Hospital Association and the National Center for Health Statistics (HealthIT.gov, n.d.). According to the report, in 2021, 96% of hospitals and 78% of office-based physicians have adopted a certified EHR as opposed to 28% of hospitals and 34% of office-based physicians in 2011. It marks a substantial 10-year progress in EHR adoption and implementation.

## CONCLUSION

Organizational design and structure are detrimental factors in enhancing the operational efficiency and long-term growth of a healthcare organization. The leadership style and its people are one of the determining factors in providing quality healthcare service. Leadership is responsible for the design and development of organizational processes. They set the vision, shape organizational culture, define decision-making authority, manage change, engage personnel in the workplace, and promote innovation and creativity, all of which are antecedents of organizational design. An effective organizational design of a healthcare organization dictates efficient resource allocation, inventory management, infrastructure development, and technology integration into processes, ensuring safe and high-quality patient-centered care. Given the increasing digitalization and rapid innovation in the field of healthcare science, it is imperative that decision-makers of the healthcare organization are technologically savvy and believe in growth mindset.

# END-OF-CHAPTER RESOURCES

## CRITICAL THINKING QUESTIONS

- How did CMS's organizational structure for Medicare beneficiaries shift from insurance companies to physicians directly?
- How would you analyze CMS's move in terms of beneficiaries?
- Why were some organizations quick and successful in adopting EHR systems, but others were not?
- How does being part of the major healthcare system affect you in adopting new technologies?

## LEARNING ACTIVITIES

**CourseConnect** >

To access self-assessment questions and interactive, competency-based learning activities for this chapter, visit www.springerpub.com/courseconnect. See inside front cover and tear-out card for CourseConnect details.

## REFERENCES

Ahmadi, E., Masel, D. T., Metcalf, A. Y., & Schuller, K. (2019). Inventory management of surgical supplies and sterile instruments in hospitals: A literature review. *Health Systems, 8*(2), 134–151. https://doi.org/10.1080/20476965.2018.1496875

Barney, J. B. (1991). The resource-based view of strategy: Origins, implications, and prospects. *Journal of Management, 17*(1), 97–211.

Bokhour, B. G., Fix, G. M., Mueller, N. M., Barker, A. M., Lavela, S. L., Hill, J. N., Solomon, J. L., & Lukas, C. V. (2018). How can healthcare organizations implement patient-centered care? Examining a large-scale cultural transformation. *BMC Health Services Research, 18*(1), 1–11. https://doi.org/10.1186/s12913-018-2949-5

Brown, C. V., & Bostrom, R. P. (1994). Organization designs for the management of end-user computing: Reexamining the contingencies. *Journal of Management Information Systems, 10*(4), 183–211. https://doi.org/10.1080/07421222.1994.11518025

Center for Medicare and Medicaid Services. (n.d.). *Accountable Care Organizations (ACOs): General Information.* https://www.cms.gov/priorities/innovation/innovation-models/aco

Center for Medicare and Medicaid Services. (2018, January 26). *2016 Medicare Electronic Health Record (EHR) incentive program payment adjustment fact sheet for critical access hospitals.* https://www.cms.gov/newsroom/fact-sheets/2016-medicare-electronic-health-record-ehr-incentive-programpayment-adjustment-fact-sheet-critical

Fiedler, F. E. (1964). A contingency model of leadership effectiveness. In L. Berkowitz (Ed.), *Advances in experimental social psychology* (Vol. 1, pp. 149–190). Academic Press.

Geller, A. B., Polsky, D. E., & Burke, S. P. (2023). *Federal policy to advance racial, ethnic, and tribal health equity.* National Academic Press.

HealthIT.gov. (n.d.). *National trends in hospital and physician adoption of electronic health records.* https://www.healthit.gov/data/quickstats/national-trends-hospital-and-physician-adoption-electronic-health-records

Hlavka, J. P., Mattke, S., & Liu, J. L. (2019). Assessing the preparedness of the health care system infrastructure in six European countries for an Alzheimer's treatment. *Rand Health Quarterly, 8*(3), 2. https://doi.org/10.7249/RR2503

Lamé, G., & Dixon-Woods, M. (2020). Using clinical simulation to study how to improve quality and safety in healthcare. *BMJ Simulation & Technology Enhanced Learning, 6*(2), 87–94. https://doi.org/10.1136/bmjstel-2018-000370

Lee, E., & Jang, I. (2020). Nurses' fatigue, job stress, organizational culture, and turnover intention: A culture-work-health model. *Western Journal of Nursing Research*, *42*(2), 108–116. https://doi.org/10.1177/0193945919839189

Misron, A., & Hee, O. C. (2021). A conceptual analysis of tech-savvy trait, emotional intelligence and customer-oriented behaviour among Malaysian nursing students. *International Journal of Academic Research in Business and Social Sciences*, *11*(2), 679–694. https://doi.org/10.6007/IJARBSS/v11-i2/8519

Oballah, D., Waiganjo, E., & Wachiuri, W. E. (2015). Effect of inventory management practices on organizational performance in Public Health Institutions in Kenya: A case study of Kenyatta National Hospital. *International Journal of Education and Research*, *3*(3), 703–714.

Satpathy, S., Khalaf, O., Kumar Shukla, D., Chowdhary, M., & Algburi, S. (2024). A collective review of Terahertz technology integrated with a newly proposed split learning based algorithm for healthcare system. *International Journal of Computing and Digital Systems*, *15*(1), 1–9.

Suprapti, S., Asbari, M., Cahyono, Y., Mufid, A., & Khasanah, N. E. (2020). Leadership style, organizational culture and innovative behavior on public health center performance during Pandemic Covid-19. *Journal of Industrial Engineering & Management Research*, *1*(2), 76–88. https://doi.org/10.7777/jiemar.v1i2.42

Turner, H. C., Archer, R. A., Downey, L. E., Isaranuwatchai, W., Chalkidou, K., Jit, M., & Teerawattananon, Y. (2021). An introduction to the main types of economic evaluations used for informing priority setting and resource allocation in healthcare: Key features, uses, and limitations. *Frontiers in Public Health*, *9*, 722927. https://doi.org/10.3389/fpubh.2021.722927

Wade, M., & Hulland, J. (2004). The resource-based view and information systems research: Review, extension, and suggestions for future research. *MIS Quarterly*, *28*(1), 107–142. https://doi.org/10.2307/25148626

Weill, P., Apel, T., Woerner, S. L., & Banner, J. S. (2019). It pays to have a digitally savvy board. *MIT Sloan Management Review*, *60*(3), 41–45. https://sloanreview.mit.edu/article/it-pays-to-have-a-digitally-savvy-board/

Wingfield, A. H., & Chavez, K. (2020). Getting in, getting hired, getting sideways looks: Organizational hierarchy and perceptions of racial discrimination. *American Sociological Review*, *85*(1), 31–57. https://doi.org/10.1177/0003122419894335

CHAPTER 6

# PUBLIC HEALTH SYSTEM IN THE UNITED STATES

Nizar K. Wehbi and Koshy Koshy

### LEARNING OBJECTIVES

- Understand the definition of public health.
- Identify the social determinants of health.
- Describe how the social determinants of health affect the overall health of individuals.
- Understand the core public health functions.
- Understand the fundamentals of Healthy People 2030.
- List key stakeholders needed for public health to function.
- Identify how public health practitioners interact to promote community health.

### KEY TERMS

There are many public health key terms that are essential to understanding the proper practice of public health. Many of the key terms relate to disease **prevention** and surveillance, determinants of health, quality and metrics, **assessment**, and access. It is important to understand and differentiate the meaning of many key words like the following:

- Endemic
- Epidemic
- Health disparities
- Health equity
- Health outcomes
- Healthcare access
- Intervention
- Pandemic
- Prevention
- Quality of care

# THE PURPOSE OF PUBLIC HEALTH

## WHAT IS PUBLIC HEALTH?

Charles-Edward A. Winslow, one of the leading figures in the field of public health, defined the "protean field of public health" using terms that are still valid and relevant today as they were in 1920. In his address as the retiring chairman of the Section on Physiology and Experimental Medicine at the Yale School of Medicine, titled "The Untilled Fields of Public Health," Winslow (1920) defined *public health* as "the science and art of preventing disease, prolonging life, and promoting physical health and efficiency through organized community efforts for the sanitation of the environment, the control of community infections, the education of the individual in principles of personal hygiene, the organization of medical and nursing service for the early diagnosis and preventive treatment of disease, and the development of the social machinery which will ensure to every individual in the community a standard of living adequate for the maintenance of health."

The Centers for Disease Control and Prevention (CDC) Foundation (n.d.) defines public health as "the science of protecting and improving the health of people and their communities." This could be achieved through the promotion of healthy lifestyles, scientific research, and injury prevention, as well as detection, **prevention**, and the proper response to infectious diseases.

The American Public Health Association (n.d.-a) recognizes that public health "promotes and protects the health of the people and their communities." According to the World Health Organization (1946), health is "a state of complete physical, mental, and social well-being and not merely the absence of disease or infirmity." Public health focuses on the health of entire populations, communities, or neighborhoods. It also aims to reduce **health disparities**, promote access to healthcare, and ensure better **quality of care**.

As such, the practice of public health could include many activities and services that are meant to ensure the safety and health of people and their communities. Such activities might include the following:

- Conducting disease surveillance and tracking outbreaks
- Providing vaccines and outreach to communities to distribute and administer vaccines
- Partaking in school nutrition programs
- Ensuring access to clean and drinkable water
- Supporting tobacco electronic nicotine delivery systems cessation programs
- Promoting exercise and healthier diets
- Ensuring clean air quality
- Ensuring food safety and inspecting restaurants
- Eliminating health disparities and ensuring access to care, among many others

## THE CORE PUBLIC HEALTH FUNCTIONS AND SERVICES

According to the American Public Health Association (n.d.-b), public health has 10 **core functions** (Table 6.1):

1. Assess and monitor population health, through continuous monitoring of the health status of communities and populations to identify problems and hazards.
2. Investigate, diagnose, and address health hazards and root causes; this can be achieved by identifying the true root causes of health issues and attempting to address them in order to alleviate hazards to the population.

## TABLE 6.1. THE 10 ESSENTIAL PUBLIC HEALTH SERVICES

| Equity | Assessment | Assess and monitor population health. |
|---|---|---|
| | | Investigate, diagnose, and address health hazards and root causes. |
| | Policy development | Communicate effectively to inform and educate. |
| | | Strengthen, support, and mobilize communities and partnerships. |
| | | Create, champion, and implement policies, plans, and laws. |
| | | Utilize legal and regulatory actions. |
| | Assurance | Enable equitable access. |
| | | Build a diverse and skilled workforce. |
| | | Improve and innovate through evaluation, research, and quality improvement. |
| | | Build and maintain a strong organizational infrastructure for public health. |

*Source:* Adapted from American Public Health Association. (n.d.). *10 essential public health services*. Retrieved August 17, 2023, from https://www.apha.org/what-is-public-health/10-essential-public-health-services.

3. Communicate effectively to inform and educate the public. This can be achieved through proper and effective communication with various populations in order to educate them and improve their health status.
4. Strengthen, support, and mobilize communities and partnerships by bridging relationships and strengthening collaborative efforts in order to improve the health of the public.
5. Create, support, and implement policies, plans, and laws that impact health.
6. Utilize legal and regulatory actions. This involves using legal and regulatory actions designed to improve and protect public health.
7. Enable equitable access to ensure that all individuals have equitable access to the health services they need.
8. Build a diverse and skilled workforce to ensure that public health needs are effectively met.
9. Improve and innovate solutions for serious illnesses by conducting research and evaluating programs for the sake of quality improvement.
10. Build and maintain a strong public health infrastructure that would allow us to meet the needs of the community and for individuals to achieve their optimal health.

These 10 core functions could be categorized into three major services:

1. **Assessment** includes the systematic collection of data related to the health status of a community, analyzing and predicting trends, investigating and addressing health issues, and undertaking protective measures to prevent or mitigate them from happening again in the future.
2. **Policy development** is based on collecting evidence-based knowledge that informs policymakers and rallies community stakeholders to build partnerships and alliances for the purposes of drafting, passing, and implementing policies that aim at improving health and reducing harm in communities and populations.
3. Assurance involves guaranteeing the public that the workforce providing necessary public health services is well trained and competent. It also includes ensuring that data is collected and evaluated to improve quality of services, innovate, and implement new **interventions** and programs that enhance public health.

Recognition of the 10 core functions of public health motivated many public health agencies and local public health departments to advocate for their inclusion in guidelines that preserve their functions and clearly articulate the services, value, and role of public health agencies. For instance, during the 2023 legislative session, the North Dakota legislators passed a bill defining the minimum core functions that a public health unit in the state should provide (North Dakota Century Code § 23-35-02, 2023). In testimony supporting the bill, it was stated that defining these core functions will ensure "that every citizen will have access to a set of basic services" (Will, 2023). The bill was signed into law and defined the functions as follows:

- Communicable disease control including disease surveillance and identification, recognition, and response to communicable diseases
- Chronic disease and injury prevention through conducting programs aimed at reducing injury and disease burden
- Environmental public health through prevention of environmental hazards, preventing and responding to any community-based environmental hazards
- Maternal, child, and family health through assessment of maternal and child health as well as implementing programs and policies that promote their health
- Access to clinical care through collaboration with healthcare system partners and facilitating linkages and referrals

# THE ROLE OF DIFFERENT STAKEHOLDERS IN THE FIELD OF PUBLIC HEALTH

## PUBLIC HEALTH STAKEHOLDERS, INFRASTRUCTURE, AND SYSTEMS

Today, public health is a dynamic, extensive, and matrixed field that concerns itself with health and wellness challenges for populations globally, nationally, and locally. An immense range of issues and aspects span across such spheres as infectious diseases, surveillance, research, monitoring, data collection, investigation, prevention and preparedness strategies, vaccination campaigns, and health education. Its scope also encompasses at-risk occurrences, such as occupational safety and health, school safety, societal trends in violence, mental health, and many other threats to individuals in these respective populations. Various socioeconomic interests and advocacy initiatives include promoting increased **healthcare access**, improving nutrition, and stopping malnutrition and starvation. Public health components include epidemiology, microbiology, immunology, toxicology, community outreach, and environmental health. There is a high level of collaboration between international public health agencies and various stakeholders, such as healthcare providers, practitioners, and community organizations.

The public health infrastructure in the United States is a multitiered system involving federal, state, and local entities. Each level plays a critical role in maintaining and improving the health of the American population.

- *Federal public health departments:* At the federal level, the primary agency is the U.S. Department of Health and Human Services (HHS). The HHS's mission is to enhance the health and well-being of all Americans. The HHS oversees the CDC, which is a part of the U.S. Public Health Service (USPHS). The CDC plays a significant role in public health at the national level (U.S.HHS, n.d.).
- *State and territorial public health departments:* Each state and territory in the United States has its own health department, responsible for the health of its residents.

These departments work in conjunction with the federal agencies to implement and manage health programs at the state level. They play a crucial role in disease prevention, health promotion, and response to health emergencies.
- *Local public health departments:* Local health departments operate at the city, county, or multicounty levels and are often the first line of defense in public health. There are approximately 3,400 local health departments across the United States. They lead efforts to prevent and reduce the effects of chronic diseases, detect and stop outbreaks of diseases, and protect children and adults from infectious diseases through immunization.

One of the most critical parts of public health is healthcare. Healthcare systems or networks provide services such as medical care, prevention and control, restoration of health, treatment of injury and illness, and the promotion of wellness to individuals in various communities. Healthcare systems typically involve a network of healthcare professionals, institutions, and resources that work together to deliver the aforementioned services. These systems generally include primary or general care, as well as specialized medical professionals who have advanced training and expertise in specific areas including cardiology, oncology, neurology, surgery, psychiatry, and many other specialties.

Various stakeholders play critical roles in protecting and improving public health and keeping communities healthy, including government agencies, medical practitioners, research institutions, pharmaceutical companies, collateral businesses, and even the media. Government agencies develop, implement, and enforce a wide range of health and safety policies and regulations. These agencies include the U.S. HHS and the U.S. Department of Labor (USDOL). By its mission, the CDC "serves as the national focus for developing and applying disease prevention and control, environmental health, and health promotion and health education activities designed to improve the health of United States citizens." The mission of USDOL-Occupational Safety and Health Administration (OSHA) is to ensure safe and healthy working conditions for people by setting and enforcing standards and by providing training, outreach, education, and assistance. The American workforce comprises nearly 167.1 million people (Bureau of Labor Statistics, USDOL, 2023). Supporting OSHA is the National Institute of Safety and Health (NIOSH), another institute of the CDC which is responsible for conducting research and providing recommendations to OSHA for advancing scientific knowledge in the field of occupational safety and health. NIOSH conducts research to better understand various workplace hazards and develops guidelines and models for safety and health standards (National Nanotechnology Coordination Office, n.d.).

Healthcare infrastructure consists of hospitals, clinics, and medical transport. These omnipresent components are central to healthcare such as emergency care, surgery, intensive care, and inpatient treatment for individuals with severe or complex medical conditions. Another aspect of healthcare is the care of long-term support facilities for individuals who have chronic illnesses, disabilities, or are unable to perform daily activities independently. These institutions include nursing homes, assisted living facilities, home healthcare services, and rehabilitation centers. Pharmaceutical distribution and research, including drug development, manufacturing, and dispensing, play a crucial role in treating and managing diseases. Health insurance and financing are almost always involved in all these services, whether private or public. Healthcare is a complex and multifaceted field that encompasses a wide range of services, professionals, and institutions. It aims to address the health needs of individuals and populations, improve **health outcomes**, and enhance community well-being through various stakeholders.

Public health practitioners serve as epidemiologists, health educators, health policy analysts, environmental health specialists, medical professionals, and administrators.

Epidemiologists study patterns of illnesses and injuries to identify their causes and develop intervention strategies. They analyze data with statisticians, investigate outbreaks, and design studies to identify risk factors. Health educators develop and implement programs to promote healthy behaviors and educate the public about potential health threats. Some of these institutions also promote community outreach and education programs that foster lifelong learning opportunities for public health practitioners, workers, and the general public.

## PUBLIC HEALTH RESPONSE IN THE PAST CENTURY

Significant global health crises and their respective responses over the past century have helped shape modern public health approaches. They point us toward a potentially more effective approach based on emerging cooperation and competition.

The Spanish flu (1918–1919) stands as one of the deadliest **pandemics** in history, infecting an estimated one third of the world's population and resulting in tens of millions of deaths worldwide across every continent. In terms of devastating impact, only the Black Death compares. The global response to this airborne communicable virus included travel restrictions, limitations on public gatherings, isolation practices, wearing face-covering masks, and educating populations through various available public campaigns (Selleck & Barnard, 2020).

Some 60 years later, public health, with more modern resources of communications and research technology, turned its attention to HIV and its immune system disorder, AIDS. HIV/AIDS is not an airborne communicable disease; it is transmitted through sexual contact, needle or syringe sharing, unsafe medical injections or blood transfusions, and organ or tissue transplantation. In many respects, it differs in its public health response approach. According to UNAIDS (the Joint United Nations Program to end HIV/AIDS), since the first HIV/AIDS case in the early 1980s, around 78 million people have become infected and 35 million have died from this illness. Public health professionals help deploy prevention strategies and informational and profile-raising campaigns, including promoting safe sex by using condoms, encouraging the use of clean needles for intravenous drug use, implementing universal precautions in healthcare and research, and combating misinformation and ignorance surrounding the stigmas and myths of the disease. These efforts are fruitful, significantly lowering HIV/AIDS's impact, and while there is still no cure, there have been advancements in antiretroviral treatment (ART), which effectively suppress the virus and keep the disease from progressing (Lokko & Stone, 2016).

The Ebola outbreaks in West Africa (2014–2016) and the Democratic Republic of Congo (2018–2020) were major public health crises. The disease, which spreads through contact with an infected person's blood or bodily fluids, such as saliva, urine, sweat, feces, or vomit—prompted urgent and large-scale public health responses during both periods. Public health response included interventions such as isolation and international collaboration, contact tracing, safe burial practices, infection prevention within healthcare settings, education, and practitioner training (Baller et al., 2022). Ebola remains contained and vaccine development appeared to show promising efficacy and has been used during outbreaks.

The COVID-19 pandemic, caused by the SARS-CoV-2 virus, has had an unprecedented impact on global health and economies. COVID-19, first identified in humans at the end of 2019, has caused millions of deaths worldwide, overwhelmed healthcare systems, and led to major social and economic disruptions. By early March 2020, most of the world had shut down all but essential activities, attempting to limit its transmission (Koshy et al., 2021). Vaccines, therapeutics, and tests were implemented to combat the spread of COVID-19. Tragically, millions of lives were lost. Through the multiyear effort to combat this pandemic, the world witnessed the need to bolster confidence in science and defend misinformation and follow science and evidence-based decisions.

While pandemics have worldwide global impact, endemic diseases occur consistently over time within a specific region or population and tend to follow predictable, relatively stable baseline rates (e.g., Lyme disease in the Northeastern and Upper Midwest of the United States). Epidemics involve sudden surges in disease cases beyond expected levels for a particular area or across jurisdictional boundaries. For example, a measles outbreak in an undervaccinated community may rise to constitute an epidemic when cases sharply exceed baseline levels.

Public health practitioners address endemic diseases through routine surveillance, targeted prevention programs—such as vaccination campaigns, vector control, and public education—and regional coordination. Conversely, epidemics require greater urgency in action, more rapid detection, emergency interventions, and collaboration across multiple overlapping jurisdictions (e.g., local, state, tribal, and federal agencies).

The opioid crisis has had a significant impact on public health and has resulted in the loss of hundreds of thousands of lives worldwide. However, the response appears minimally effective since the crisis continues to grow. Opioid-related overdoses are the leading cause of drug-related deaths globally. In the United States, according to the CDC, over 70% of drug overdose deaths involved opioids and nearly 110,000 people died from its use in 2022 (Mattson et al., 2021). Various public health initiatives including addiction prevention programs and prescription drug monitoring systems, have helped by supporting clinical decision-making and identifying potentially inappropriate prescribing practices. Other such interventions include evidence-based addiction treatment with drugs like methadone, buprenorphine, and naltrexone and improving access to naloxone, an overdose-reversal medication. Various harm reduction strategies also exist such as establishing supervised injection sites and implementing needle exchange programs. These strategies reduce the transmission of infectious diseases, which also increase HIV/AIDS risk.

## EMERGING CHALLENGES

Changes in the world will inevitably bring changes in public health that may bring the emergence of strategies to face new collective risks. While we will undoubtedly continue to face existing issues, as discussed previously, including many noncommunicable health issues such as cardiovascular diseases, cancer, diabetes, obesity, and mental health, we must also anticipate the future risks and consider possible interventions.

Deductively, some new challenges may loom on the horizon and turn public health in an unexpected direction. The rise of antimicrobial resistance through the overuse and misuse of antibiotics and other antimicrobial drugs has led to resistant bacteria, making infections more difficult to treat. Climate change coupled with a wider spread of environmental pollutants and chemical exposures can further contaminate ecosystems and pose serious risks to public health. Socioeconomic health disparities and inequalities remain persistent challenges. From a communication perspective, limited health literacy skills can hinder populations' collective ability to understand and act upon health information, contributing to vaccination hesitancy; disinformation and misinformation related to health; and by extension, geopolitical uncertainty. The proliferation of false or misleading health information challenges public health messaging and interventions.

## DETERMINANTS OF HEALTH AND THEIR IMPACT

In 1974, Henrik Blum (Blum, 1974) proposed the model of health determinants, referring to four major forces having varied levels of impact on the health status of an individual. These forces are heredity, lifestyle, environment, and medical access.

- Heredity refers to the genetic components that influence an individual's health. These are inheriting aspects that are passed on from one generation to another and are not controlled by the individual. Nonetheless, with the advancement in science and gene therapy, there might be ways to alter the expression of these genes and thus modify the level heredity influences overall health or the manifestation of diseases.
- Lifestyle refers to the behaviors and attitudes that an individual adopts, which have an impact on health. These can be influenced by individual choices or a variety of external interactions with others. For example, individuals typically have no control over decisions—whether beneficial or harmful—made by their parents, such as the type of food fed to them as infants or exposure to secondhand smoke and other adverse childhood experiences that affect their lives. On the other hand, tobacco use and nutrition choices by adults are aspects that are controlled by the individual. Lifestyle forces are thought to be the most influential on individuals' health and thus might be the most impactful when addressing health issues.
- Environment has a big influence on health. This refers to a multitude of factors including the physical environment where a person lives, socioeconomic status, education, employment, built environment, air and water quality, and so forth. For example, poor housing conditions might be dependent on employment and income levels and can significantly impact the health status of the individual. Likewise, poor air and water quality negatively affects an individual's health and respiratory system. Easy access to trails, bike lanes, parks, and safe neighborhoods might allow and encourage physical activity.
- Medical services refer to the availability and ease of access to health services, including clinics, hospitals, preventative care, and rehabilitation. These are important components that ensure the health and well-being of individuals and address diseases if and when they happen, thus highlighting the impact on health when barriers to access exist. For instance, urban areas might have easy access to medical care facilities that have an abundance of preventative and specialty care services; on the other hand, medical facilities in rural areas might be more remote and lack many specialty services.

**Social determinants of health** are those factors that are nonmedical, yet they affect health outcomes. They might include income, socioeconomic status, level of education, access to healthcare services, living environment, access to food, housing location, and so forth. Social determinants of health that eventually impact an individual's health status could be classified into five domains (Figure 6.1; Artiga & Hinton, 2018; U.S. HHS, n.d.).

1. Economic stability includes socioeconomic status, employment, level of income, and financial debt. Having steady jobs and steady income results in better health outcomes. Income greatly influences housing, education, food choices, and medical care, among others.
2. Physical environment and neighborhood constitute housing, transportation, parks, safe neighborhoods, clean water, and so forth. The term "built environment" refers to human constructed features, such as walkability and amenities, that influence health choices and behaviors.
3. Education constitutes early childhood education, high school, higher education, and vocational training. Higher educational attainment is correlated with higher income and healthier and longer lives.
4. Community support system includes community engagement, food security, and access to healthier alternatives. Social interactions and relationships with family, friends, coworkers, and community have a major impact on the physical and mental health of individuals.

**FIGURE 6.1.** Social determinants of health.

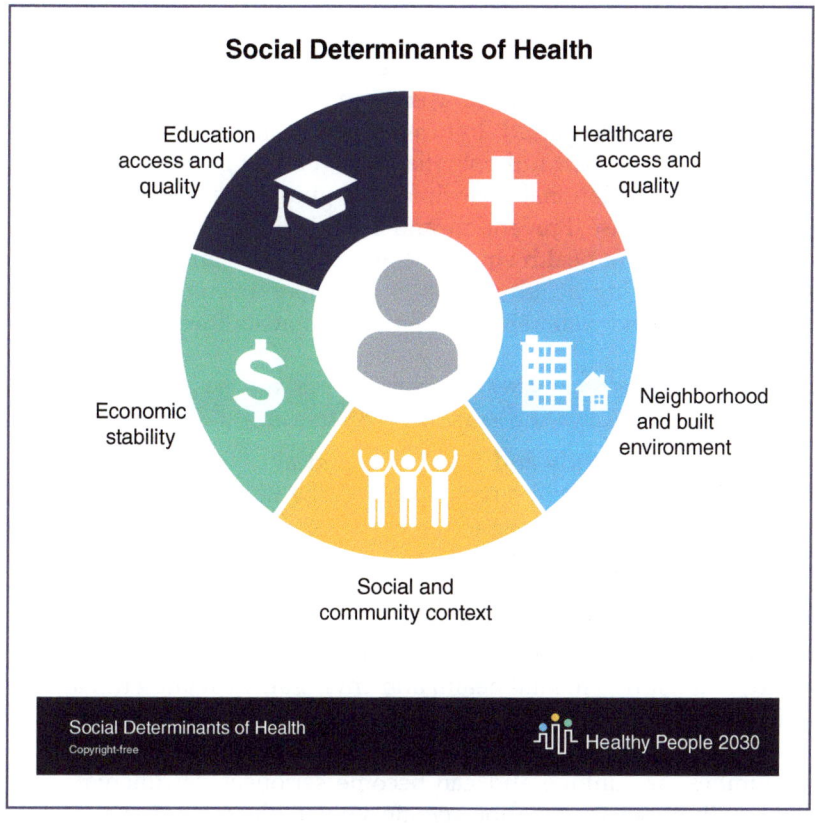

*Source:* U.S. Department of Health and Human Services, Office of Disease Prevention and Health Promotion. (2020). Social determinants of health. *Healthy People 2030.* Retrieved February 15, 2025, from https://odphp.health.gov/healthypeople/objectives-and-data/social-determinants-health.

5. The healthcare system includes access to care, availability of specialty care, health insurance, and quality of care. Access to healthcare, affordability and availability of healthcare services, and easy access to providers and specialists affect the health status and health outcomes of individuals.

## HEALTHY PEOPLE 2030

### BUILDING A HEALTHY FUTURE

On August 18, 2020, the U.S. HHS (U.S.HHS, Office of Disease Prevention and Health Promotion, n.d.-a) released the **Healthy People 2030** Initiative (HP2030). This *road map*, in its fifth iteration of the Healthy People Initiative, provides a set of goals for creating a healthy community. It focuses on addressing the most critical public health challenges and prioritizes strategies for improving the health of all Americans. HP2030 focuses on creating **health equity** for all people by addressing inequalities and historical injustices such as the lack of simple language information on health and well-being. HP2030 also focuses on reducing the incidence of chronic diseases, including heart disease, diabetes, and high blood pressure. Other aspects of HP2030 include promoting healthy eating habits, increasing physical activity, and reducing the rate of obesity to improve the lives of all people.

Around 12 million people worldwide die each year from working or living in an unhealthy environment; HP2030 strives to increase awareness about how environmental contaminants impact human health (Prüss-Ustün et al., 2016). Exposures to air, soil, and water contaminants influence an individual's respiration system, cause heart disease, and may lead to some types of cancer. Tracking environmental pollutants is key to identifying where and how people are exposed. Improving the health and well-being of *all* people will help everyone achieve their full potential and well-being across their lifespan.

HP2030 adopted foundational principles to guide the decision-making process (U.S.HHS, Office of Disease Prevention and Health Promotion, n.d.-a). These principles are based on achieving health equity; promoting health and well-being; eliminating health disparities; achieving healthy physical, social, and economic environments; and recognizing that health and well-being are shared responsibilities among all stakeholders.

## CONCLUSION

Public health, as a field of study and practice, is critical to the holistic management and perpetuation of community well-being throughout the world. To achieve their objective, practitioners utilize scientific research, data analysis, epidemiology, biostatistics, and other approaches to identify risk factors to health, develop interventions, and evaluate the effectiveness of related programs and policies. Constantly evolving, this effort is often collaborative and cooperative, and over the past several decades, the field has expanded to address a large range of socioeconomic concerns, promote healthcare access, combat food insecurity, and address mental health and environment-related threats.

The future course of public health faces many new challenges, but those associated with technology and the reliability of information, which is dispersed instantly to most global communities, are unique and can become seriously detrimental. The accuracy, efficacy, and credibility of information remain vulnerable. Governmental outlets, social networking platforms, a growing reliance on artificial intelligence, and traditional media all play a significant role in disseminating information. Viewing public health from the context of its prehistory, history, emergence, evolution, and structure will assuredly help quiet some of modernity's noisy confusion. Like any course or journey, a path forward is always more direct and faithful if we know our goals, actions, and the means to fulfill our purposes.

# END-OF-CHAPTER RESOURCES

## CRITICAL THINKING QUESTIONS

- Considering the five domains of the social determinants of health, which one might have the biggest impact on health status?
- Looking at public health from an emergence perspective, what are the next steps needed to further develop a comprehensive system to detect, respond, and implement effective mitigation strategies for emerging infectious diseases and enhance global preparedness?
- Transitioning to agricultural societies increased the risk of zoonotic disease transmission from animals to humans. What are the ecological, cultural, and technological factors that played a role in this phenomenon? What are some strategies to mitigate health risk in modern agricultural practices?
- How did the emergence of epidemiology in the 1800s revolutionize our understanding of pathogens and their role in shaping society and public health?
- What obstacles can potentially affect our current public health models and what systemic controls can we use to offset these challenges?

## LEARNING ACTIVITIES

**CourseConnect >**

To access self-assessment questions and interactive, competency-based learning activities for this chapter, visit www.springerpub.com/courseconnect. See inside front cover and tear-out card for CourseConnect details.

## REFERENCES

American Public Health Association. (n.d.-a). *What is public health?* Retrieved August 8, 2023, from https://www.apha.org/what-is-public-health

American Public Health Association. (n.d.-b). *10 essential public health services*. Retrieved August 17, 2023, from https://www.apha.org/what-is-public-health/10-essential-public-health-services

Artiga, S., & Hinton, E. (2018, May 10). *Beyond health care: The role of social determinants in promoting health and health equity*. https://files.kff.org/attachment/issue-brief-beyond-health-care

Baller, A., Padoveze, M. C., Mirindi, P., Hazim, C. E., Lotemo, J., Pfaffmann, J., Ndiaye, A., Carter, S., Degail Chabrat, M. A., Mangala, S., Banzua, B., Umutoni, C., Niang, N. R., Kabego, L., Ouedraogo, A., Houdjo, B., Mwesha, D., Ousman, K. B., Kolwaite, A., … Fall, I. S. (2022). Ebola virus disease nosocomial infections in the Democratic Republic of the Congo: A descriptive study of cases during the 2018–2020 outbreak. *International Journal of Infectious Diseases, 115*, 126–133. https://doi.org/10.1016/j.ijid.2021.11.039

Blum, H. L. (1974). *Planning for health: Development and application of social change theory*. Human Sciences Press.

Bureau of Labor Statistics, U.S. Department of Labor. (2023). *The employment situation—August 2023*. https://www.bls.gov/news.release/pdf/empsit.pdf

Centers for Disease Control and Prevention (CDC) Foundation. (n.d.). *What is public health?* Retrieved August 8, 2023, from https://www.cdcfoundation.org/what-public-health

Koshy, K., Shendell, D. G., & Presutti, M. J. (2021). Perspectives of region II OSHA authorized safety and health trainers about initial COVID-19 response programs. *Safety Science, 138*, 105193. https://doi.org/10.1016/j.ssci.2021.105193

Lokko, H. N., & Stone, V. E. (2016). Stigma and prejudice in patients with HIV/AIDS. In R. Parekh & E. W. Childs (Eds.), *Stigma and prejudice: Touchstones in understanding diversity in healthcare* (pp. 167–182). Humana Press/Springer Nature. https://doi.org/10.1007/978-3-319-27580-2_10

Mattson, C. L., Tanz, L. J., Quinn, K., Kariisa, M., Patel, P., & Davis, N. L. (2021). Trends and geographic patterns in drug and synthetic opioid overdose deaths—United States, 2013–2019. *Morbidity and Mortality Weekly Report, 70*(6), 202–207. https://doi.org/10.15585/mmwr.mm7006a4

National Nanotechnology Coordination Office. (n.d.). *National Institute for Occupational Safety and Health (NIOSH)*. https://www.nano.gov/NIOSH

North Dakota Century Code § 23-35-02. (2023). *Chapter 23–35 public health units*. Retrieved September 6, 2023, from https://www.ndlegis.gov/cencode/t23c35.pdf

Prüss-Üstün, A., Wolf, J., Corvalán, C. F., Bos, R., & Neira, M. P., (2016). *Preventing disease through healthy environments: a global assessment of the burden of disease from environmental risks*. World Health Organization. Retrieved from https://iris.who.int/handle/10665/204585

Selleck, P., & Barnard, R. (2020). The 1918 Spanish influenza pandemic: *Plus ça change, plus c'est la même chose*. *Microbiology Australia, 41*, 177–182. https://doi.org/10.1071/MA20049

U.S. Department of Health and Human Services. (n.d.). *Mission statement of the Department of Health and Human Services*. Retrieved March 27, 2023, from https://www.hhs.gov/about/index.html

U.S. Department of Health and Human Services, Office of Disease Prevention and Health Promotion. (n.d.-a). *Healthy People 2030 framework*. https://health.gov/healthypeople/about/healthy-people-2030-framework

U.S. Department of Health and Human Services, Office of Disease Prevention and Health Promotion. (2020). *Social determinants of health*. Healthy People 2030. Retrieved August 21, 2023, from https://health.gov/healthypeople/objectives-and-data/social-determinants-health

Will, T. (2023, January 18). *Testimony by Theresa Will, RN, Administrator/Executive Officer, City-County Health District-Valley City*. https://www.ndlegis.gov/assembly/68-2023/testimony/SHUMSER-2153-20230118-14229-F-WILL_THERESA.pdf

Winslow, C. E. (1920). The untilled fields of public health. *Science, 51*(1306), 23–33. https://doi.org/10.1126/science.51.1306.23

World Health Organization. (1946). *Preamble to the Constitution of WHO as adopted by the International Health Conference, New York, 19 June - 22 July 1946; signed on 22 July 1946 by the representatives of 61 States (Official Records of WHO, no. 2, p. 100) and entered into force on 7 April 1948*. World Health Organization. https://apps.who.int/gb/bd/pdf/bd47/en/constitution-en.pdf

# CHAPTER 7

# INTRODUCTION TO HEALTH POLICY AND HEALTHCARE REFORM

Mark Bonica and Peter Wright

## LEARNING OBJECTIVES

- Define the phrase "health policy."
- Understand how the federal structure and divided government affect the policymaking process.
- Understand the components of the policy cycle.
- Define the phrase "market failure."
- Explain why health reform is necessary.

## KEY TERMS

- Federalism
- Health policy
- Health reform
- Market failure
- Policy cycle

## WHAT IS HEALTH POLICY?

*Public policy* can be defined as "authoritative decisions made in the legislative, executive, or judicial branches of government intended to direct or influence the actions, behaviors, or decisions of others" (Longest, 2010). These decisions shape the behavior of private actors (individuals and firms) by setting rules about what can and cannot be done, as well as creating incentives that nudge private actors toward one sort of action or another.

The World Health Organization (WHO) defines *health* as "a state of complete physical, mental and social well-being and not merely the absence of disease or infirmity" (WHO, n.d.). We can think of **health policy** as the subset of government decisions meant to influence the health of society. Given the expansive WHO definition, health policy encompasses decisions that not only include the delivery of care and the payment for those services, which we typically think of as addressing "disease and infirmity," but also policies that influence the social determinants of health, such as access to grocery stores, schooling, transportation, and affordable housing (Healthy People 2030, n.d.).

The U.S. healthcare system is generally regarded as complex, fragmented, and incomplete, and it is so because of the nature of health policy in the United States. Two factors distinguish the U.S. healthcare system from other economically developed countries: the lack of universal insurance for all citizens and the high cost of care. The U.S. healthcare system is not designed by a central authority. Power is highly decentralized in the United States, and the complexity of the U.S. healthcare system reflects that decentralization. In this chapter, we consider how the structure of the U.S. government affects health policymaking in the United States specifically, as well as structural forces that affect policymaking in general both in the United States and internationally. We will then turn to health reform in the United States and efforts to rationalize health policy.

## FEDERALISM AND DIVIDED GOVERNMENT

Health policy varies by country and depends on the size and governmental structure of the country, at the state and local levels. Government structure in the United States strongly influences the way policy is made and what is possible, especially at the national level. The U.S. Constitution, which dictates the structure of the Federal government and its relationship with the states, was explicitly designed to limit the Federal government's policymaking capabilities by adopting a federalist structure and devolving extensive policymaking powers to the states (Hickey et al., 2023).

### FEDERALISM

A federal structure, **federalism** is a system in which a single political entity, such as a country, is divided into multiple levels of government, each with its own set of powers and responsibilities. The United States has the federal government at the national level and state, county, and city/town governments at the local levels. Other countries with a federal system include Canada, Germany, and Switzerland. Most countries are unitary states (France, the UK, and Japan), where local governments only have the authority granted to them by the national government and do not have independent authority. Local governments in unitary states are essentially local offices of the national government, and they derive their authority from the national government (Elazar, 1997). In the United States, state governments are not subordinate to the federal government; they are semiautonomous governments with their authorities. Thus, an individual U.S. citizen is subject to overlapping jurisdictions: required to obey the laws and regulations of the federal government on matters that it is authorized to control while also subject to the laws and regulations of state, county, and city/town governments, each of which has limited scopes of authority. This overlap and semiautonomy can lead to policy fragmentation, redundancy, and even conflict, as each level of government seeks to improve its policy set (Figure 7.1).

State governments are smaller than the federal government, but they play a vital role in creating the policies that govern their citizens. The Constitution enumerates the federal government's rights and privileges, including responsibilities such as providing for a national military and negotiating with other countries. However, it leaves the majority of economic policy to the states, limiting the ability of the federal government to directly regulate businesses, including healthcare delivery, unless the business crosses state lines.

**FIGURE 7.1.** Federalism and overlapping levels of jurisdiction.

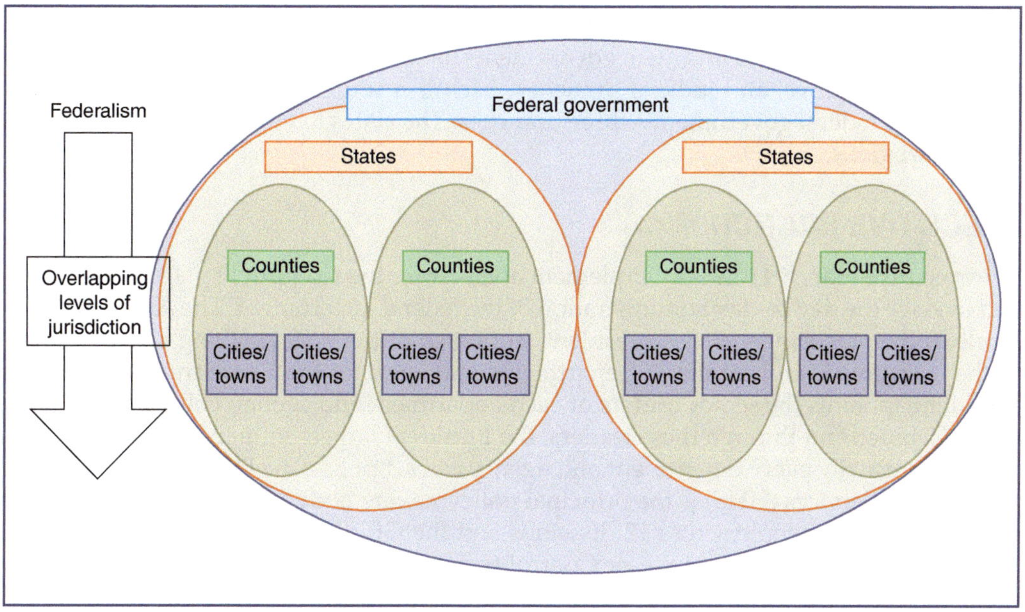

Although healthcare delivery within a state is primarily under the regulatory control of the states, the federal government still exerts significant control at the state level. It does so through the Medicare program. Most hospitals and other providers receive a significant portion of their revenue from participating in the Medicare program. To participate, providers must meet the Centers for Medicare & Medicaid Services (CMS) conditions of participation (CoPs; CMS.gov, n.d.-a). By manipulating the CoPs, CMS can impose policy mandates on participating providers at the state level.

The three levels of government each have principal policymaking roles (Table 7.1), but they also interact because of their overlapping jurisdictions and act as a check on each other's power.

### TABLE 7.1. POLICY BY LEVEL OF GOVERNMENT

|  |  |
|---|---|
| **Federal** | • The federal government is the single largest payor for healthcare through Medicare, Medicaid, the Veterans Administration, and other programs. It influences policy through payment.<br>• It regulates the production of pharmaceuticals, medical equipment and devices, and other services.<br>• It regulates and funds various programs: critical access hospitals, federally qualified health clinics, community mental health clinics, rural health clinics, and more. |
| **State** | • It regulates the licensing of individual providers (physicians, nurses, etc.).<br>• It regulates the licensing of organizations such as hospitals, nursing homes, and others.<br>• It regulates the health insurance within the state.<br>• It regulates the implementation, payment, and coverage guidelines of Medicaid. |
| **Local** | • It is responsible for the primary regulation of *social determinants of health*, such as the built environment, sanitation, and education system citizens live in on a day-to-day basis. |

## DIVIDED GOVERNMENT

In addition to a federal structure with power shared between the federal government and the states, the federal and state governments have internally divided structures, with legislative, executive, and judicial branches. Each is a source of policymaking. We will examine the federal government's three branches. The states have similar structures with minor variations.

## EXECUTIVE BRANCH

The executive branch's role is to implement and enforce the laws put in place by Congress and oversee the day-to-day administration of the federal government. The American public elects the president and vice president, but much of the policymaking activity occurs in the executive branch of the 15 departments and agencies the President oversees. The President appoints the senior leaders of each department and agency, collectively known as the Cabinet, and through these leaders, the President largely influences policy.

While virtually every department and agency can set policy, the Department of Health and Human Services (HHS) is the principal policymaking body for health. HHS employs more than 80,000 people across 12 divisions and the Office of the Secretary. These divisions include the Centers for Disease Control and Prevention, the Food and Drug Administration (FDA), the CMS, and others (see complete organization structure here: https://www.hhs.gov/about/agencies/orgchart/index.html).

One of the important ways departments like HHS make policy is within the context of legislation passed by Congress that includes a delegation of rulemaking authority from Congress to the secretary. Congressional leaders often work on complex topics, especially when they are legislating healthcare delivery. Congress will often pass laws that provide a broad outline of intention and then instruct the secretary to take charge of filling in the specific details. This is called delegating rulemaking authority, and it allows the department to propose regulations that will define how the law is implemented (Kerwin & Furlong, 2018).

When the HHS engages in rulemaking, it must follow a process that includes notifying the public of proposed regulations. After the public has had a chance to comment, the department must provide reasoned responses to significant comments. Once revisions are made, the final rule is published in the Federal Register and ultimately incorporated into the Code of Federal Regulations, a comprehensive collection of all federal regulations carrying the force of law.

## LEGISLATIVE BRANCH

Congress, composed of the House of Representatives and the Senate, constitutes the legislative branch of the federal government. Envisioned by the authors of the Constitution as the most powerful branch, the executive and judiciary branches were granted powers to check it (Madison, 1788). Congress has the power to pass laws within the scope authorized in the Constitution. It has the authority to create executive departments and the structure of the judicial branch below the Supreme Court. It also has the power to tax and authorize the spending of the federal government. The executive branch is responsible for spending most of the federal government's money, but it can only spend on things and programs Congress has authorized and appropriated.

Congress and state legislatures are constantly involved in making health policy. For example, the 2010 Patient Protection and Affordable Care Act (PPACA) passed by the U.S. Congress is one of the most influential laws addressing health since the creation of Medicare and Medicaid in 1965.

## JUDICIAL BRANCH

Even after rulemaking processes, laws may still be ambiguous or unclear. Courts often interpret and clarify laws passed by legislatures using established legal principles and precedents to the specific facts of a case. A court's decision will become part of how the law is enforced. For example, the Supreme Court case *Roe v. Wade* (1973) made it legal across the United States for a woman to have an abortion. This was a judicial decision, not the result of a law passed by Congress, but had the force of law preventing the states from passing laws that prohibited abortion. In 2022, *Dobbs v. Jackson Women's Health Organization* reversed this decision, with the court declaring that access to abortion was a state-level matter and there was not a constitutional right to abortion at the federal level. Courts can also overturn laws passed by Congress if they determine that the law violates the Constitution. This is a powerful check provided to the judiciary to prevent abuses of power (Boudreaux & Pritchard, 1994).

While the federal judiciary handles high-level cases, such as challenges to *Roe* and *Dobbs*, state courts deal with more mundane but important cases, such as malpractice suits. State courts interpret and enforce policies at the state level about malpractice, health insurance, and other healthcare-related rights through their decisions.

## POLICY EMERGENCE

### SUPPLY AND DEMAND FOR POLICY

Policy suppliers, such as members of Congress, supply policy to demanders in exchange for support of their election to office (Tollison, 1988). The demand for the policy comes from citizens, corporations, lobbying firms, and other groups who continuously seek changes throughout the cycle from government actors, such as new laws from Congress, changes and modifications to regulations by executive agencies, or through legal action in the court system. There is almost always tension between demanders of policy, even when both parties are well intentioned. For example, pharmaceutical manufacturers might seek policy changes to the FDA approval process that make the process less burdensome and increase their ability to bring more potentially life-saving drugs to market more quickly, while patient advocates may seek stricter regulations to ensure patient safety. The challenge to policymakers is to balance those interests with the public good. Policies emerge from the interaction between various suppliers and demanders through a series of compromises, depending on each party's relative power.

### THE POLICY CYCLE

The process of policy development tends to follow a cyclical pattern (Figure 7.2) with questions and actions at each step:

1. *Issue identification*. What is the issue of concern? A clear articulation of the problem to be addressed by government action. Establish a clear goal of the policy.
2. *Policy analysis*. What facts are known? Which constituencies will support the policy goal identified? What level and branch of government would be the appropriate target for policymaking? Clarify the goal of the policymaking effort.
3. *Policy formulation*. What incentives, prohibitions, or mandates would support the goal of the policy? Consider the interests of a coalition to support the policy.
4. *Policy enactment*. Build a coalition of interested parties to convince the appropriate government branch to adopt the policy.

**FIGURE 7.2.** The policy cycle.

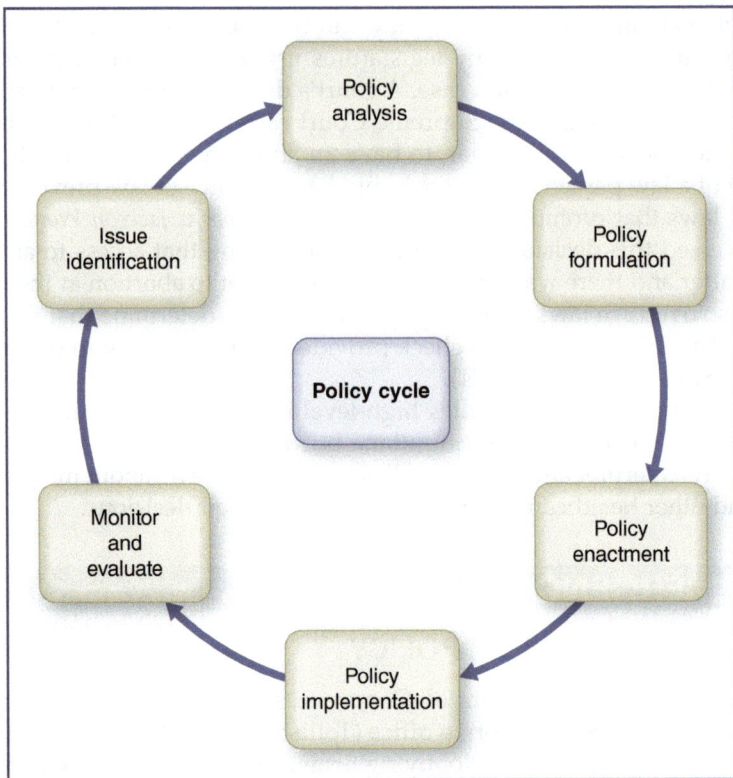

5. **Policy implementation**. Translate the policy into actionable rules to achieve the intended goals.
6. **Monitor and evaluate**. Are the actors following the rules developed during implementation? Are the expected results of the new rules consistent with the goals?

The policy cycle is continuous. Demanders are always identifying new issues where they believe changes in policy can result in improvements to their interests.

## MARKET FAILURE

The United States has a more individualist culture than most countries and is characterized by a default preference for market-based rather than government-planned solutions (Pew Research Center, 2011). The term *markets* in this context refers to the interaction between individuals with each other and individuals with corporations or interactions between corporations to acquire goods and services. Markets naturally emerge wherever people are free to trade (McMillan, 2003). Most of the time, markets are an engine for prosperity and generally are responsible for bringing innovative quality products and services at lower costs. However, markets do not always yield socially optimal outcomes. When market processes do not yield the socially optimal outcome, this is called **market failure** (Randall, 1983). Government policymakers can sometimes improve outcomes by regulating how a market functions. Because of the nature of healthcare, it can be particularly vulnerable to market failure (Fabes et al., 2022).

*Information asymmetry* is perhaps the most important cause of market failure in healthcare markets. Information asymmetry means that one party to a transaction has more information than the other. Patients often lack the medical expertise to assess their needs effectively, leaving them dependent on healthcare providers' information. Providers may have financial incentives misaligned with patient welfare, potentially leading to overutilization or inappropriate treatments. Hidden costs and opaque pricing add further confusion, while the uncertainty of health outcomes complicates decision-making. Government regulation can sometimes address some market failures arising from information asymmetry.

One specific way markets often fail is they may not provide the socially optimal quantity of *public goods*. Public goods are goods or services that are nonexcludable and nonrivalrous. Nonexcludable means that individuals cannot be easily excluded from using or benefiting from the good or service, and nonrivalrous means that one person's use or consumption of the good does not diminish its availability or benefits for others. Most public health programs are public goods. Public health measures, such as clean air and water, disease monitoring, or vaccination programs, benefit everyone in a community. If one person in a community is vaccinated, it does not reduce the ability of others to be vaccinated, and everyone benefits from reduced disease spread. Similarly, efforts to ensure clean air and water benefit all community members without exclusion or rivalry, making public health a clear example of a public good.

### CASE STUDY 7.1: THE RURAL EMERGENCY HOSPITAL MODEL

Over the past 10 to 15 years, healthcare policy has increasingly focused on delivery in the rural environment. With nearly 200 rural hospital closures since 2005, many small rural hospitals (50 beds or less) were dealing with a declining inpatient census yet needing to maintain the fixed costs of inpatient care. After years of studying the need, Congress created a new program for rural hospitals. The rural emergency hospital (REH) was designed to reduce the number of rural hospital closures through innovative payment reform and prioritizing close alignment between outpatient services and rural community healthcare needs (Schaefer et al., 2023). The rules governing the REH were published in the 2023 Hospital Outpatient Prospective Payment System and Ambulatory Surgical Center final rule on November 23, 2022.

A facility can enroll as an REH if it is a critical access hospital (CAH) or a rural hospital with 50 beds or less as of December 27, 2020. The benefits of converting to REH are highly dependent on the circumstances of the hospital. Rural hospitals facing closure may benefit from enhanced payments. REHs receive the Outpatient Prospective Payment System rate plus an additional 5% for REH-covered services. Non-REH services (such as laboratory, distinct part skilled nursing facility services) are paid according to the facility's respective fee schedule and do not qualify for the added 5%. In addition, REHs received a monthly facility payment of $272,866 in 2023, with annual increases determined by CMS. As the REH provider designation became active for Medicare on January 1, 2023, states have varied legislative and regulatory responses to recognizing the provider type.

## HEALTHCARE REFORM—AN ATTEMPT TO RATIONALIZE UNITED STATES HEALTHCARE

The two main challenges to the U.S. healthcare system are a lack of universal insurance coverage and high costs. Health reform is meant to address these two issues. Because of the cost of modern healthcare, most individuals need health insurance to pay for care.

However, health insurance is expensive in the private market. A recent survey showed that employer-sponsored health insurance in 2023 costs an average of $8,435 for single coverage and $23,968 for family coverage (Kaiser Family Foundation, 2023). Employers typically share this cost with employees, but this can be a major financial burden for individuals without an employer who can share the cost. While Medicare covers individuals over the age of 65, Medicaid covers some individuals with low incomes, and there are other government programs that provide coverage for other specific groups, some people are still not able to afford health insurance. This is an example of an important market failure. It is one of the market failures that health reform in the United States has tried to address.

Rising costs in the U.S. healthcare system cause rising health insurance rates. The National Health Expenditures Account (NHE) measures all spending on health, including healthcare, research, training, and other elements contributing to health. In 1960, the NHE was estimated to be $27.1B. In 2021, it rose to $4.3T. This represents about 18% of gross domestic product, a measure of all spending in the United States. Spending on health grew at approximately 8.6% per year during that period, much faster than the consumer price index (CPI), a measure of inflation, which grew at an annual rate of approximately 3.7% per year. Had health spending grown at the same rate as the CPI, health spending in 2021 would have been approximately $248B, about one seventeenth of what it was (Figure 7.3).

Growth in the cost of the Medicare and Medicaid programs mirrors the overall national health expenditure (Figure 7.4). In 2021, expenditures on these two programs represent almost 40% of all healthcare costs in the United States and roughly one quarter of all expenditures by the federal government (figures exclude state spending on Medicaid). With such a large portion of the federal budget allocated to medical care, this constrains what else the federal government can afford, such as funding national defense, education, infrastructure, and more.

**FIGURE 7.3.** NHE rate of growth versus CPI rate of growth (1960 = 100).

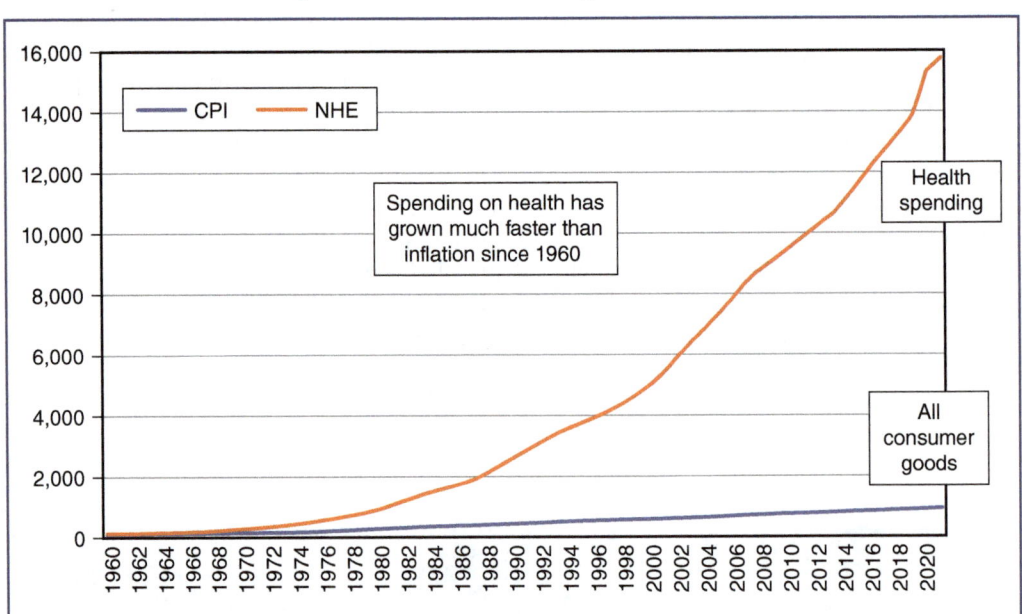

CPI, consumer price index; NHE, national health expenditure.
*Source:* Data from U.S. Bureau of Labor Statistics, Consumer Price Index for All Urban Consumers; CMS National Health Expenditure Data, 1960–2021.

**FIGURE 7.4.** Growth of Medicare and Medicaid expenditures (in $B).

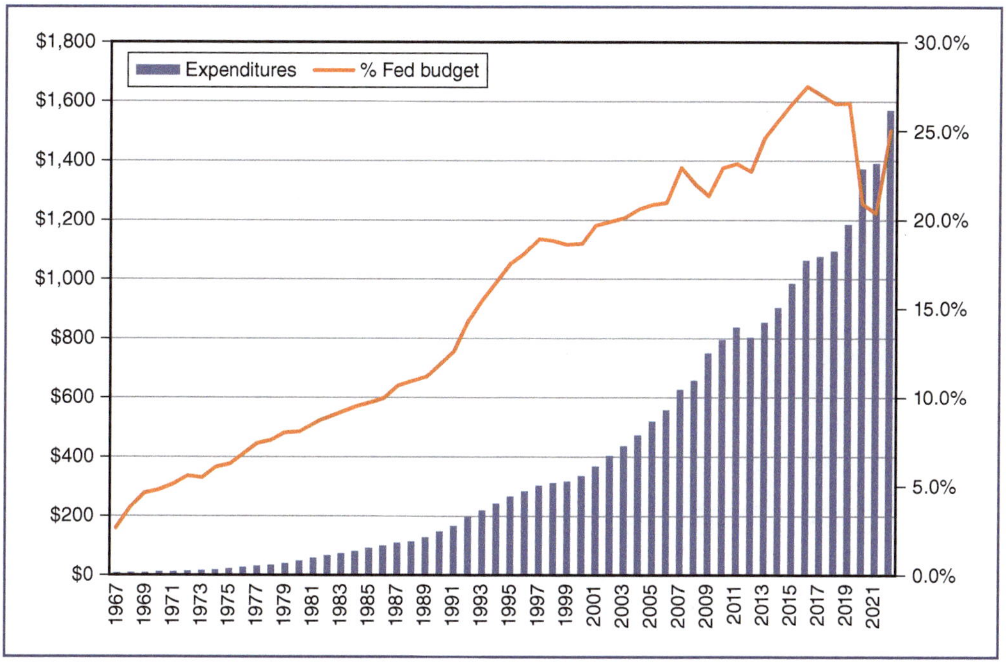

*Source:* Data from Congressional Budget Office. (2023). *The Budget and Economic Outlook: 2023 to 2033.*

Some of the increases in cost over time come from improvements in quality. The improvements in what healthcare can do today compared to what it could in 1960 are similar to comparing a 1960 rotary telephone to today's smartphone. While both can be used to make voice calls, the product is fundamentally different in many ways, and those improvements justify some of the additional cost. Technological advances like minimally invasive robotic surgery that allow patients to go home the same day as opposed to enduring weeks of recovery in a hospital and fewer complications are hard to compare. Nevertheless, **health reform** seeks to make healthcare more affordable and, therefore, more accessible to all while continuing to improve quality.

## THE 2010 PATIENT PROTECTION AND AFFORDABLE CARE ACT

The PPACA is part of the health reform movement and one of the most far-reaching pieces of legislation since the creation of Medicare and Medicaid. While cost control was an important part of the PPACA, improvement to quality and coordination across the care continuum was also central to the reforms in the law. The PPACA emphasizes value-based care, moving the U.S. health system from the traditional, volume-based, transactional fee-for-service system to improve quality and reduce costs (Buehler et al., 2018). The law further focuses on enhancing the patient experience by expanding access and promoting transparency.

Some tools that the PPACA created to encourage movement toward value-based care included the introduction of the Medicare Shared Savings Program and accountable care organizations to incentivize healthcare providers to deliver high-quality care at lower costs (CMS.gov., n.d.-b). The goal of value-based care is to better align reimbursement to healthcare providers with patient health outcomes, which will help with market failures based on asymmetry of information, while reducing cost (Hodges, 2015).

**FIGURE 7.5.** The U.S. uninsured population.

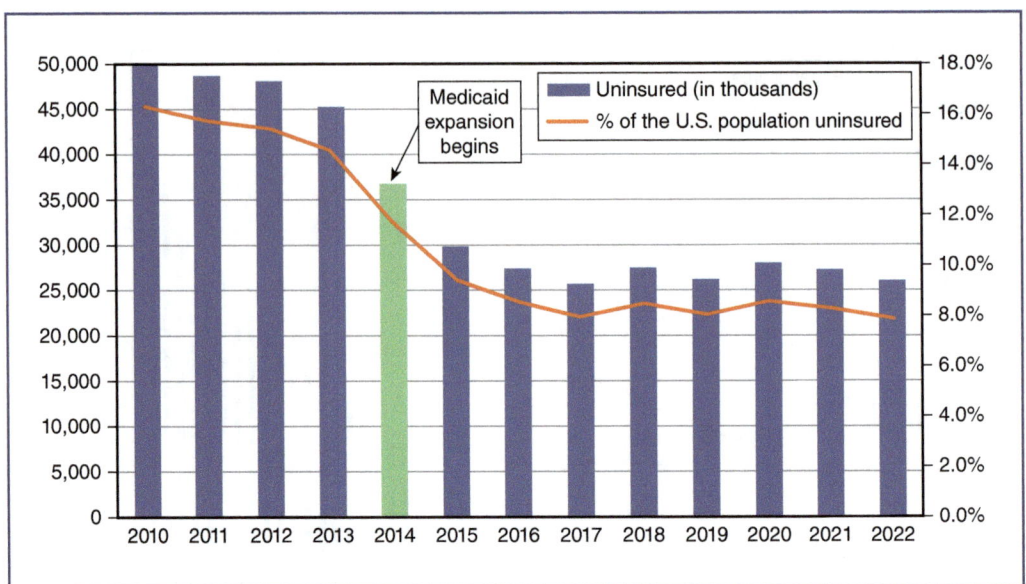

*Source:* Data from 2023 US Census Bureau Current Population Survey.

The PPACA also sought to enhance the patient experience by introducing policies to improve access and quality of care. It mandated coverage of essential health benefits, including preventive services, with no cost-sharing for patients. Furthermore, the law prohibited insurance companies from denying coverage based on preexisting conditions, ensuring patients could access insurance when needed. It also allowed young adults to stay on their parents' insurance plans until age 26, providing greater financial security for young individuals. Patient experience was further addressed through initiatives that encouraged greater transparency in healthcare pricing and quality, empowering patients to make more informed decisions about their care.

Finally, the PPACA focused on extending healthcare coverage to a broader segment of the population. It introduced Health Insurance Marketplaces to help individuals and families purchase private health insurance plans, often with subsidies based on income. Medicaid expansion allowed states to increase eligibility for low-income adults.

Although the implementation of the PPACA has been controversial, one of the major successes of the law has been the expansion of Medicaid. Medicaid expansion took effect in 2014 and has significantly contributed to reducing the number of uninsured Americans since the policy went into effect (Figure 7.5). Many of the other policies have had mixed results.

## POLICY AREAS DEVELOPING NOW

It is a thrilling time to be thinking about health policy. We have recently emerged from the first truly global pandemic in a century and that has shown us many areas where policy could be improved. We also face the demographic challenges of an aging society and, consequently, an aging workforce. We also see new, transformational technologies emerging and stand poised to see changes in healthcare delivery. Some areas to watch:

**Artificial intelligence (AI).** AI can substitute some human labor and provide complements for other aspects (Krakowski et al., 2023). Like the automation of assembly lines in the 20th century, routine processes are likely to be turned over to AI. Routine review of imaging scans and pathological samples are likely to be done by AI. On the administrative side, coding of patient records and the preparation of bills will likely be automated with AI interfaces, replacing human labor. AI will likely be used as a complement to providers during the diagnostic process (Zhang & Kamel Boulos, 2023). In research, AI will help researchers look for patterns in data from individuals to potentially find new approaches to treatment that have eluded humans. The policy challenges for AI in healthcare include issues such as liability. If a radiology practice employs an AI to read scans and the AI misses a diagnosis, who is at fault? The practice or the developer who sold the practice the AI?

**Telehealth**. Telehealth proved invaluable during the pandemic. It reduced costs, provided patient access, improved patient experience, and reduced health disparities (Garfan et al., 2021). Communication technology will continue to improve, allowing more remote interactions that are closer to being in person. Some of the regulatory fragmentation imposed by federalism, such as state-level licensing of providers, reduces the efficacy of telehealth since the provider must have a license to practice in the state where the patient is physically sitting. Furthermore, most insurance plans do not pay the same for a virtual visit as an in-person visit. Both barriers were removed temporarily during the pandemic, allowing widespread use of the technology, but permanent policy solutions are necessary. Addressing regulatory issues such as licensing across state lines and equitable reimbursement of providers will be the policy challenges for the continued growth of telehealth.

**Workforce development**. Healthcare is a human service. Most healthcare organizations spend nearly half of their budget on salaries and wages (Definitive Healthcare, 2022). As the population ages, we will need more healthcare workers, particularly in long-term care (Gruber & McGarry, 2023). With technological change, we will need workers who can partner with AI and other emerging technologies. Finally, the healthcare workforce itself is aging.

The policy challenges for workforce development will continue to be finding ways to attract top talent to all aspects of the field, providing efficient training, and ensuring that the training is not financially prohibitive.

## CONCLUSION

The U.S. healthcare system is complex, fragmented, and incomplete. The complexity of the U.S. healthcare system is explained in part by the structure of government. With the interaction of the levels of government in a federal system and divided government at each level, as well as the interests of private actors, policymaking is a complicated and multifaceted process. The result has been a system where exceptional healthcare is coupled with high costs and lack of access for many citizens. The PPACA was an attempt to rationalize the system and move toward one that rewards value over volume. While it has not brought about universal coverage or a significant decrease in cost, it has helped many Americans gain access to the healthcare system. As the healthcare landscape evolves with emerging technologies and demographic shifts, ongoing policy efforts must navigate complexities to ensure equitable access, sustainable financing, and a responsive healthcare workforce. Amid these challenges lies the opportunity for innovative policy solutions that prioritize public health and individual well-being.

## END-OF-CHAPTER RESOURCES

### LEARNING ACTIVITIES

**CourseConnect >**

To access self-assessment questions and interactive, competency-based learning activities for this chapter, visit www.springerpub.com/courseconnect. See inside front cover and tear-out card for CourseConnect details.

### REFERENCES

Boudreaux, D. J., & Pritchard, A. C. (1994). Reassessing the role of the independent judiciary in enforcing interest-group bargains. *Constitutional Political Economy*, 5, 1–21. https://doi.org/10.1007/BF02393253

Buehler, J. W., Snyder, R. L., Freeman, S. L., Carson, S. R., & Ortega, A. N. (2018). It's not just insurance: The Affordable Care Act and population health. *Public Health Reports*, 133(1), 34–38. https://doi.org/10.1177/0033354917743499

CMS.gov. (n.d.-a). *Conditions for Coverage (CfCs) & Conditions of Participation (CoPs)*. https://www.cms.gov/medicare/health-safety-standards/conditions-coverage-participation

CMS.gov. (n.d.-b). *Shared savings program*. https://www.cms.gov/medicare/payment/fee-for-service-providers/shared-savings-program-ssp-acos

Definitive Healthcare. (2022). *Average salary expense at U.S. hospitals*. https://www.definitivehc.com/resources/healthcare-insights/average-salary-expense-us-hospitals

Elazar, D. J. (1997). Contrasting unitary and federal systems. *International Political Science Review*, 18(3), 237–251. https://www.jstor.org/stable/1601342

Fabes, J., Avşar, T. S., Spiro, J., Fernandez, T., Eilers, H., Evans, S., Hessheimer, A., Lorgelly, P., Spiro, M., & Health Economics Survey Group. (2022). Information asymmetry in hospitals: Evidence of the lack of cost awareness in clinicians. *Applied Health Economics and Health Policy*, 20(5), 693–706. https://doi.org/10.1007/s40258-022-00736-x

Garfan, S., Alamoodi, A. H., Zaidan, B. B., Al-Zobbi, M., Hamid, R. A., Alwan, J. K., & Momani, F. (2021). Telehealth utilization during the Covid-19 pandemic: A systematic review. *Computers in Biology and Medicine*, 138, 104878. https://doi.org/10.1016/j.compbiomed.2021.104878

Gruber, J., & McGarry, K. M. (2023). *Long-term care in the United States (No. w31881)*. National Bureau of Economic Research.

Healthy People 2030. (n.d.). *Social determinants of health*. https://health.gov/healthypeople/priority-areas/social-determinants-health

Hickey, K., Adkins, B., Novak, W., & Sykes, J. (2023). *Federalism-based limitations on congressional power: An overview*. Congressional Research Service.

Hodges, N. (2015). Accountable care organizations: Realigning the incentive problems in the U.S. Health Care System. *University of Florida Journal of Law and Public Policy*, 26, 99. https://scholarship.law.ufl.edu/jlpp/vol26/iss2/1

Kaiser Family Foundation. (2023, October 18). *2023 employer health benefits survey*. https://www.kff.org/report-section/ehbs-2023-section-1-cost-of-health-insurance/

Kerwin, C. M., & Furlong, S. R. (2018). *Rulemaking: How government agencies write law and make policy*. CQ Press.

Krakowski, S., Luger, J., & Raisch, S. (2023). Artificial intelligence and the changing sources of competitive advantage. *Strategic Management Journal*, 44(6), 1425–1452. https://doi.org/10.1002/smj.3387

Longest, B. (2010). *Health policymaking in the United States* (5th ed.). Health Administration Press.

Madison, J. (1788). The Federalist Papers: No. 48. *The Federalist Papers*, 134. https://guides.loc.gov/federalist-papers/text-41-50

McMillan, J. (2003). *Reinventing the bazaar: A natural history of markets*. WW Norton.

Pew Research Center. (2011). *The American-Western European values gap*. Pew Research Center's Global Attitudes Project. https://www.pewresearch.org/global/2011/11/17/the-american-western-european-values-gap/

Randall, Alan. (1983). The problem of market failure. *Natural Resources Journal, 23*(1), 131–148. https://digitalrepository.unm.edu/nrj/vol23/iss1/9

Schaefer, S. L., Mullens, C. L., & Ibrahim, A. M. (2023). The emergence of rural emergency hospitals: Safely implementing new models of care. *JAMA, 329*(13), 1059–1060. https://doi.org/10.1001/jama.2023.1956

Tollison, R. D. (1988). Public choice and legislation. *Virginia Law Review, 74*(2), 339–371. https://doi.org/10.2307/1073146

World Health Organization. (n.d.). *Constitution.* https://www.who.int/about/governance/constitution

Zhang, P., & Kamel Boulos, M. N. (2023). Generative AI in medicine and healthcare: Promises, opportunities and challenges. *Future Internet, 15*(9), 286. https://doi.org/10.3390/fi15090286

# CHAPTER 8

# COMMUNITY AND POPULATION HEALTH MANAGEMENT

Christopher E. Johnson, Thomas Walton, and Mary Curnutte

## LEARNING OBJECTIVES

- Describe the County Health Rankings & Roadmaps program and Robert Wood Johnson Foundation Culture of Health Prize.
- Define health equity and describe the five priorities for the 2022 to 2023 Centers for Medicare & Medicaid Services (CMS) Framework for Health Equity.
- Describe the role of the social determinants of health (SDOH)/health-related social needs on community and population health.
- Describe the types of multistakeholder collaboratives working to improve community and population health and the role of health leaders in collaboratives.
- Understand the requirement, preparation, and use of community health needs assessments and their role in community and population health initiatives.
- Describe the impact of emerging payment models and technologies on community and population health.

## KEY TERMS

- Alternative payment models
- Health disparities
- Health equity
- Needs assessments
- Population health
- Social determinants of health

## WHAT IS POPULATION HEALTH?

When we think of healthcare, we are generally thinking about the interaction between clinicians and patients at the micro-level where patients are diagnosed, treatments are determined, and health (hopefully) improves or is maintained. Under this medical model of healthcare, healthcare delivery is a micro-event, and to improve health, clinicians focus on sick, high-risk patients with improved care management and care coordination. These actions lead to health improvements, but is this the best way to achieve macro-level impacts on the health delivery system?

For example, let us consider an underserved portion of an urban community where its inhabitants are receiving excellent healthcare within its community clinics. If these citizens were surveyed, they would say great things about the hardworking doctors and nurses. However, the overall health outcomes within this community are very poor compared to other parts of this city, despite the excellent care in these clinics. How can the community and its healthcare providers improve the overall healthcare outcomes for the entire community so that they are at the same level as more affluent parts of the city? Figure 8.1 outlines how policy interventions can impact determinants of health and health outcomes.

We first need to think about what we mean by "community health" and the implications for healthcare delivery when we adjust our thinking to a more macro level. The American Hospital Association (AHA) states "Community health refers to nonclinical approaches for improving health, preventing disease and reducing health disparities through addressing social, behavioral, environmental, economic and medical determinants of health in a geographically defined population" (AHA Center for Health Innovation, 2024).

This community-level view of the healthcare delivery system requires a different way of strategizing about improving populations' health beyond clinical interventions with high-risk groups. Rose (1992) argued that "medical thinking has been largely concerned with the needs of sick individuals." The question that policymakers and healthcare delivery systems need to consider is as follows: by focusing exclusively on healthcare at the medical level, are we missing opportunities to prevent health-related problems from

**FIGURE 8.1.** How policy interventions can impact determinants of health and health outcomes.

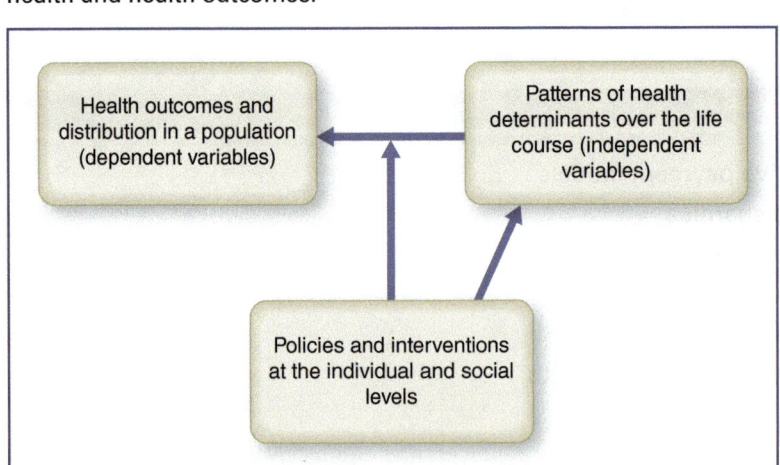

*Source:* Kindig, D., & Stoddart, G. (2003). What is population health? American Journal of Public Health, 93(3), 380–383. https://doi.org/10.2105/ajph.93.3.380.

**FIGURE 8.2.** Traditional healthcare, public health, and interventions.

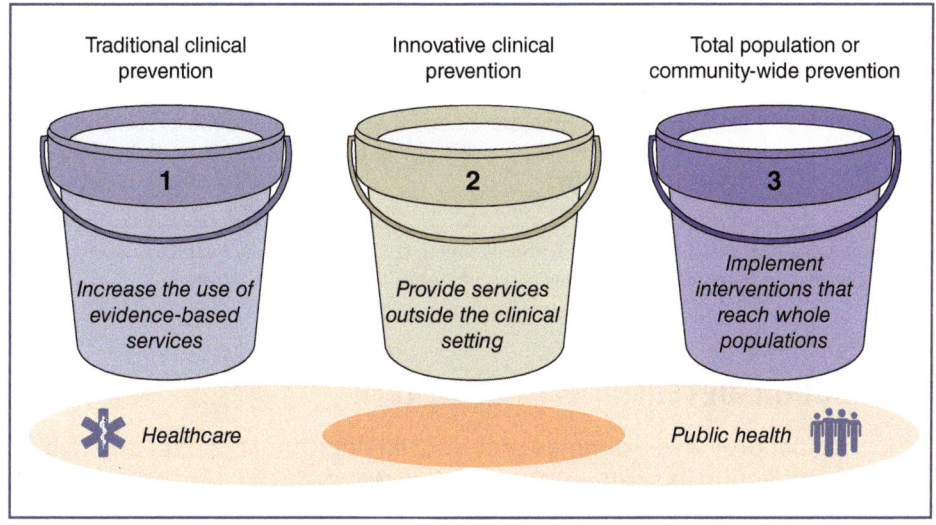

Source: DeSalvo, K. B., Wang, Y. C., Harris, A., Auerbach, J., Koo, D., & O'Carroll, P. (2017). Public Health 3.0: A call to action for public health to meet the challenges of the 21st century. *Preventing Chronic Disease*, *14*, E78. https://doi.org/10.5888/pcd14.170017.

occurring in the first place? If a patient has to delay care because they do not have health insurance coverage, cannot leave work in time to seek primary care assistance, is not eating a healthy or nutritious diet, and lives in an area known to contain biohazards, could this patient's presence in a hospital have been prevented by population health interventions to address these harmful effects? The Institutes of Medicine (2000) go so far as to say that personal healthcare is potentially the least powerful determinant of an individual's health. Designing interventions that can impact these macro-health determinants requires new interventions that include healthcare delivery systems, local communities, and state and federal resources.

The Centers for Disease Control and Prevention (CDC) developed its own conceptual model of this relationship between traditional medicine and population-level interventions. Figure 8.2 outlines the critical relationship between traditional healthcare, public health, and the interventions at different levels to impact the individual and the community. The CDC "views **population health** as an interdisciplinary, customizable approach that allows health departments to connect practice to policy for change to happen locally." This approach utilizes nontraditional partnerships among different community sectors—public health, industry, academia, healthcare, local government entities, and so forth—to achieve positive health outcomes (CDC, 2023).

## SOCIAL DETERMINANTS OF HEALTH AND HEALTH EQUITY

Public health researchers have long hypothesized that there are nonbiological factors that impact the health of communities.

Table 8.1 outlines this critical relationship and how it impacts healthcare outcomes. According to the Office of Disease Prevention and Health Promotion, "**social determinants of health** (SDOH) are the conditions in the environments where people are born, live, learn, work, play, worship, and age that affect a wide range of health, functioning,

**TABLE 8.1. NONBIOLOGICAL FACTORS THAT IMPACT THE HEALTH OF COMMUNITIES**

| SYSTEM | COMMUNITY | PERSON |
| --- | --- | --- |
| Systemic causes: The fundamental causes of the social inequities that lead to poor health | Social determinants of health: Underlying social and economic conditions that influence people's ability to be healthy | Social needs: Individuals' nonmedical, social, or economic circumstances that hinder their ability to stay healthy and/or recover from illness |

*Source:* Adapted from AHA Community Health Improvement. (2024). Community health assessment toolkit. https://www.healthycommunities.org/resources/community-health-assessment-toolkit.

---

### BOX 8.1: SOCIAL DETERMINANTS OF HEALTH

The following list provides examples of the social determinants of health, which can influence health equity in positive and negative ways:

- Income and social protection
- Education
- Unemployment and job insecurity
- Working life conditions
- Food insecurity
- Housing, basic amenities, and the environment
- Early childhood development
- Social inclusion and nondiscrimination
- Structural conflict
- Access to affordable health services of decent quality

---

and quality-of-life outcomes and risks. These factors influence health outcomes but are not medical conditions and include economic policies, social norms, social policies, and political systems" (Healthy People 2030, 2023; Box 8.1).

The World Health Organization estimates that SDOHs "... account for 30% to 55% of health outcomes. In addition, estimates show that the contribution of sectors outside health to population health outcomes exceeds that of the health sector" (World Health Organization, 2024). This means that hospital administrators ignoring SDOH may not be accounting for the significant impact they have on the health of the population their organizations serve.

Figure 8.3 outlines the key dimensions the CDC has identified as the nonmedical SDOH factors that can impact health outcomes. Given these impacts, how can healthcare delivery systems and communities influence these macro-level influences? Housing interventions designed to provide adequate space and living conditions for those with chronic conditions have been shown to improve healthcare conditions and, in some cases, reduce healthcare costs. Similarly, interventions that create healthy food environments and improve access to higher quality and nutritious foods benefit recipients.

Transportation plays a key role in communities and how populations can access employment and the healthcare system. The availability of public transit systems and other infrastructure improvements gives all community members better access to nonemergency healthcare. Studies have shown the great importance of social and economic mobility on positive health outcomes. Better education at all ages leads to better

**FIGURE 8.3.** Nonmedical SDOH factors.

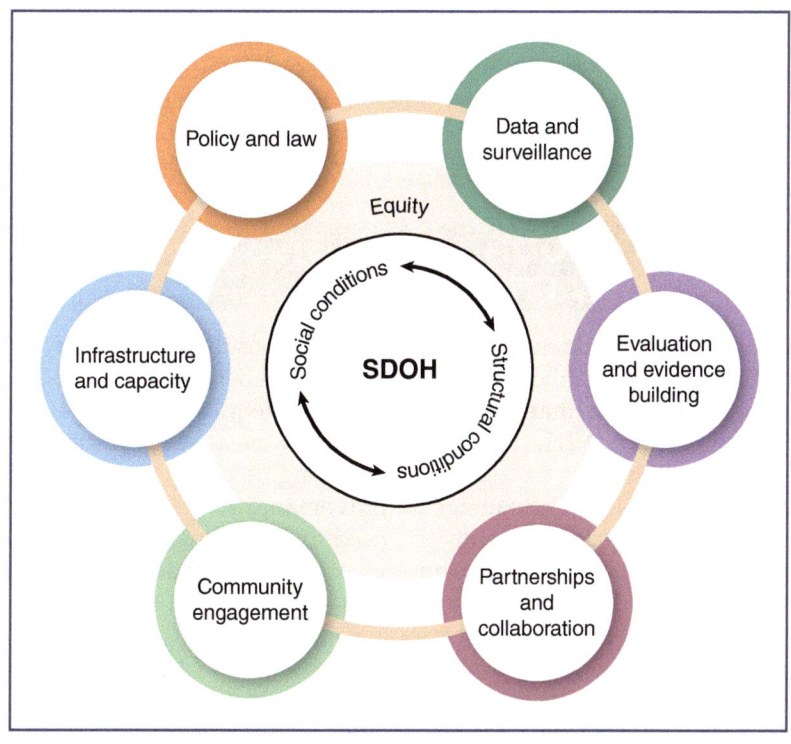

*Source:* Centers for Disease Control and Prevention. (2022, December 8). Social determinants of health (SDOH) at CDC. https://www.cdc.gov/about/sdoh/index.html.

employment opportunities and access to employer-sponsored health insurance, among other benefits (Whitman et al., 2022). The AHA has identified the importance of improving and managing SDOH. The AHA is "...working to support hospitals and health systems as they address social determinants of health, eliminate healthcare disparities and provide comprehensive care to every patient in every community—all of which improve community health" (AHA, 2024b).

With the switch from the International Classification of Diseases, 9th Revision, Clinical Modification (ICD-9-CM) to ICD-10-CM codes, policymakers were able to add new coding opportunities to track SDOH as part of the medical provision of healthcare. These new codes were designed to capture data on the social needs of a healthcare system's patient population. These new ICD-10-CM codes are included in categories Z55 to Z65 ("Z codes"), identifying nonmedical factors that may influence a patient's health status. Z codes can capture information about a patient's socioeconomic situation, including education and literacy; employment; housing; lack of adequate food or water; and occupational exposure to risk factors like dust, radiation, or toxic agents (AHA, 2022). Unfortunately, hospitals have not widely adopted the use of Z codes. According to the AHA, "...adoption has been limited due to a lack of clarity on who can document a patient's social needs, absence of operational processes for documenting and coding social needs, and unfamiliarity with Z codes." Given that there is also a resource commitment required to capture these codes, many health systems have not prioritized this activity (AHA, 2024a).

The AHA encourages health systems to use various tools that will help identify and improve SDOH. "Guiding Care Teams to Engage Patients" is a tool from "The Value Initiative" designed to help healthcare delivery systems initiate sensitive conversations with patients that may be uncomfortable or awkward for medical professionals. Healthcare delivery systems should also seek input from community stakeholders about perceived unmet needs or ways to improve the community-hospital partnerships to better serve patients. According to the AHA, "...the tool includes strategic considerations for implementing a screening program, tips for tailoring screenings to hospitals' unique communities, case examples and a list of national organizations that can help connect patients with local resources" (AHA, 2019).

## THE FIVE HEALTH EQUITY PRIORITIES FOR REDUCING DISPARITIES IN HEALTH

The federal government has identified policy interventions that should impact an important aspect of SDOH—the healthcare disparities that exist between various socioeconomic groups within communities that produce healthcare inequity for populations. The National Institutes of Health (NIH) defines **health equity** as "...social justice in health (i.e., no one is denied the possibility to be healthy for belonging to a group that has historically been economically/socially disadvantaged" (Braveman, 2014).

Therefore, **health disparities** are a metric used to determine the gap in health equity within society. These disparities range from lack of access to medical care, to affordability of these services, and to differences in health outcomes based on the communities within which patients live. CMS identified five priorities that will guide developing policies and interventions to reduce health disparities and improve health equity, thereby operationalizing each priority to achieve health equity and eliminate disparities. This integrated approach was driven by input from CMS stakeholders about how the organization can most effectively reduce disparities and improve health equity in the United States (Box 8.2).

One difficulty with identifying health disparities is that a great deal of accurate and population-level data is required to pinpoint the disparity and the best intervention to solve the problem. CMS recognizes this problem and prioritizes the use of "...comprehensive, interoperable, standardized individual-level demographic and social determinants of health (SDOH) data, including race, ethnicity, language, gender identity, sex, sexual orientation, disability status, and SDOH" (CMS, 2023b). The availability of this data will allow a much better success rate in identifying social risk factors that may impact a community's health outcomes. The availability of good data will enable CMS to measure the impacts that policy interventions have on health equity and disparity reduction.

### BOX 8.2: CMS FIVE HEALTH EQUITY PRIORITIES FOR REDUCING DISPARITIES

Priority 1: Expand the collection, reporting, and analysis of standardized data.

Priority 2: Assess causes of disparities within CMS programs and address inequities in policies and operations to close gaps.

Priority 3: Build capacity of healthcare organizations and the workforce to reduce health and healthcare disparities.

Priority 4: Advance language access, health literacy, and the provision of culturally tailored services.

Priority 5: Increase all forms of accessibility to healthcare services and coverage.

CMS, Centers for Medicare & Medicaid Services

CMS prioritized supporting healthcare systems that serve traditionally lower socioeconomic areas for resource allocation and policy interventions that promote the highest quality of care. This approach means that healthcare professionals will receive targeted support to ensure equitable access to healthcare services for all patients within a community. Health literacy additionally plays a vital role in healthcare quality. Many communities require tailored culturally appropriate services to remove disparities in patient safety and experience. Ensuring that language is not a barrier to care has been shown to improve patient health outcomes and the quality of care delivery (CMS, 2023b). Finally, CMS must increase access to healthcare services and coverage. They seek to "…direct feedback from individuals with disabilities, including physical, sensory and communication, intellectual disabilities, and other forms of disability, to understand their experiences navigating CMS-supported benefits, services, and coverage and tailor our programs and policies to ensure equitable access and quality" (CMS, 2023b).

## COMMUNITY NEEDS ASSESSMENT

Given the importance of SDOH and CMS and other healthcare professional organizations' focus on health equity and disparities, communities are engaged in assessing the access, cost, and quality of health services to assess the ability of the healthcare infrastructure to adequately meet the needs of communities. Public health departments and healthcare delivery systems conduct most of these community **needs assessments**. Many public health departments are required to perform these community needs assessments to analyze where the public health system is meeting service demands and where unmet needs exist within communities. The Patient Protection and Affordable Care Act (ACA) added section 501(r) to the Internal Revenue Code that requires all not-for-profit health systems with a 501(c)(3) tax-exempt status to conduct community health needs assessment (CHNA; Box 8.3) to maintain their not-for-profit status.

If healthcare delivery systems and CMS already collect data on the services patients use, why is it necessary to conduct a "needs assessment"? This assessment is necessary to determine if the health services provided within communities and their healthcare delivery systems are aligned with the health conditions prevalent within the population served. For example, there could be healthcare conditions within unhoused populations

---

### BOX 8.3: THE COMMUNITY HEALTH NEEDS ASSESSMENT TO MAINTAIN NOT-FOR-PROFIT STATUS

1. Map development process.
2. Build relationships.
3. Develop community profile.
4. Increase equity with data.
5. Prioritize needs and assets.
6. Document and communicate results.
7. Plan equity strategy.
8. Develop action plan.
9. Evaluate progress.

*Source:* Adapted from AHA Community Health Improvement. (2024). *Community health assessment toolkit.* https://www.healthycommunities.org/resources/community-health-assessment-toolkit

that would not be captured by healthcare visits within traditional settings but could have a significant impact on a community's health. Data collection and analysis must be done to objectively ascertain if the needs of a population are being met by its healthcare community. The data collection requires epidemiological, qualitative, and comparative methods to describe the health problems of a population and then to determine priorities for services given the resources available within the area (Wright et al., 1998).

These CHNAs are completed every 3 years by healthcare delivery systems that operate one or more hospitals that have the 501(c)(3) tax-exempt status. Healthcare systems self-define the geographic region of their community, with the exception that they may not exclude medically underserved communities within the region. Healthcare delivery systems have flexibility over their definition of a significant healthcare need in their communities. Still, they must seek and receive input from community stakeholders and public health experts about their CHNA findings and conclusions (American Lung Association, 2022; Box 8.4).

The Internal Revenue Service (IRS) provides specific guidance around how healthcare systems need to define their geography served, the target populations (elderly, children, etc.), and principal specialty areas or targeted diseases. However, a hospital facility may not define its community in a way that excludes medically underserved, low-income, or minority populations who live in the geographic areas from which it draws its patients (unless such populations are not part of the hospital facility's target population or affected by its principal functions) or otherwise should be included based on the method the hospital facility uses to define its community. According to the IRS,

> "Medically underserved populations include populations experiencing health disparities or that are at risk of not receiving adequate medical care because of being uninsured or underinsured, or due to geographic, language, financial, or other barriers. Populations with language barriers include those with limited English proficiency. Medically underserved populations also include those living within a hospital facility's service area but not receiving adequate medical care from the facility because of cost, transportation difficulties, stigma, or other barriers" (IRS, 2024).

An essential part of the CHNA process is identifying a community's significant health needs. The hospital in the report determines which needs are the highest priority. However, the healthcare delivery system must also make recommendations to resolve these problems and identify resources that can be used to alleviate the community needs. According to the IRS, it can include the need to "…address financial and other barriers to accessing care, prevent illness, ensure adequate nutrition, or address social, behavioral, and environmental factors that influence health in the community" (IRS, 2024).

## BOX 8.4: STEPS TO CONDUCT A CHNA

To conduct a CHNA, a hospital facility must complete the following steps:

1. Define the community it serves.
2. Assess the health needs of that community.
3. In assessing the community's health needs, solicit and take into account input received from persons who represent the broad interests of that community, including those with special knowledge of or expertise in public health.
4. Document the CHNA in a written report (CHNA report) that is adopted for the hospital facility by an authorized body of the hospital facility.
5. Make the CHNA report widely available to the public.

CHNA, community health needs assessment

*Source:* Example Community Health Needs Assessment: https://www.mhsystem.org/community/health-needs-assessment/; https://www.mhsystem.org/wp-content/uploads/2023/08/Community-Health-Needs-Assessment-Final-9-30-21.pdf.

> **BOX 8.5: COMMUNITY STAKEHOLDERS**
>
> - Healthcare consumers and consumer advocates
> - Nonprofit and community-based organizations
> - Academic experts
> - Local government officials
> - Local school districts
> - Healthcare providers and community health centers
> - Health insurance and managed care organizations
> - Private businesses
> - Labor and workforce representatives

The significance of the health need is determined by the hospital's analysis of the need's seriousness, the interventions required to address it, the ability to reduce health disparities if the need is met, and the importance placed on the problem within the local community and its stakeholders.

The IRS is very specific about what types of state, local, tribal, and public health departments, as well as state offices of rural health, that must be included in the input required for CHNA. Written comments about the health system's CHNA must be included from these groups as well as members of underserved communities and other community stakeholders within the geographic region (Box 8.5).

The ultimate purpose of the CHNA is for communities to devise strategies to address unmet needs and to reduce disparities in access to care and healthcare outcomes. One example of the impact of CHNA on community health is in Florida where Gruber et al. (2019) studied the impact of CHNA on pediatric healthcare planning. The authors found that "…results indicated that CHNAs do have the potential to identify and compare key health priorities across Florida by engaging community stakeholders and utilizing relevant databases." CHNAs were used to monitor and track changes in community health status postpandemic. Molella et al. (2022) found that communities used CHNA surveys to compare prepandemic with postpandemic data, which showed decreased well-being and increased substance use and financial stress.

## COMMUNITY AND POPULATION HEALTH MODELS

### PAYMENT MODELS

Financial models within healthcare are being adjusted to align financing with incentives to increase community and population health. Prior to the ACA, the major payment model used by insurance companies was based on a volume-based (fee-for-service) method. Population health proponents argued that simply paying for the volume of service without an expectation that community health outcomes were high quality and meeting patient needs was not beneficial to society. These types of financial systems tied to expected high-quality outcomes became known as **alternative payment models**. CMS's value-based programs aimed to link quality and value measures to provider payment. The four original programs were the Hospital Value-Based Purchasing (HVBP) Program, the Hospital Readmission Reduction (HRR) Program, the Value Modifier (VM) Program, and the Hospital-Acquired Conditions (HAC) Program. Table 8.2 provides a brief overview of the programs. Subsequently, other more specialized value-based programs have been developed, including the End-Stage Renal Disease (ESRD) Quality Initiative Program, the Skilled Nursing Facility Value-Based Purchasing (SNF VBP) Program, and the Home Health Value-Based Purchasing (HHVBP) Model (CMS, 2023a).

### TABLE 8.2. OVERVIEW OF THE CMS VALUE-BASED PROGRAMS

| PROGRAM | PURPOSE | IMPORTANCE |
| --- | --- | --- |
| Hospital Value-Based Purchasing Program | Rewards acute care hospitals with incentive payments for the quality of care they give to Medicare beneficiaries | Promotes better clinical outcomes for hospitalized patients and makes their care experience better during hospital stays |
| Hospital Readmission Reduction Program | Provides financial incentives to hospitals to reduce costly and unnecessary hospital readmissions (within 30 days) | Improves healthcare for Medicare beneficiaries by linking what we pay hospitals to the quality of care, not just the quantity |
| Value Modifier Program (or Physician Value-Based Modifier) | Measures the quality and cost of care under the Medicare Physician Fee Schedule | Determines the amount of Medicare payments to physicians based on performance on specified quality and cost measures |
| Hospital-Acquired Condition Reduction Program | Reduces what we pay to hospitals that rank worst for how often patients get hospital-acquired conditions | Encourages hospitals to improve patient safety and reduce the number of hospital-acquired conditions |

CMS, Centers for Medicare & Medicaid Services.
*Source:* Centers for Medicare & Medicaid Services. (2023, September 6). *What are the value-based programs?* https://www.cms.gov/medicare/quality/value-based-programs.

The general push to tie quality and value to payment for services is codified through CMS's revision of the Medicare payment system. CMS implemented the Medicare Access and Children's Health Insurance Program (CHIP) Reauthorization Act of 2015 (MACRA). This legislation reforms Medicare payment by linking quality and value to provider payments to those who provide care to its beneficiaries. These changes create a Quality Payment Program (QPP). First, the QPP ends the sustainable growth rate formula that was used to determine Medicare payments for provider services. Second, it creates a new framework for rewarding providers for providing better care, not just more care. Finally, it combines the existing CMS quality reporting programs into a new system. The MACRA QPP would implement these changes through one of two pathways: the Merit-Based Incentive Payment System (MIPS) or the Advanced Alternative Payment Models (APMs). Currently, Medicare measures value and quality of care through a patchwork of programs, which includes the Physician Quality Reporting System, the Value Modifier Program, and the Medicare Electronic Health Record Incentive Program. With MIPS, these programs are improved and streamlined into a single system. Providers and other eligible professionals would then be measured through MIPS on quality, resource use, clinical practice improvement, and meaningful use of certified electronic health record (EHR) technology (Medicare Access and CHIP Reauthorization Act of 2015: Quality Payment Program, 2016).

The Advanced APMs, on the other hand, focus on care transformation. Providers who choose to participate in Advanced APMs to a sufficient extent would be exempt from MIPS payment adjustments. They would also qualify for a 5% Medicare Part B incentive payment. Some examples of APMs include CMS Innovation Center models, Shared Savings Program tracks, or statutorily required demonstrations of two-sided risk models. These can take the form of Accountable Care Organizations (ACOs), patient-centered medical homes, and bundled payment models if they meet a list of criteria given by CMS (Medicare Access and CHIP Reauthorization Act of 2015, 2015).

# ROBERT WOOD JOHNSON FOUNDATION AND THE CULTURE OF HEALTH

The Robert Wood Johnson Foundation (RWJF) actively funds and evaluates interventions designed to improve community and population health. The County Health Rankings & Roadmaps (CHR&R) is one such program that brings "actionable data, evidence, guidance and stories to support community-led efforts to grow community power and improve health equity" (CHR&R, 2024). This CHR&R is run by the University of Wisconsin Population Health Institute (UWPHI).

RWJF also sponsors a Culture of Health Prize. This award is provided to communities that are addressing structural racism and other structural injustices to create conditions that advance health equity. Other ward criteria include the following:

- Committing to sustainable policy, systems, environmental, and cultural changes
- Working alongside partners across sectors and elevating the expertise and solutions held by people with firsthand experiences of health inequities
- Engaging in cultural work that envisions and advances a more just future
- Making the most of available community resources and fostering sustainability
- Measuring and sharing qualitative and quantitative indicators of progress in culturally relevant ways. Nine communities across the United States received this annual award in 2023 (RWJF, 2024)

# EMERGING TECHNOLOGIES AND COMMUNITY AND POPULATION HEALTH

To understand the impact of SDOH at the community and population level, new technologies need to be used to track and gather data necessary to measure at a macro level. EHRs, wearable technology, geographic information systems, remote patient monitoring, and data analytics are being used to provide SDOH-driven data. For example, tracking behavioral health community-level needs is enhanced by modifying EHRs to include mental health and behavioral health tracking. Wearable technology like smartwatches, wristbands, eyewear, and clothing can provide physical assessment data. Artificial intelligence (AI) and data analytics can take this individual-level data and conduct community-level analyses to impact health outcomes (Hartman Executive Advisors, 2023). Geographic information systems (GIS) can be used to map and visualize data for things like food deserts (lack of grocery store access), pharmacy deserts (lack of pharmacy access), travel distance to providers, access to providers, and many other key SDOH-data elements. Remote patient monitoring, technology that significantly improved during the COVID-19 pandemic, allows patients to be monitored outside of the clinic walls and can provide real-time data about various health conditions. Finally, the collection of medical records, electronic documents, unstructured emails, social and demographic data, and environmental factors allows data analytics and AI to find SDOH patterns that need to be addressed within communities (Hartman Executive Advisors, 2023).

## CASE STUDY 8.1: ENGAGING MULTIPLE STAKEHOLDERS

A community-wide health advisory board has representatives from local government, health systems, public and private health plans, community-based organizations (CBOs), advocacy organizations, an employer coalition, philanthropy, and educational institutions. The advisory board utilizes the expertise of people with lived experience (e.g., people living without shelter) and credentials (e.g., organizational leaders, academic degrees) to inform its work.

The advisory board has three workstreams: increase screening for unmet basic needs; improve navigation pathways to resources to meet unmet needs; and increase the community's capacity to meet the needs in food, housing, transportation, and digital connectivity. To improve screening for unmet needs, the advisory board evaluates and recommends assessment tools, encourages organizations to screen for multiple unmet needs versus one need (e.g., a food pantry screening for food insecurity), and promotes the utilization of a CBO's electronic referral system.

To improve navigation, the advisory board played a role in identifying a backbone CBO to implement and operate an electronic referral system. The board also catalogs other referral systems operated by various organizations, including Medicaid Managed Care Organizations (MCOs), Medicare Advantage Plans, state government, and CBOs. The unmet needs data from these referral systems is used to inform public agencies, and health system CHNAs and develop a community-wide shared understanding of resource capacity gaps.

To reduce navigation complexity, the advisory board focuses on linking the work of organizations and coalitions to create the ability for client-facing organizations to multisolve for the unmet needs of individuals and families they serve.

Organizations can screen and navigate; however, if a community does not have the resources to make a difference in an individual's or family's life, the work is wasted. To increase the community's capacity in the areas of food, housing, transportation, and digital connectivity, the advisory board focuses on changing organizational and governmental policies. (Note: A panel of lived experience experts identified the areas of food, housing, transportation, and digital connectivity. Organizational policies include advocating for anchor institutions [e.g., education, healthcare, and government] and MCOs to invest in housing, creation of community land trusts, etc. Government policies include inclusive zoning, eviction expungement, etc.)

The advisory board continues to identify, evaluate, and recommend interventions to address all three workstreams. For example, the board is exploring the creation of a community care cub (CCH) to provide a shared administrative infrastructure which makes it possible for multiple neighborhood-based community organizations to contract with health plans, health systems, and governments to meet health-related social needs.

The board is also developing a methodology to calculate the financial return on investment (ROI) in programs to address health-related social needs for organizations and the community. At the organization level, the methodology asks, "What is the ROI for an MCO if it funds a medically tailored meal program for its members with type 2 diabetes?"

The community-wide methodology asks, "In addition to the ROI for each organization that participates in a multiorganization program, what is the community-wide ROI?" In other words, since the sum is greater than the parts, how does a community determine the sum? For example, if the community develops a multiorganization program to reduce visits to its emergency departments for nonmedically necessary care for people experiencing homelessness, there may be a financial impact on emergency medical services, police departments, jails, shelters, hospitals, health plans, and so forth. Other factors to be considered in a community-wide ROI may include the public's perception of downtown areas, impact on commerce, and so forth.

A related consideration is the "wrong pocket problem." For example, if a hospital invests in a care management program for people experiencing homelessness, will the hospital incur the expense while the patient's health plan sees a positive financial impact?

## CONCLUSION

Community and population health focus on improving health outcomes at a macro level as opposed to medicine's micro-level intervention. With payment models changing to hold healthcare delivery systems accountable for population-level outcomes, health administrators must understand how local environments impact community health, how to design interventions to improve population health, and what data is necessary to be collected to determine community health service needs outside of a hospital's walls. Healthcare systems cannot rely solely on decision-makers within their organizations. They must involve multiple community stakeholders, departments of public health, and support service agencies to thoroughly understand the best places to expend resources to solve population health problems. Not-for-profit health systems are required by the IRS to collect and analyze community health data to maintain their tax-exempt status.

Community and population health improvement requires taking a very strategic and long-run vision for providing healthcare services within markets. This was a difficult transition for many healthcare delivery systems focusing on episodic care. NIH, CMS, and state health departments provided guidance and data analytic policies that helped with this transition. The ACA codified population health as an important function of the healthcare delivery system and it will continue to be monitored and improved in the years to come.

## END-OF-CHAPTER RESOURCES

### CRITICAL THINKING QUESTIONS

- What are the advantages and disadvantages to the people and organizations in a community to create one community-wide referral network or a network of referral networks? Specifically, address the potential impact on population health.
- What are the barriers to multiple organizations collaborating to improve the health and well-being of a community?
- How might the data from a referral network be used in a CHNA conducted by a health system? Conducted by a public health agency and conducted by a Medicaid MCO?
- Describe ways a health system might engage lived experience experts in its CHNA and in its quality improvement processes.
- Describe data sources, governance structures, organizational goals, and so forth, which should be addressed in developing organizational and community-wide ROI discussions and calculations.

### LEARNING ACTIVITIES

**CourseConnect >**

To access self-assessment questions and interactive, competency-based learning activities for this chapter, visit www.springerpub.com/courseconnect. See inside front cover and tear-out card for CourseConnect details.

### REFERENCES

AHA Center for Health Innovation. (2024). *Community health & well-being*. https://www.aha.org/center/community-health-well-being

American Hospital Association. (2019). *Screening for social needs: Guiding care teams to engage patients*. https://www.aha.org/toolkitsmethodology/2019-06-05-screening-social-needs-guiding-care-teams-engage-patients

American Hospital Association. (2022, January). *Resource on ICD-10-CM coding for social determinants of health*. https://www.aha.org/system/files/2018-04/value-initiative-icd-10-code-social-determinants-of-health.pdf

American Hospital Association. (2024a). *Resource on ICD-10-CM coding for social determinants of health*. https://www.aha.org/dataset/2018-04-10-resource-icd-10-cm-coding-social-determinants-health

American Hospital Association. (2024b). *Social determinants of health series*. https://www.aha.org/social-determinants-health/populationcommunity-health/community-partnerships

American Lung Association. (2022, November 17). *What is a community health needs assessment (CHNA)?* https://www.lung.org/policy-advocacy/tobacco/cessation/technical-assistance/hospital-community-benefits/what-is-a-community-health-needs-assessment

Braveman, P. (2014). What are health disparities and health equity? We need to be clear. *Public Health Report*, *129*(Suppl. 2), 5–8. https://doi.org/10.1177/00333549141291S203

Centers for Disease Control and Prevention. (2023, July 20). *What is population health?* https://archive.cdc.gov/#/details?url=https://www.cdc.gov/pophealthtraining/whatis.html

Centers for Medicare & Medicaid Services. (2023a, September 6). *What are the value-based programs?* https://www.cms.gov/medicare/quality/value-based-programs

Centers for Medicare & Medicaid Services. (2023b, December 18). *CMS framework for healthy communities*. https://www.cms.gov/priorities/health-equity/minority-health/equity-programs/framework

County Health Rankings & Roadmaps. (2024). *2023 County health rankings national findings report*. https://www.countyhealthrankings.org/findings-and-insights/2023-county-health-rankings-national-findings-report

Gruber, J., Wang, W., Quittner, A., Salyakina, D., & McCafferty-Fernandez, J. (2019). Utilizing community health needs assessments (CHNAs) in nonprofit hospitals to guide population-centered outcomes research for pediatric patients: New recommendations for CHNA reporting. *Population Health Management, 22*(1), 25–31. https://doi.org/10.1089/pop.2018.0049

Hartman Executive Advisors. (2023, April 21). *The role of technology in tracking social determinants of health to improve outcomes.* https://hartmanadvisors.com/the-role-of-technology-in-tracking-social-determinants-of-health-to-improve-outcomes/

Healthy People 2030. (2023). *Social determinants of health.* https://health.gov/healthypeople/priority-areas/social-determinants-health

Institute of Medicine (US) Committee on Quality of Health Care in America, Kohn, L. T., Corrigan, J. M., & Donaldson, M. S. (Eds.). (2000). *To err is human: Building a safer health system.* National Academies Press. https://doi.org/10.17226/9728

Internal Revenue Service. (2024, March 21). *Community health needs assessment for Charitable Hospital Organizations—Section 501(r)(3).* https://www.irs.gov/charities-non-profits/community-health-needs-assessment-for-charitable-hospital-organizations-section-501r3

Medicare Access and CHIP Reauthorization Act of 2015, Pub. L. No. 114-10, 129 Stat. 87 (2015).

Molella, R., Murad, A. L., Sherden, M., Fritz, D., Sadecki, E., Briggs, G., Wang, Z., & Murad, M. H. (2022). Community health needs assessment data and community recovery from COVID-19. *American Journal of Preventive Medicine, 63*(2), 273–276. https://doi.org/10.1016/j.amepre.2022.02.010

Robert Wood Johnson Foundation. (2024). *RWJF culture of health prize: Communities leading the way.* https://www.rwjf.org/en/grants/grantee-stories/culture-of-health-prize.html

Rose, G. (1992). *The strategy of preventive medicine.* Oxford University Press.

Whitman, A., De Lew, N., Chappel, A., Aysola, V., Zuckerman, R., & Sommers, B. D. (2022). Addressing social determinants of health: Examples of successful evidence-based strategies and current federal efforts. *Office of Health Policy.*

World Health Organization. (2024). *Social determinants of health.* https://www.who.int/health-topics/social-determinants-of-health#tab=tab_1

Wright, J., Williams, R., & Wilkinson, J. R. (1998). Development and importance of health needs assessment. *British Medical Journal, 316*(7140), 1310–1313. https://doi.org/10.1136/bmj.316.7140.1310

**CHAPTER 9**

# CASE: POPULATION/ COMMUNITY HEALTH IMPROVEMENT: IMPROVING MATERNAL AND CHILD HEALTH IN RURAL AMERICA

Rocco Gonzalez, Nathalie Occean, and Kashif Khan

### LEARNING OBJECTIVES

- Summarize the different types of health disparities.
- Develop ways to address health disparities in practice.
- Identify socioeconomic challenges and demographic shifts that impact effective workforce planning and organizational transformation in healthcare.
- Name social determinants of health (SDOH) that impact access to and management of healthcare.
- Apply knowledge in effective strategies to positively influence maternal and child health in rural areas.

### KEY TERMS

- Access to healthcare consolidation
- Community health needs assessment (CHNA)
- Demographics
- Health disparities
- Organizational transformation
- Social determinants of health (SDOH)
- Socioeconomic challenges
- Workforce planning

## INTRODUCTION

This case focuses on improving access to care and improving health outcomes. It centers around enhancing maternal and child health in rural America.

## MAJOR CHALLENGES AND DILEMMA

Public transportation is fragmented and unreliable. Rideshare services are often spotty, making it challenging to find drivers who are willing to be patient with Elise Washington and her two kids. In addition to seeking general maternal care-related services, Elise is temporarily wheelchair-bound after suffering a recent injury to her legs. Elise is also a Medicaid beneficiary who qualifies for nonemergency medical transportation benefit, yet she still experiences challenges getting to and from critical appointments.

Elise's community hospital provides a wide range of inpatient and outpatient services, including general surgery, emergency care, maternity care, and primary care. The community's health needs are diverse, but there are some specific challenges that are common to rural areas. For example, the community has a higher rate of chronic diseases than urban areas, and many residents have limited access to healthcare providers. The community hospital plays a vital role in providing healthcare to the residents, but it faces challenges due to its limited resources and the high cost of providing care in a rural setting.

Elise's town is in a rural area with a strong sense of community. The residents are generally conservative and religious. The town has a strong agricultural economy. There are few job opportunities outside of agriculture and manufacturing. The town is located far from major urban centers, which can make it difficult for residents to access specialized medical care.

## ORGANIZATIONAL OVERVIEW

Reynolds County Medical Center (RCMC) is a critical access hospital located in rural Missouri. It is approximately 2 hours away from the nearest acute care facility, which makes RCMC the closest medical resource in the region. Due to the wide geographic area between facilities, community members must travel long distances to access needed healthcare. Economic development remains a struggle with a higher prevalence of families under the federal poverty line living in the county. The cultural stigma against any form of clinical care remains from the COVID-19 pandemic, thus breaking the trust between patient and provider.

As a nonprofit hospital, RCMC performs a community health needs assessment (CHNA) every 3 years. This process looks at internal medical data and external public health information and engages local community stakeholders' voices to pinpoint the most pressing needs. The newly developed CHNA has shown three key priorities:

1. *Maternal and child health:* Focus on health issues concerning women, children, and families, including access to prenatal care, infant and maternal mortality prevention, newborn screening, and child nutrition.
2. *Transportation access:* Focus on transportation availability for both medical and daily living activities, including access to healthcare providers, employers, and grocery stores.
3. *Food security:* Focus on access to enough food for an active, healthy life, including affordable produce and close proximity stores.

The CHNA was facilitated through a collaborative approach with other impactful nonprofit organizations serving the patients through food, housing, and other social services.

Of the dozen organizations engaged, the most influential and outspoken organizations were as follows:

- *United Way of Reynold County:* Main funding organization of the region
- *Faithful Food Bank:* Main food provider for the underserved of the region
- *Reynold County Public Health Department:* Main communicator of key initiatives/ programs for the underserved of the region

Over five million people across the United States either miss or delay medical care due to lack of reliable transportation, which costs the U.S. healthcare system over $150 billion annually. Understanding how transportation has presented a barrier for patients, the RCMC team has secured grant funding to support the distribution of bus vouchers at no cost to their patients.

Community Demographics:

- Population: 5,000 residents
- Age Distribution:
  - 18–64 years old: 70% (3,500 residents)
  - 65 and older: 30% (1,500 residents)

Ethnicity:

- White: 80% (4,000 residents)
- Hispanic/Latinx: 15% (750 residents)
- Black: 5% (250 residents)

Education Level:

- High school diploma or equivalent: 65% (3,250 residents)
- Some college or associate's degree: 30% (1,500 residents)
- Bachelor's degree or higher: 5% (250 residents)

Occupational Distribution:

- Farming/agriculture: 20% (1,000 residents)
- Manufacturing: 15% (750 residents)
- Healthcare: 10% (500 residents)
- Retail/services: 35% (1,750 residents)
- Government/education: 10% (500 residents)

Healthcare Status:

- Medicare beneficiaries: 40% (2,000 residents)
- Medicaid beneficiaries: 10% (500 residents)
- Uninsured: 15% (750 residents)
- Private health insurance: 35% (1,750 residents)

## LEVERAGING PERSON-CENTERED CARE

As the Centers for Medicare & Medicaid states, doctors and other healthcare professionals who provide person-centered care (PCC) help patients manage their healthcare by providing tools and services that align with their patients' preferences and values so they can reach their health goals. Ensuring your healthcare organization prioritizes this approach will assist in addressing health disparities and improving outcomes.

Key features of PCC include the following:
- Care that is guided and informed by patients' goals, preferences, and values
- Success measured by patient-reported outcomes
- Integrated and coordinated care across health systems, providers, and care settings
- Management of chronic and complex conditions
- Relationships built on trust and a commitment to long-term well-being

In a value-based healthcare system, doctors and other healthcare providers deliver high-quality care using a PCC approach. This differs from a traditional fee-for-service system where patients get their healthcare from multiple, siloed specialists who focus on a specific health issue rather than patients' comprehensive, long-term needs.

## END-OF-CHAPTER RESOURCES

### CASE OBJECTIVES

1. How can RCMC collaborate with local community leaders and organizations to address economic development challenges and improve access to healthcare for families living under the federal poverty line?
2. What innovative telemedicine solutions could be implemented to provide healthcare services remotely, especially for routine check-ups and prenatal care, minimizing the burden of travel for rural residents?
3. How can RCMC create a culturally sensitive workforce that is representative of the community, fostering a more inclusive and trusting relationship between healthcare providers and residents?
4. In what ways do social determinants (or drivers) of health impact not only the patient but also their caregivers and the healthcare organizations from which they are seeking care?
5. What strategies can be implemented to overcome the geographic barriers between RCMC and the nearest acute care facility, ensuring that pregnant women and children receive timely and adequate medical attention?
6. How might RCMC collaborate with local schools and community organizations to implement health education programs that specifically target maternal and child health, emphasizing preventive care and healthy lifestyle choices?

### LEARNING ACTIVITIES

**CourseConnect >**

To access self-assessment questions and interactive, competency-based learning activities for this chapter, visit www.springerpub.com/courseconnect. See inside front cover and tear-out card for CourseConnect details.

# SECTION II: HEALTHCARE MANAGEMENT: THEORIES AND APPLICATIONS

# CHAPTER 10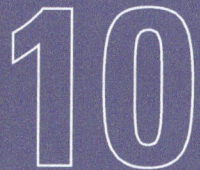

# STRATEGIC PLANNING

Nalin Johri and Kenneth M. Morris, Jr.

## LEARNING OBJECTIVES

- Appreciate the origins of strategic planning.
- Define strategic planning.
- Develop strategic planning elements more comprehensively.
- Identify key trends in healthcare landscape that impact strategic planning.
- Apply strategic planning framework.
- Understand unique aspects of strategic planning in healthcare.
- Identify pitfalls in and benefits of strategic planning.

## KEY TERMS

- Alternative strategies
- Equity
- Long-term goals
- Social determinants of health
- Strategic control
- Strategic direction
- Strategic framework
- Strategic planning

## INTRODUCTION

The root of the word strategy runs deep and is traced to the Greek *strategos*, "an elected general in ancient Athens. The *strategoi* were mainly military leaders with combined political and military authority, which is the essence of strategy" (Cohen, 2023). From being inextricably linked to war, the battlefield for strategy expanded to include nonmilitary references to chess, politics, business, and more. Using the analogy of strategy to chess also clarifies that strategy is not the individual moves that the chess pieces make but rather a collection of these moves that has a larger purpose that aims to neutralize, say the rook or bishop, or the ultimate checkmate.

## BOX 10.1: STRATEGIES TO ADDRESS GLOBAL HEALTHCARE WORKFORCE SHORTAGE

In a recent opinion piece on CNN, Amanda, an RN and leader of a global team, provides advice on strategies to address the global healthcare workforce shortage by "address(ing) the key factors pulling healthcare workers away from their home countries in the first place, including low salaries, unsafe working conditions, and a lack of an adequate social safety net" (McClelland, 2023). These are strategic choices that need to be made over a longer time horizon. Choices and long-time horizon are integral to strategy.

For businesses, "strategic management describes efforts to guide organizations in an integrated manner, and to do so with purpose and over a long-time horizon" (Harrison & Thompson, 2014, p. 4). Applying strategy in a business context then implies that we are not focused on the day-to-day operations of the business but rather a longer time horizon that is focused on goal(s). With its focus on goals of the organization, there is also implicit within strategy an element of control. Kyriazoglou describes the purpose of **strategic control** is to "establish, motivate and reward achievement of general goals, and specific objectives of the organization by its management and employees. Also stimulate organizational learning, growth and development of new ideas and strategies" (2020, pp. 3–4). In his book, Kyriazoglou describes strategic controls being achieved through strategic planning committees, plans, budgets, implementation plans, and performance frameworks (Box 10.1).

**Strategic planning** can take place at various levels of an organization as well as governments (federal, state, and local). At any level, effective strategic (planning) entails both a process and a way of thinking. The strategic (planning) process includes activities such as analysis of the firm and its environment, establishment of a **strategic direction**, evaluation of **alternative strategies** the firm might pursue to achieve this direction, and implementation planning (Harrison & Thompson, 2014, p. 4). Thus, strategic planning is a very systematic process that is rooted in the internal assessment of the organization as to its current state and its brand. This assessment then expands to the external market and environment (social, political, economic, etc.) that the organization operates in. These internal and external assessments provide the basis to establish strategic directions or long-term goals that the organization seeks to achieve. To reach these strategic directions, there are alternative approaches that the organization might choose. Each of these alternative approaches has its pros and cons that need to be understood to decide the approach to be adopted. Inherent in the weighing of alternative approaches is a choice of what approach is taken and equally which is not. Additionally, because of limited resources, choosing one approach means that resources are committed and hence not available for alternative approaches. Once the approach is chosen, the task of planning for the implementation of this approach begins in right earnest. An integral part of implementation planning is also evaluation of the approach adopted—to assess if the goals are met.

## CASE STUDY 10.1: STRATEGIC MANAGEMENT

Consider strategic management at St. Joseph's University Medical Center (SJUMC) as they weighed options to address frequent use of emergency department services.

SJUMC is the flagship facility within the St. Joseph's Health (SJH) system. It is a major academic medical/trauma center and a five-time Magnet® Recognized Catholic Medical Center.

The Medical Center is also the major anchor institution in its host city and a major safety-net provider in northern New Jersey, with primary Medicaid, Medicare, and charity care patients in its case mix.

In 2023, the emergency department at St. Joseph's University averaged over 175,000 visits. Many of these visits were repeat patients who had little or no access to primary care and were uninsured or underinsured, with the majority seeking care for chronic health conditions, such as asthma, chronic obstructive pulmonary disease (COPD), diabetes, hypertension, and obesity. Reducing the cost associated with this population's frequent use of emergency department services was aligned with SJUMC's strategy to reduce overutilization of its emergency department to reduce consumer costs, focus efforts on addressing the lack of access to primary care services, and enhance the overall patient experience of this population.

SJUMC thoroughly analyzed internal and external environmental factors, including the cost associated with the overutilization of costly emergency services and the level of reimbursement the hospital received from its payers. In addition, it surveyed emergency department users on social indicators such as housing, access to primary care, clinics, childcare, public transportation, trust in the healthcare system, and public safety.

The analysis revealed a crucial finding: housing insecurity, specifically the lack of high-quality, safe, affordable housing, was directly linked to many patients' inability to effectively manage their chronic health conditions. This, in turn, led to an overutilization of the hospital's emergency department, resulting in costly care and a lack of long-term health management for these patients.

Executive leadership recognized that developing affordable housing was outside St. Joseph's core business. Yet, its unquestionable link to population health and chronic disease management made creating affordable, high-quality housing an essential strategic priority.

SJUMC began to explore working with housing developers to build affordable housing near its campus and partnering with community agencies that assist low-income families in acquiring affordable housing. SJUMC also attempted to work with the Center for Medicaid Services to amend the 1115 waiver to allow housing vouchers for vulnerable populations so they could obtain affordable housing. These options proved to be either too costly, would not address the healthcare needs of the targeted population, or too difficult from a regulatory standpoint.

Ultimately, the best strategic option was for SJUMC to partner with the New Jersey Housing and Mortgage Finance Agency (HMFA). In concert with the 4% low-income housing credit, this partnership leveraged the hospital's equity to create a supportive affordable housing development near the hospital campus.

SJUMC owned a shovel-ready site that was approximately 100 yards west of the front of the hospital along the main access road leading to the hospital. The property was ideally located near public transportation. In addition, the site was located close to the Garden State Parkway and Routes 80, 46, and 19. Tenants could access downtown Paterson's New Jersey Transit railway, approximately one mile away. St. Joseph's highly skilled physicians; Magnet-recognized nurses; and clinical, administrative, and health professional staff pride themselves on providing highly responsive healthcare with a "patients first" approach. St. Joseph's unique caring culture epitomizes its mission, vision, and values. SJUMC's decision to follow this strategic direction to address housing insecurity allowed SJUMC to address a social need while simultaneously healing the body, mind, and spirit of the tenants who would occupy the project.

In this example from SJUMC on addressing overuse of its emergency department, strategic management included analyzing the root causes not only from its perspective but also including social indicators. This analysis brought up the key role that affordable housing plays in their patients' inability to effectively manage chronic health conditions. This led SJUMC to weigh various tried and trusted options to develop affordable housing which was outside the ambit of its core business. Eventually, they zeroed in on a partnership that pooled resources, including hospital equity to build affordable housing for its patients. Here, because SJUMC has committed resources to addressing overuse of emergency department services, the pool of available resources has shrunk. Since affordable housing has only just been opened, SJUMC will need to plan evaluations over a suitable time horizon to assess how this strategic choice affects the overuse of its emergency department services. Later in this chapter, a case study provides more details of SJUMC's approach to addressing overuse of emergency services through building affordable housing.

## ELEMENTS OF STRATEGIC PLANNING

The systematic process of strategic planning, as outlined by Harrison and Thompson, is a great start to making sure that an approach to strategic planning includes due consideration of these processes. This systematic approach is a great start. Building on this initial approach is a more comprehensive and inclusive approach to strategic planning.

To understand strategic planning more comprehensively, consider the example of the U.S. National Strategy for Eliminating Hepatitis B and C (National Academies of Sciences et al., 2017). This strategy draws upon the World Health Organization's (WHO) Strategic Directions from the Global Health Sector Strategy on Viral Hepatitis (WHO, 2016). This global health sector strategy is well captured in Figure 10.1 and described here:

1. What is the situation? Understanding the prevailing situation helps to provide information for focused action. Here, the emphasis is on the problem at hand and response as a basis for advocacy, political commitment, national planning, resource mobilization and allocation, implementation, and program improvement.
2. What services should be delivered? Prioritizing services helps to choose interventions that will impact the problem. Describe the essential package of interventions that need to be delivered to reach targets established for strategic goals.

**FIGURE 10.1.** Framework for strategic planning.

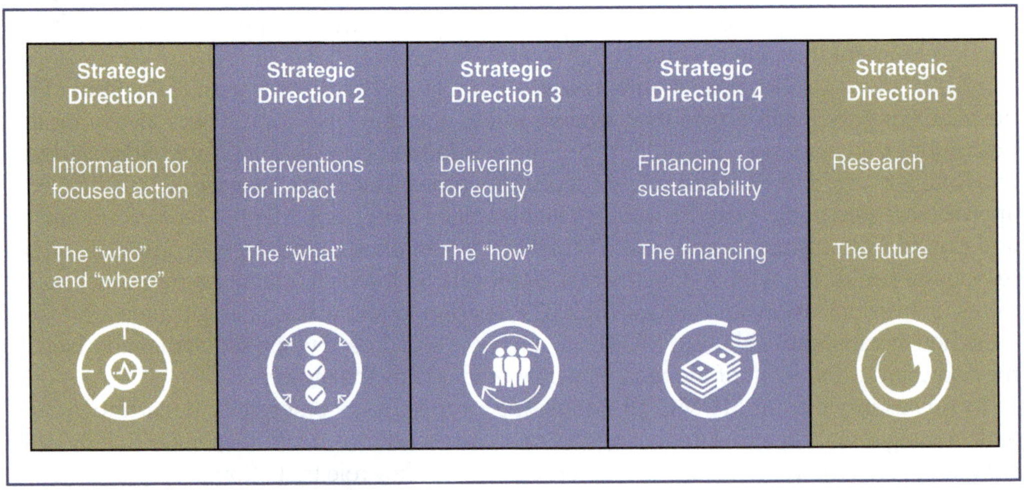

| Strategic Direction 1 | Strategic Direction 2 | Strategic Direction 3 | Strategic Direction 4 | Strategic Direction 5 |
|---|---|---|---|---|
| Information for focused action | Interventions for impact | Delivering for equity | Financing for sustainability | Research |
| The "who" and "where" | The "what" | The "how" | The financing | The future |

*Source:* Adapted from World Health Organization. (2016). *Global health sector strategy on viral hepatitis, 2016–2021: Towards ending viral hepatitis.* Retrieved July 19, 2016, from http://apps.who.int/iris/bitstream/10665/246177/1/WHO-HIV-2016.06-eng.pdf.

3. How can these services be delivered? Identify the best methods for delivering the continuum of services to different populations in different locations, to achieve equity, maximize impact, and ensure quality.
4. How can the costs of delivering the package of services be met? Identify sustainable and innovative models for the financing of interventions and approaches for reducing costs so that people can access the necessary services without incurring financial hardship.
5. How can the trajectory of responses be changed? Research and identify where there are major gaps in knowledge and technologies, where innovation is required to shift the trajectory of response for those responses to be accelerated for targets to be achieved.

This framework for strategic planning was developed and used for strategic planning around viral hepatitis at the global and national levels. However, just like the strategic planning process can occur at various levels of organizations and governments, this framework has ready application for healthcare organizations, too, and builds on the approach to strategic planning by Harrison and Thompson. It specifically includes an emphasis on equity, financing for sustainability, and a research component to make sure that any gaps in knowledge related to the prioritized interventions and established targets are monitored. There is much truth to the saying "You get what you inspect, not what you expect." Under this framework, ideas of equity, financing sustainability, and research are inspected and not left to expectation. Thus, including these concepts as an integral part of the strategic planning process ensures that these critical concepts are not left to chance but specifically considered in the strategic planning process.

Dimensions of **equity** and inclusivity are only now being recognized in the strategic planning process. In reviewing the literature on strategies to promote equity and inclusivity in sexual and reproductive health among marginalized populations, Schaaf et al. concluded that "garnering support from communities involved, health system actors, and local politicians" is a first step. In addition, strategies that have clear linkages to legal accountability, budgets, or organizational processes as well as making conscious and genuine efforts to include marginalized groups through specific roles in the program go a long way in promoting health equity and inclusivity (Schaaf et al., 2022). A strategy to make mental health more accessible and equitable appears in Box 10.2.

To gain an understanding of the effective strategic planning, consider the following examples from the European Commission, the Office of U.S. Global AIDS Coordinator, and National Defense Strategy.

The European Commission's Global Health Strategy provides an agenda through 2030. This strategy has three priorities:

1. Deliver better health and well-being of people across the life course;
2. Strengthen health systems and advance universal health coverage; and
3. Prevent and combat health threats, including pandemics.

### BOX 10.2: OUT-OF-THE-BOX STRATEGIZING FOR MENTAL HEALTH

The never-ending healthcare workforce shortage, especially in mental health, requires some out-of-the-box strategizing. According to Wells, the use of health coregulation—a positive way to deal with social and health challenges—through a health coach, would be a good start. While coregulation would not substitute for a qualified mental health professional, it would make mental health more accessible even with a shortage of mental health professionals (Wells, 2023).

Underpinning these strategies are "twenty guiding principles to shape global health and then make concrete lines of action for operationalization of the principles. To assess progress and ensure the accountability of the EU's global health action, permanent monitoring and assessment will be set up" (Viberg et al., 2023, p. 553). The European Commission's strategy relates directly to the long-term nature of strategy, its planning, and ongoing monitoring and evaluation.

Similarly, the Office of U.S. Global AIDS Coordinator, uses a **strategic framework** that includes use of data, prevention, access to treatment, and partnerships for sustainability to address the problem of HIV/AIDS across the globe (Functional Bureau Strategy, 2018).

As part of the National Defense Strategy of 2018, there were efforts to ensure that the Military Health System is ready for the changing landscape of war. Strategically, this included casualty care on the battlefield, enhancing treatment options, prepositioning medical assets, and improving resilience of medical logistics (RAND Corporation, 2021). This strategy shows how changes in the external environment drive weighing options to strategically respond to these changes.

Without due consideration of strategic planning, things can go wrong, which is what happened with the merger of the insurer Unum Group with Provident in 1999 as the first company to offer group disability coverage under employee benefits. Even after spending huge sums of money on training and integration, the environments of the two companies were too different, leading to a breakup in less than a decade (Achieveit, 2021). Here, it is likely that a detailed internal assessment of the two organizations might have been perfunctory and may have glossed over the prevailing cultural differences in the two organizations.

If saving costs in U.S. healthcare is a strategic goal, this requires a strategy that is focused on the primary drivers of poor health which requires increasing resources directed to wellness (not sickness), nutrition, prevention (not treatment), and patient education. However, analysis of federal resources dedicated to nutrition research is seen to be one fortieth of those devoted to drugs, biotech, and medical devices (Smack, 2019). In this example, there appears to be a failure to completely evaluate the different approaches—wellness, nutrition, prevention—to achieving the strategic goal of saving costs in U.S. healthcare.

## UNIQUE ASPECTS OF STRATEGIC PLANNING IN HEALTH

Strategic planning in health needs due consideration of two unique aspects of health compared to other businesses. For starters, health includes direct interaction between providers and patients or clients. Secondly, health has proximate and distant determinants in health and nonhealth sectors, an approach that is well captured through the **social determinants of health** (SDOH). Examples of how strategic planning in health takes cognizance of these unique aspects are provided here.

### DIRECT INTERACTIONS WITH PATIENTS

Strategy in healthcare is built around patients and requires insights about patients. These insights are gleaned from "market data, understanding treatment algorithms and paradigms, all with an effort to understand the situation the patient is in" (Haimowitz, 2011, p. 97). In another example, the Department of Defense sought inputs from warfighters about their priorities and concerns regarding brain health and developed a strategic approach as a "framework for deliberate, prioritized, and rapid development of end-to-end solutions" (DOD, 2021, p. 3).

## SOCIAL DETERMINANTS OF HEALTH

The United States National Pain Strategy was developed by the National Institutes of Health based on a 2011 Institute of Medicine (IOM) report. This strategy encompassed "population research, prevention and care, disparities, service delivery and reimbursements, professional education and training, and public awareness and communication" (Interagency Pain Research Coordinating Committee, n.d., p. 3). Integral to the National Pain Strategy was a recognition of SDOH through population research, prevention, disparities, and others.

Post–COVID-19 pandemic, several countries, especially low- and middle-income countries, have been grappling with additional adverse impacts on their existing malnutrition challenges among women and children. In these countries, evidence-based strategic initiatives focused on food insecurity, social protection programs, access to healthcare, educational programs, and safe and healthy household community environments that cut across health and nonhealth sectors are seen as the best way to sustainably address the determinants directly and indirectly linked to these challenges, given the unique country situations (Akseer et al., 2020). The need for healthcare strategies to cut across health and nonhealth sectors is also underscored by experiences in Canada where strategies to address determinants of health across sectors is seen to be most beneficial (Salmond & Mahato, 2021).

In reviewing strategies to respond to the COVID-19 pandemic, Monti et al. noted that we need to include digital exclusion as well as essential workers into an expanded understanding of SDOH (Monti et al., 2021). Given the lessons learned from COVID-19, there is also a recognition now to adopt multisector strategies, especially for zoonotic diseases (Gorji et al., 2022).

Overdose Response Strategy (ORS) is a partnership between public health and public safety to reduce drug overdoses in local communities. This strategy is reliant on the sharing of data, intelligence, and evidence-based and innovative responses to overdose. Strategies such as ORS are ripe for replication in other health and safety issues such as gun violence or bioterrorism that require coordination between public health and public safety (Wolff et al., 2022).

The need for multisector strategic approaches to health is very well brought out in managing chronic conditions and diseases. Airhihenbuwa and others have collected and analyzed 15 articles on strategies to address chronic diseases that were published between 2017 and 2020 to identify unique and common strategies across the world. They found that strategies to address chronic disease prevention and management are unique to local settings across the world. However, across the world, sharing challenges and opportunities for innovation in evidence-based approaches is essential to improving population-based health strategies for chronic disease prevention and management. Preventing and managing chronic diseases reinforce the value that individual experiences hold lessons in both promises and challenges that can be shared globally (Airhihenbuwa et al., 2021). Box 10.3 provides a description of strategies (health and nonhealth) that are being used to better manage diabetes in communities.

At the same time, in our rush to ensure that strategic initiatives are addressing SDOH that cut across different sectors of the economy, there is still not a shared understanding and definition of what constitutes SDOH across health and nonhealth sectors. Greater clarity of the language as well as concepts underlying these determinants can aid their planning, implementation, and evaluation (Alderwick & Gottlieb, 2019).

## BOX 10.3: HEALTH STRATEGIES TO ADDRESS CHRONIC CONDITIONS

Continuing with the theme of strategies to address chronic conditions, a study by Gunter and others on population health innovations and payments for diabetes management found that organizations are using the following strategies to address medical and social needs:

- Supplemented staffing models to support high-risk patients with diabetes (e.g., community health workers, behavioral health specialists)
- Innovations in information technology (e.g., software for social needs referrals)
- Protocols to identify high-risk populations with gaps in care
- Identify and address social needs (e.g., food insecurity, housing)
- Invest in human capital to support social needs referrals and coordination (e.g., embedding social service employees in clinics)
- Work with organizations to connect to community resources

In their study, Gunter et al. found that value-based payment mechanisms are usually biased toward rewarding clinical performance metrics rather than measures of population health or social needs interventions.

*Source:* Data from Gunter, K. E., Peek, M. E., Tanumihardjo, J. P., Carbrey, E., Crespo, R. D., Johnson, T. W., Rueda-Yamashita, B., Schwartz, E. I., Sol, C., Wilkinson, C. M., Wilson, J., Loehmer, E., & Chin, M. H. (2021). Population health innovations and payment to address social needs among patients and communities with diabetes. *The Milbank Quarterly, 99*(4), 928–973. https://doi.org/10.1111/1468-0009.12522.

## APPLICATION OF STRATEGIC PLANNING

Consider an application of the elements of strategic planning to the case study. Refer to the case study 10.2 that follows.

## CASE STUDY 10.2: HOW AN INNER-CITY ACUTE CARE MEDICAL CENTER ADDRESSED HOUSING INSECURITY AMONG FREQUENT USERS OF EMERGENCY SERVICES

### INTRODUCTION

Safe, affordable, and supportive housing is crucial for good health. However, poor housing, combined with little or no available services that support vulnerable families, results in chronic health conditions such as COPD, asthma, increased risk of cardiovascular disease, and the spread of diseases like tuberoses and other respiratory infections. Families in substandard housing are also often forced to live in overcrowded conditions, which directly correlates to increased mental illness and stress. All these factors lead to increased healthcare costs for consumers and care providers.

This case study outlines strategic considerations and steps SJH took to design and construct an effective, affordable, supportive housing project. This step-by-step process is illustrated in Figure 10.2.

### BACKGROUND

In 2008, Paterson, New Jersey, designated 244 acres around the SJUMC campus as an area needing redevelopment. As a trusted anchor institution, SJUMC—the flagship acute care hospital in the SJH hospital and healthcare system—was named the master developer of this

**FIGURE 10.2.** Step-by-step process in planning affordable housing development.

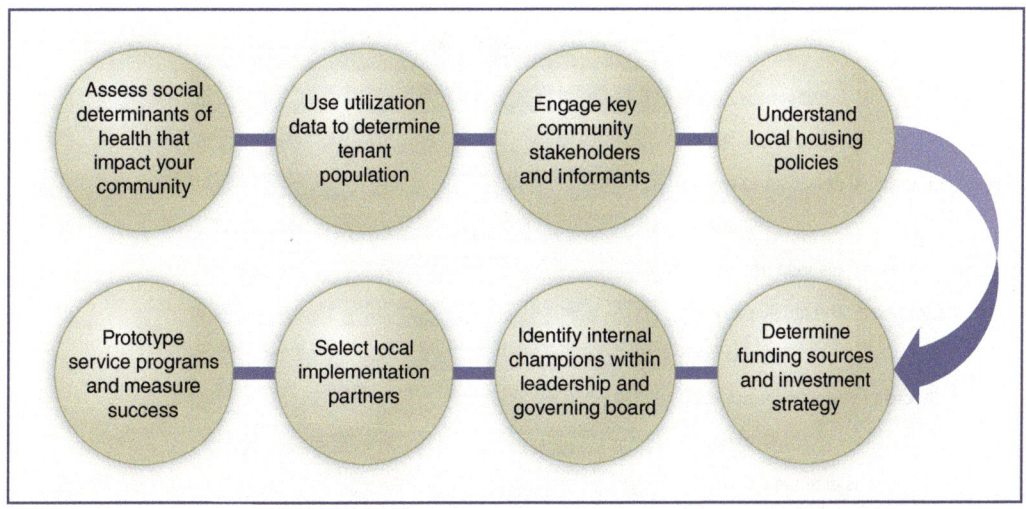

newly designated redevelopment area. Recognizing that housing insecurity is a significant driver of poor health outcomes, SJH partnered with the State of New Jersey, New Jersey Community Development Corporation (NJCDC), and Community Asset Preservation Corporation (CAPC) to design, build, and operate a 56-unit supportive housing project for people who frequently utilize the hospital's emergency services.

This $26.4 million project mixes capital from the low-income housing tax credit program (syndicated by Enterprise Housing Credit Investments), the New Jersey Housing and Mortgage Finance Agency, TD Bank, and St. Joseph's contribution of $6.4 million in cash and land. Ten of the 56 units will be designated for people with behavioral health needs. Units will be a mix of one-, two-, and three-bedroom units affordable to families and hospital employees. All residents will be offered medical care through SJH and social services through community-based social service providers and partners to help reduce unnecessary use of the emergency department.

The Barclay Street housing project will also include space for social, health, and wellness services that address SDOH, including employment services, parenting/coaching and life skills, mental health services, and financial literacy. All services provided in the development will be tenant determined.

## ASSESS SOCIAL DETERMINANTS OF HEALTH THAT IMPACT YOUR COMMUNITY: USE UTILIZATION DATA TO DETERMINE TENANT POPULATION

Utilization data from SJUMC's emergency department showed that many patients used the emergency department as their primary care provider. Additionally, these patients were uninsured or underinsured. Data from electronic medical records, using collection tools like PREPARE (Protocol for Responding to and Assessing Patients' Assets, Risks, and Experiences) and ICD-10 SDOH Z-codes, indicated that frequent users of SJUMC emergency services were experiencing severe housing insecurity. Survey results from SJH's most recent community health needs assessment (CHNA) also showed that mental health, diabetes, and access to healthcare services were rated as moderate to significant problems in the community (Figure 10.3).

SJH convened a group of community stakeholders who represented a cross-section of community-based agencies and organizations to evaluate and prioritize health issues that

**FIGURE 10.3.** Key informants: Relative positions of health topics as problems in the community.

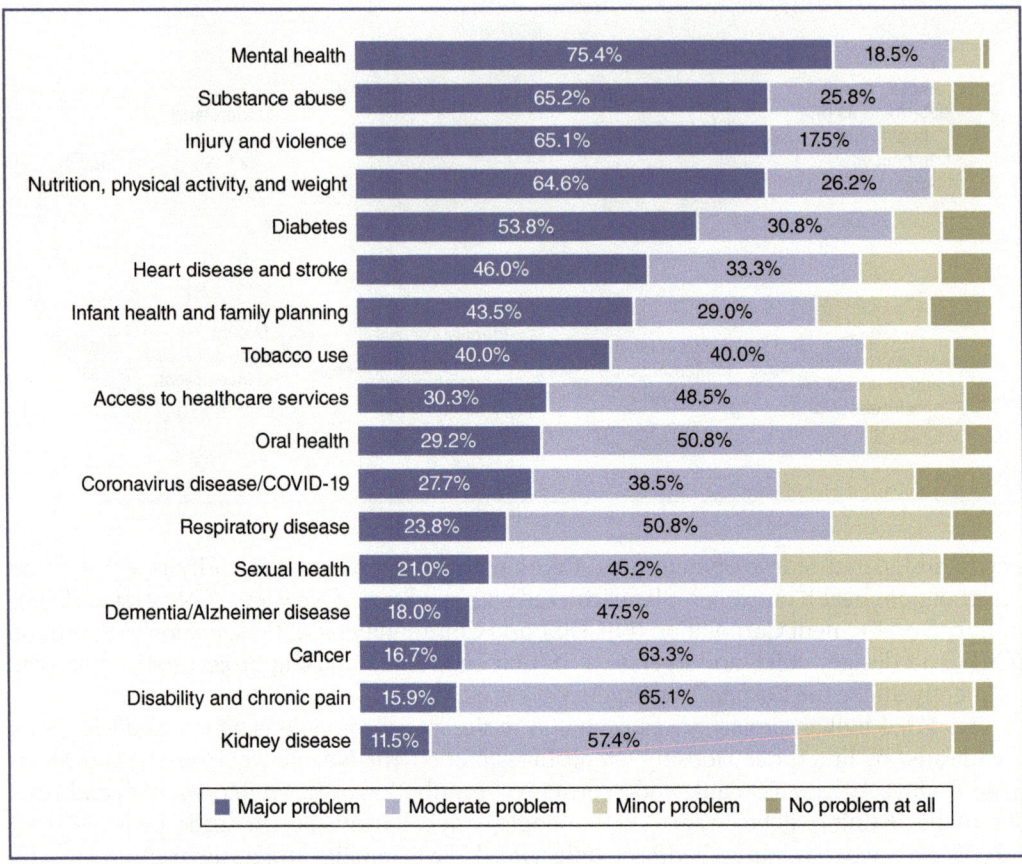

*Source:* Data from *2022 Community Health Needs Assessment*, Southern Passaic County, NJ. Professional Research Consultants (PRC), December 2022.

impacted SJH's service areas. Based on the findings of the CHNA, housing was ranked seventh out of 15. Furthermore, 32% of residents living around the Paterson campus had a severe housing problem, coupled with existing housing being overpriced and overcrowded and the majority lacking adequate kitchens, having poor plumbing, and littered with multiple asthma triggers. Rents for the area were also high, with the cost to rent a one-bedroom unit at $1,475 per month and a three-bedroom unit as high as $2,475 per month.

## ENGAGE KEY COMMUNITY STAKEHOLDERS AND INFORMANTS: UNDERSTANDING LOCAL HOUSING POLICIES

SJH engaged its community early and often to understand how to respond to their needs by leveraging the strengths of its organization to provide a transformational healing presence in collaboration with those who share their values, understood its mission, and desire to foster health equity.

The success of the supportive housing project depended heavily on developing critical partnerships and stakeholder support. NJCDC was identified and brought on as the project developer. NJCDC has a successful history of mission-driven work and has completed over 24 projects, from building housing for people experiencing homelessness and youth aging out of foster care to full services in community schools and youth centers. New Jersey Community Capital (NJCC) is one of New Jersey's leading community development financial institutions.

New Jersey Community Capital has invested nearly $650 million in underserved communities, rehabilitated over 10,000 housing units in neighborhoods heavily impacted by foreclosures, and developed multifamily housing and condominiums throughout New Jersey. Their parent organization, NJCC, has extensive experience in syndicating low-interest tax credits, a significant funding source for this project. Other key constituencies were local elected officials. Local officials needed to approve a PILOT (Payment In Lieu of Taxes) agreement for the project financing. Local elected leaders and the councilperson representing the ward where the project would be built were engaged early in the process. They were provided regular updates as the project progressed. The ward councilperson also facilitated interactions with the local authority boards, such as the planning, zoning, and historic preservation boards. Having a strong advocate in local government is critical to the success of any affordable housing project.

## DETERMINE FUNDING SOURCES AND INVESTMENT STRATEGY

The project was structured using 4% low-income housing tax credit equity, tax-exempt debt, and a $4.8 million contribution from the hospital. The HMFA provided subsidy funding up to $4 million. HMFA financing was structured as a cash flow loan payable in full at the end of the mortgage term. SJH's contributed land valued at $1.6 million, not included in the subsidy contribution from the hospital discussed earlier. The capital funding stack shows all funding sources (Figure 10.4). This project is mission aligned and enhances employee wellness and care management. The project builds trust and partnership with valued employees and the Paterson community while stabilizing the neighborhood around the SJUMC campus.

**FIGURE 10.4.** Project cost and financing for supportive housing project.

| Uses | |
|---|---|
| Acquisiton costs | $350,000 |
| Construction | $17,095,012 |
| Dev fee | $3,258,000 |
| Prof services | $1,298,949 |
| Preoperational expenses | $164,675 |
| Carrying, financing, and escrows | $4,301,065 |
| Total | $26,467,701 |

| Sources | |
|---|---|
| NJHMFA tax exempt bond | $3,846,362 |
| HMFA hospital subsidy PILOT program | $4,500,000 |
| St. Joseph health project contribution/loan | $4,500,000 |
| NJHMFA special needs housing trust fund | $1,000,000 |
| Deferred dev fee | $1,590,509 |
| LIHTC equity investor proceeds | $11,030,830 |
| Total | $26,467,701 |

HMFA, Housing and Mortgage Finance Agency; LIHTC, low-income housing tax credit; NJHMFA, New Jersey Housing and Mortgage Finance Agency; PILOT, Payment In Lieu of Taxes.

## PROGRAM DESIGN AND MEASURES

SJUMC serves as the primary social service provider for the project. SJUMC entered into an agreement with the NJCDC for the latter to provide service coordination/case management staff to the project for a minimum of 20 hours per week.

The 10 supportive housing units will have State Rental Assistance Program rental vouchers through the New Jersey Department of Community Affairs. Residents in these units will pay up to 30% of their household income toward rent and utility costs.

Barclay Place will provide residents with access to a comprehensive array of supportive services focused on helping them improve their health status and reduce health inequity. These services will include case management; linkages to mainstream resources; and access, linkages, and ongoing follow-up to existing community resources that include but are not limited to the following:

- Employment programs, including job training and job search assistance
- Education programs, including general educational development (GED) tutoring, literacy training, and linkages to higher education
- Financial management training from a qualified provider and ongoing budget support
- Linkage and ongoing follow-up services to healthcare, including dental care, physical health, and primary healthcare prevention services
- Other services, including mental healthcare, addiction services, social skills training, and wellness programs
- On-call crisis response 24 hours per day, 7 days per week

Services will be provided on-site at Barclay Place, SJUMC, and other locations throughout Paterson, such as the One-Stop Career Center, Greater Paterson Opportunities Industrial Center, Eva's Village, and New Destiny Family Success Center. All services will be available to residents voluntarily and will not be a condition of residency. Individual service plans will be reassessed periodically and updated to reflect the residents' changing needs. Additionally, residents will not have out-of-pocket expenses for supportive or case management services. The case manager will coordinate supportive services for residents through the use of the Health Coalition of Passaic County's Pathways to Success program and the Unite US platform, which includes developing individualized service plans, providing linkages to available support services on-site and in the community, and ongoing follow-up and assessment.

## CONCLUSION

Modern-day hospitals, particularly those in urban centers, are anchor institutions by definition and geographic scope. They are rooted in place and significantly impact their neighborhood and communities.

The Barclay Street Housing project, known as Barclay Place, consists of 56 affordable one- and three-bedroom rental units for area residents. Rents will range between $1,161 for a one-bedroom unit and $1,598 for a three-bedroom unit. The entire first floor of the project will house an array of on-site services that address SDOH, including a commercial kitchen, community meeting space, and a state-of-the-art fitness center. Of the 56 units, there will be 46 units for families with low to moderate incomes and 10 permanent, supportive units for individuals with mental illness.

SJH's investment in this project aligned community investments with activities that address neighborhood and environmental conditions. By improving sustainable housing in the community and offering support services, SJH developed a true partnership with those it serves to improve health equity.

### TABLE 10.1. APPLYING FRAMEWORK FOR STRATEGIC PLANNING TO CASE STUDY

| ELEMENT DESCRIPTION | APPLICATION TO CASE STUDY |
|---|---|
| Information for focused action | • Anchor institution named as master developer for area around hospital needing redevelopment<br>• Housing insecurity is a significant driver of poor health outcomes<br>• Data from emergency department utilization and CHNA |
| Interventions for impact | • Safe, affordable, and supportive housing<br>• Services to support vulnerable families—medical service through St. Joseph's Health and social services through community partners<br>• On-site services address SDOH |
| Delivering for equity | • 56 units—10 designated for people with behavioral health needs<br>• 10 supportive units have NJ Rental Assistance Program vouchers<br>• 46 units for families with low to moderate income |
| Financing for sustainability | • $26.4 million project—low-income housing tax credit, NJ Housing & Mortgage Finance, TD Bank and St. Joseph ($6.4 million = cash + land)<br>• Rents—$1,161 (1 bedroom) to $1,598 (3 bedroom) |
| Research | • Poor housing and lack of services results in chronic conditions and increased risk of disease and infections<br>• Substandard/Overcrowded housing correlates to increased mental illness and stress |

CHNA, community health needs assessment; SDOH, social determinants of health.

The case study provides background and context to the strategic decision by SJUMC in Paterson, New Jersey, to address SDOH. Table 10.1 identifies each of the elements of strategic planning from this case study.

## INFORMATION FOR FOCUSED ACTION

As an anchor institution, SJUMC was in a trusted position to take on the role of master developer for the redevelopment of the area around its flagship acute care hospital. Utilization and other data from its emergency department confirmed that many patients were uninsured or underinsured and used the emergency department as their primary care provider and were experiencing severe housing insecurity. Survey results from its most recent CHNA highlighted mental health, diabetes, and access to healthcare services as problems.

## INTERVENTIONS FOR IMPACT

Even though housing was ranked seventh based on the CHNA, a third of residents living near SJUMC had severe housing problems and rents were costly: $1,475 per month for one bedroom and $2,475 for three bedrooms. By engaging key community partners and critical stakeholder support, including local elected and government officials, the intervention was focused on safe, affordable, and supportive housing, called Barclay Place. At Barclay Place, medical services would be provided through SJUMC and a variety of social services through community partners, including linkage to mainstream and community resources to address SDOH.

## DELIVERING FOR EQUITY

Barclay Place is a 56-unit affordable housing project. Of these, 10 units were designated for vulnerable populations with behavioral health needs. At the same time, 46 units were for use by families with low to moderate income and 10 units were supported through NJ Rental Assistance Program vouchers.

## FINANCING FOR SUSTAINABILITY

The total project cost of $26.4 million was structured using 4% low-income housing tax credit, tax-exempt debt, and a $4.8 million contribution from SJUMC. In addition, NJHMFA provided subsidy funding up to $4 million and SJUMC also contributed land valued at $1.6 million. Local officials also approved a PILOT agreement for project financing. The Barclay Place project was thus able to provide rental units at $1,161 per month for one-bedroom and $1,598 for three-bedroom units.

## RESEARCH

Research into affordable housing confirmed that poor housing and lack of services result in chronic health conditions and increased risk of cardiovascular diseases, as well as respiratory infections. Living in overcrowded and unsafe conditions is also directly correlated with increased mental illness and stress.

Applying the elements of strategic planning to this case study shows that these elements are very relevant to the real world. SJUMC's Barclay Place project opened earlier in 2023. The conceptualization of this project, working with community partners and stakeholders, as well as championing this affordable housing project by a hospital as an anchor institution, also showcases how hospitals can go about strategically addressing SDOH and work across health and nonhealth sectors.

## NEED FOR HEALTHCARE STRATEGIC PLANNING

The Society for Healthcare Strategy and Market Development of the American Hospital Association brought out in 2017 its second edition of *Bridging Worlds: The Future Role of the Healthcare Strategist* (Society for Healthcare Strategy and Market Development, 2017). This book outlines several facets of the evolving health landscape that have implications for healthcare strategy:

- *Changing utilization patterns*: Changes in reimbursement are making it imperative that services and procedures that were earlier identified solely with hospitals are delivered in very different settings. This leads to dramatic changes in volume in inpatient, outpatient, and ambulatory settings.
- *Advanced science of medicine*: Advances in medicine and technology are rapidly translating to the practice of medicine exponentially changing. These advances create strategic competitive advantages for organizations.
- *Technology*: Innovations in technology in the hospital, wearable on patients, and remote monitoring far outpace their deployment. These innovations are a game changer for healthcare.
- *Big data*: Healthcare organizations are sitting on a treasure trove of data. The use of artificial intelligence and predictive models is making more of this data actionable.
- *Uncertainty in payment models and policy*: The transition from volume to value-based payments is underway. However, till this transition plays out, there is lingering

uncertainty that also needs to contend with concerns about the rising cost of healthcare.
- *New competition*: Mergers and acquisitions are leading to new competition in healthcare as well as newer entrants from payors, pharmacy chains, and online retailers are making healthcare even more competitive.
- *Partners and collaborators*: With increasing pressures on the bottom line, healthcare organizations need to seek out partners and collaborators to work with to provide care rather than do everything for all patients.
- *Consumerism and retailization*: The increasing presence of retail stores in delivering care is bringing the focus on patients as consumers. This is a strategic shift from the conventional thinking of healthcare and hospitals.
- *Engagement and behavior change*: This is the new buzz in healthcare and a generational change. With the penetration of social media and changes in how consumers experience other sectors of the economy, the need to emphasize engagement and behavior change as integral to the patient experience is paramount.
- *Holistic view of population health*: Population health is becoming more mainstream and with financial incentives now pushing this idea in healthcare, there is more of an urgency at considering upstream and downstream effects in health.

Taken together, these facets paint the picture of a rapidly changing healthcare landscape and point to the need to be ever vigilant as organizations undertake strategic planning. Ignoring these facets can only be to the peril of these organizations.

## TOOLS TO GUIDE STRATEGIC PLANNING

The elements of strategic planning and its application (see "Application of Strategic Planning") outlines the process of strategic planning. Throughout this process, a variety of tools can be used to guide strategic planning. Some of the tools are outlined here (Jesse, 2023; Seirawan, 2023):

- **S**trengths, **W**eaknesses, **O**pportunities, and **T**hreats (SWOT) analysis helps identify internal and external elements that impact an organization.
- Performance prism model and its five perspectives: stakeholder satisfaction, stakeholder contribution, strategies, processes, and capabilities
- European Foundation for Quality Management (EFQM) excellence model and its three elements: fundamental concepts of excellence, criteria, and Radar chart to understand cause and effect
- Balanced scorecard balances four perspectives: finances, customers, internal processes, and learning and growth.
- Capability analysis helps identify capabilities as sources of competitive strengths and weaknesses.
- Market analysis helps identify trends and insights into the industry and market.
- Brand vision strategy helps define and track objectives aligned with the overall mission and vision.
- Brand prioritization framework helps to prioritize initiatives that impact your brand with the attendant level of effort.
- Patient journey strategy facilitates mapping the various touch points in a patient's journey throughout their patient experience.
- Risk assessment matrix assesses the need to address potential threats to business.

## PITFALLS TO AVOID IN HEALTHCARE STRATEGIC PLANNING

Common pitfalls in strategic planning can lead to avoidable and costly (time, money, or resources) implications. Some of these pitfalls (Jesse, 2023; Seirawan, 2023) are as follows:

- Disregarding branding efforts leading to misalignment between strategy and brand
- Selecting operational key performance indicators (KPIs) instead of strategic KPIs—making sure that KPIs are linked to strategic and not operational goals
- Too many metrics—remember, you get what you inspect, not what you expect, so focus on a few metrics that can be measured and tracked
- Not having support from champions and leaders who can help to drive strategy
- Making unrealistic plans that cannot be completed in a timely manner
- Unclear roles and responsibilities within the strategy development and execution team

## BENEFITS OF STRATEGIC PLANNING

A well-thought-through and implemented organizational strategic plan can have several benefits. These benefits include the following (Strata, 2019):

- Improvement in company culture by acting on areas that strengthen the future of the organization
- Revising goals and objectives to better meet foreseeable challenges
- Appropriate budgeting to ensure that strategic priorities are funded
- Informed service line decisions that meet strategic goals
- Established capital planning for strategic investments
- Informed long-range forecasting that is data driven

## CONCLUSION

The origins of strategic planning can be traced to wars. In businesses such as healthcare, strategic planning is about making informed choices to achieve long-term goals at various levels of organizations and government. At a minimum, strategic planning includes analysis of the internal and external environment, agreeing on a strategic direction, assessing alternatives, and a plan to implement the chosen alternative(s) to achieve this strategic direction. Several key changes in the healthcare landscape driving the need for strategic planning include changing utilization patterns, advances in medicine, technology, uncertainty in payment models, consumerism, and expanded view of population health. A more intentional approach to strategic planning builds on the minimalist approach and definition of strategic planning to ensure focus on equity, sustainability, and research in this process. Two unique aspects of healthcare—direct interaction between patients and providers and SDOH (health and nonhealth sectors)—have direct implication for strategic planning, and several examples show how organizations are directly addressing these unique aspects in their strategic planning. The case study of SJUMC and its affordable housing project, Barclay Place, shows how the intentional and comprehensive strategic planning framework is used in healthcare. There are several tools that are available to aid strategic planning, and several organizations have forayed into providing services for healthcare strategic planning. Paying attention to the elements of strategic planning helps to minimize the pitfalls (brand alignment, too many metrics, unrealistic plans, unclear roles, etc.) and reap the many benefits (improvement in culture, appropriate budgeting, informed long-range forecasting, etc.) of this planning.

# END-OF-CHAPTER RESOURCES

## CRITICAL THINKING QUESTIONS

- Much is made of the longer time horizon for strategic management and planning. In the fast-paced and ever-changing healthcare landscape where outcomes and results take longer to present, what are your thoughts on appropriate time frame for strategic planning?
- How would you ensure that strategic planning is focused on the goals of the healthcare organization?
- The definition of strategic planning by Harrison and Thompson includes several activities from analysis of firm through implementation planning. If you were to choose one of these activities as being critical to strategic planning, which would it be? Justify your choice.
- In your opinion, is saving costs a strategic goal for the U.S. healthcare system? Why or why not?
- Refer to the framework for strategic planning included in this chapter. How is equity addressed in this framework?
- Much is made of the two unique aspects of health—direct interaction between providers and patients and determinants in health and nonhealth sectors—compared to other businesses. How are these unique aspects addressed in strategic planning for health?
- Pick two from the "Tools to Guide Strategic Planning" section and discuss their advantages and disadvantages for the strategic planning process.
- Several organizations have ventured into the business of healthcare strategic planning. What are your thoughts on the use of these organizations for strategic planning by healthcare organizations?
- There are several pitfalls to avoid in healthcare strategic planning. Of these pitfalls, which do you consider to be the most critical? Why?
- If you were to pitch strategic planning to a healthcare organization, which would be the top two benefits of strategic planning that you would highlight? Why?

## LEARNING ACTIVITIES

### CourseConnect ▶

To access self-assessment questions and interactive, competency-based learning activities for this chapter, visit www.springerpub.com/courseconnect. See inside front cover and tear-out card for CourseConnect details.

## REFERENCES

Achieveit. (2021, November 24). *13 notorious examples of strategic planning failure*. https://www.achieveit.com/resources/blog/13-notorious-examples-of-strategic-planning-failure/

Airhihenbuwa, C. O., Tseng, T.-S., Sutton, V. D., & Price, L. (2021). Global perspectives on improving chronic disease prevention and management in diverse settings. *Preventing Chronic Disease*, *18*, 210055. https://doi.org/10.5888/pcd18.210055

Akseer, N., Kandru, G., Keats, E. C., & Bhutta, Z. A. (2020). COVID-19 pandemic and mitigation strategies: Implications for maternal and child health and nutrition. *The American Journal of Clinical Nutrition*, *112*(2), 251–256. https://doi.org/10.1093/ajcn/nqaa171

Alderwick, H., & Gottlieb, L. M. (2019). Meanings and misunderstandings: A social determinants of health lexicon for health care systems. *The Milbank Quarterly, 97*(2), 407–419. https://doi.org/10.1111/1468-0009.12390

Cohen, E. A. (2023, December 18). Strategy *Britannica*. https://www.britannica.com/topic/strategy-military

Department of Defense, United States of America. (2021). *Department of Defense Warfighter Brain Health Initiative: Strategy and Action Plan*. https://permanent.fdlp.gov/gpo186696/DOD-WARFIGHTER-BRAIN-HEALTH-INITIATIVE-STRATEGY-AND-ACTION-PLAN.PDF

Functional Bureau Strategy. (2018, September 24). *Office of the U.S. Global AIDS Coordinator and Health Diplomacy*. https://permanent.fdlp.gov/gpo150168/FBS-SGAC_UNCLASS_508.pdf

Gorji, H. A., Ghanbari, M. K., Behzadifar, M., Shoghli, A., & Martini, M. (2022). Strategic planning, components and evolution in zoonotic diseases frameworks: One health approach and public health ethics. *Journal of Preventive Medicine and Hygiene, 62*, E981–E987. https://doi.org/10.15167/2421-4248/JPMH2021.62.4.2323

Haimowitz, I. J. (2011). *Healthcare relationship marketing: Strategy, design and measurement*. Taylor & Francis Group. https://www.taylorfrancis.com/books/mono/10.4324/9781315586380/healthcare-relationship-marketing-ira-haimowitz

Harrison, J. S., & Thompson, S. M. (2014). *Strategic management of healthcare organizations: A stakeholder management approach*. Business Expert Press.

Interagency Pain Research Coordinating Committee. (n.d.). *National pain strategy—A comprehensive population health-level strategy for pain*. https://www.ninds.nih.gov/sites/default/files/documents/NationalPainStrategy_508C.pdf

Jesse, T. (2023, April 19). Strategic planning in healthcare: An in-depth guide for executives. *ClearPoint Strategy*. https://www.clearpointstrategy.com/blog/healthcare-strategic-plan

Kyriazoglou, J. (2020). *Strategic management controls*. https://www.researchgate.net/publication/347520596_Strategic_Management_Controls

McClelland, A. (2023, December 7). Opinion: How can the world solve its shortage of health workers? *CNN*. https://www.cnn.com/2023/12/07/health/opinion-how-can-the-world-solve-its-shortage-of-health-workers/index.html

Monti, M., Torbica, A., Mossialos, E., & McKee, M. (2021). A new strategy for health and sustainable development in the light of the COVID-19 pandemic. *The Lancet, 398*(10305), 1029–1031. https://doi.org/10.1016/S0140-6736(21)01995-4

National Academies of Sciences, Engineering, and Medicine, Health and Medicine Division, Board on Population Health and Public Health Practice, Committee on a National Strategy for the Elimination of Hepatitis B and C, Brian L. Strom, & Gillian J. Buckley. (2017). *A national strategy for the elimination of hepatitis B and C: Phase two report*. National Academies Press.

RAND Corporation. (2021). *The future of combat casualty care: Is the military health system ready?* https://www.jstor.org/stable/pdf/resrep34083.pdf?refreqid=fastly-default%3A4df8aa61bf62e7415ff1657c70c112d6&ab_segments=&origin=&initiator=&acceptTC=1

Salmond, K. K., & Mahato, S. (2021). Linking to and addressing the determinants of health: A review of the Innovation Strategy experience. *Canadian Journal of Public Health, 112*(S2), 220–230. https://doi.org/10.17269/s41997-021-00518-3

Schaaf, M., Arnott, G., Chilufya, K. M., Khanna, R., Khanal, R. C., Monga, T., Otema, C., & Wegs, C. (2022). Social accountability as a strategy to promote sexual and reproductive health entitlements for stigmatized issues and populations. *International Journal for Equity in Health, 21*(S1), 19. https://doi.org/10.1186/s12939-021-01597-x

Seirawan, S. (2023). Strategic planning in healthcare: 2023 guide + examples. *Unnus*. https://unnus.com/medical/healthcare-strategic-planning/

Smack, K. (2019, June 21). *6 business strategy examples for healthcare*. https://www.esmgrp.com/blog/6-business-strategy-examples-for-healthcare

Society for Healthcare Strategy and Market Development. (2017). *Bridging worlds: The future role of the healthcare strategist*. https://www.aha.org/system/files/2018-06/bridging-worlds-shsmd.pdf

Strata. (2019). *How strategic planning benefits hospitals & healthcare systems in 2019*. https://www.stratadecision.com/blog/why-strategic-planning-is-important-in-healthcare

Viberg, N., Wanyenze, R., Nordenstedt, H., Gitahi, G., & Peterson, S. S. (2023). EU Global Health strategy: What are the challenges? *European Journal of Public Health*, *33*(4), 553–553. https://doi.org/10.1093/eurpub/ckad081

Wells, K. (2023, October 6). Addressing mental health crisis: Co-regulation as a solution. *The American Journal of Healthcare Strategy*. https://ajhcs.org/current-issue-1/f/addressing-mental-health-crisis-co-regulation-as-a-solution

Wolff, J., Gitukui, S., O'Brien, M., Mital, S., & Noonan, R. K. (2022). The overdose response strategy: Reducing drug overdose deaths through strategic partnership between public health and public safety. *Journal of Public Health Management and Practice*, *28*(Supplement 6), S359–S366. https://doi.org/10.1097/PHH.0000000000001580

World Health Organization. (2016). *Global health sector strategy on viral hepatitis 2016-2021*. Towards ending viral hepatitis. https://www.who.int/publications-detail-redirect/WHO-HIV-2016.06

# CHAPTER 11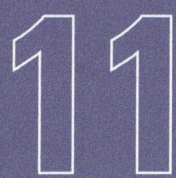

# HEALTHCARE FINANCIAL MANAGEMENT

Kevin D. Broom and Joseph C. (Chris) Rheney

### LEARNING OBJECTIVES

- Understand the major components of the field of healthcare finance.
- Discuss the role of a financial manager within the health industry context.
- Distinguish between financial management, financial accounting, and managerial accounting.
- Explain the purposes of financial statements
- Describe the use of managerial accounting concepts

### KEY TERMS

- Budgeting
- Chief financial officer
- Cost accounting
- Financial accounting
- Financial management
- Investment capital
- Managerial accounting

## INTRODUCTION TO THE FIELD OF HEALTHCARE FINANCE

This chapter provides a broad overview to the field of healthcare financial management. In the health industry, the field of "healthcare finance" is broadly defined to contain most major issues involving dollar signs. However, the domain of healthcare finance can be broken down into multiple unique business disciplines that can be treated separately (and those disciplines do often overlap). Healthcare finance typically includes a wide range of topics such as long-term financial decision-making, short-term financial decision-making, financial accounting concepts, managerial accounting techniques, pricing concepts, and the financial planning process. For the purpose of this overview chapter, we narrow the focus onto traditional financial management content and accounting content. Chapter 16, "Healthcare Marketing," introduces readers to pricing content, while the financial planning process is better aligned with Chapter 10, "Strategic Planning," as it is a nested component of the strategic management process.

## DEFINITIONS

**Financial management** is a business discipline focused on short-term and long-term decision-making aimed at achieving the overall goal of optimizing an organization's efficiency and profitability. The financial management process is broken down into short-term and long-term decisions, with the 1-year mark delineating between the two. Decisions involving business operations within a year are categorized as short term, whereas decisions involving business operations beyond a year are categorized as long term.

**Financial accounting** is a business discipline that involves the recording and reporting of an organization's financial information using a standardized set of guidelines known as *generally accepted accounting principles* (GAAP). The standardized guidelines enable external reviewers to interpret the financial health of an organization and compare it with similar organizations using the same financial information reported under the same standardized guidelines, helping them make optimal investment decisions. Likewise, financial accounting information is useful to the organization's management team in that it helps ensure proper stewardship on behalf of the organization's ownership.

**Managerial accounting** is a business discipline involving the measurement, analysis, and interpretation of accounting information that is useful in helping managers make optimal leadership decisions. Unlike financial accounting, managerial accounting does not involve using a standardized set of guidelines. Managerial accounting techniques can be customized to the organization's unique needs, thereby enabling it to make management decisions.

The remainder of the chapter provides more insight on each of these three business disciplines. We also provide some examples that can be explored in much greater depth in follow-on courses that focus exclusively on the domain of healthcare financial management.

## ROLE(S) OF THE CHIEF FINANCIAL OFFICER

The **chief financial officer** (CFO) is the top functional area expert within the organization. The CFO's primary role involves managing the financial resources of the organization, reporting the financial health of the organization, and advising the top management team on decisions of strategic importance. The CFO normally reports to the role of chief operating officer or chief of staff. However, the CFO will normally have a direct line of communication with the chief executive officer (CEO), since most major decisions will have financial implications. The CFO leads the financial planning process, is responsible for the day-to-day financial operations, analyzes the company's financial strengths and weaknesses, and advises top executives on long-term investment decisions.

## MAJOR FINANCIAL ISSUES IN THE HEALTH INDUSTRY

At societal level, one only needs to look at the sizes of the U.S. economy and the federal budget to see the financial significance of the industry. As of 2022, the health industry comprised $4.5 trillion, which is over 17% of the U.S. economy (Centers for Medicare & Medicaid Services [CMS], 2023a). Additionally, the federal government spends over $1.9 trillion—nearly 30% of all government expenditures—in support of healthcare (Figure 11.1; Kaiser Family Foundation, 2023). With this much money flowing through the health industry, societal pressures place a significant strain on it.

**FIGURE 11.1.** Federal spending on domestic and global health programs and services accounted for 29% of the net federal outlays in FY 2023.

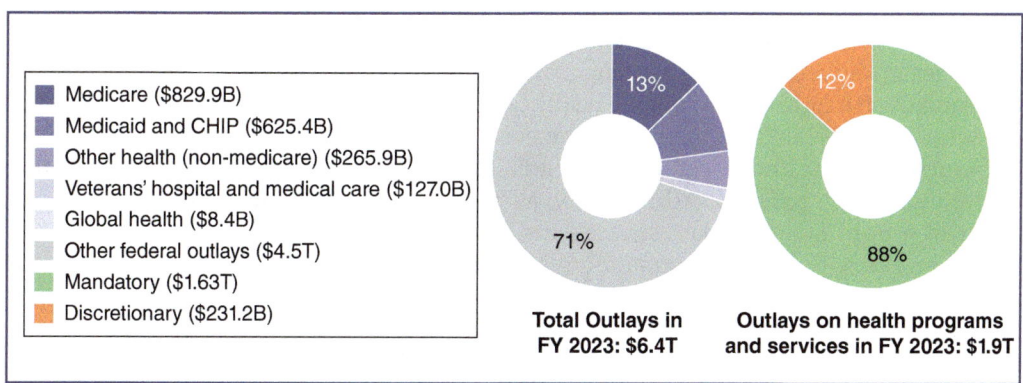

Note: Mandatory spending accounted for 88% of outlays on health programs and services.
Source: Kaiser Family Foundation. (2023). *FAQs on health spending, the federal budget, and budget enforcement tools*. https://www.kff.org/medicare/issue-brief/faqs-on-health-spending-the-federal-budget-and-budget-enforcement-tools/.

Focusing on the health industry, several pressing challenges are converging to shape it. Rising healthcare costs continue to strain budgets, necessitating innovative approaches to cost containment and revenue generation. At the same time, reimbursement challenges and the transition to value-based care models (CMS, 2023b) are reshaping payment structures. These trends require healthcare organizations to adapt their financial strategies and find new ways to control costs and maximize revenue. In addition, workforce shortages pose a significant obstacle to delivering quality care while also maintaining financial stability. Finally, cybersecurity threats loom large over healthcare financial management, with data breaches and ransomware attacks posing substantial risks to patient data security and financial integrity.

Rising healthcare costs pose a significant challenge for organizations focused on healthcare delivery. As costs rise, healthcare organizations face pressure from payers (both government and private insurance) to deliver higher quality care through value-based payment systems that reward better quality care while reducing unnecessary cost (i.e., "better value"). Meanwhile, the health insurance industry struggles to balance affordable coverage options with the escalating costs of medical treatments and services, often passing some of the burden onto consumers through higher premiums and deductibles. Addressing this highly complex issue requires collaborative efforts among policymakers, healthcare providers, insurers, and patients to ensure financially sustainable and equitable access to healthcare services without compromising quality.

Similarly, reimbursement issues create strong headwinds for healthcare providers. Medicare reimbursement rates often fall below the actual cost of providing care, particularly for specialized services, leading to questions of viability for healthcare providers. This can be especially burdensome for private practices, where operating costs are high and profit margins can be narrow. Furthermore, negotiating reimbursement rates with health insurance companies can be arduous, as insurers seek to control costs while providers strive to maintain positive profit margins. Delays and denials in reimbursement further exacerbate the situation, disrupting cash flow and hindering the ability of healthcare organizations to deliver timely and effective care. As a result, healthcare providers must navigate a risky reimbursement landscape, balancing the desire to provide quality care with the financial realities of the multi-payer model currently used in the United States that lacks transparency across the system.

Healthcare workforce challenges represent another trend driving financial challenges to our healthcare system. Many healthcare organizations face workforce issues such as shortages of qualified personnel, employee burnout, and suboptimal employee retention, all of which have significant implications for healthcare financial management. Shortages in key areas such as nursing staff, primary care, and specialized medical fields have an adverse impact on available healthcare services (Hallett et al., 2024; Markit, 2017; Rosseter, 2024), while also increasing the costs of recruitment and retention. Moreover, burnout among healthcare professionals adversely affects employee well-being, productivity, and risk to patients. Additionally, as health industry organizations compete for talent in a tight labor market, salaries and benefits may increase to attract and retain skilled workers. Effectively managing these workforce challenges is crucial to financial sustainability.

Recent cybersecurity threats in healthcare, such as ransomware attacks targeting healthcare organizations, underscore the critical importance of robust cybersecurity measures (Adler, 2024). These attacks can have far-reaching consequences, not only compromising patient data and disrupting healthcare services but also significantly impacting a healthcare organization's ability to provide care and its financial position (Neprash et al., 2022). For example, in 2023, a major hospital network experienced a ransomware attack that forced them to shut down systems and divert patients to other facilities, resulting in substantial revenue losses from canceled appointments and procedures. With incidents like this on the rise (Figure 11.2), the costs associated with remediation efforts, including restoring systems, implementing enhanced security measures, and potential legal liabilities, can further strain a hospital's finances. The reputational damage incurred from a cybersecurity breach can lead to decreased patient trust and a loss of business, compounding the financial impact on the organization. Thus, investing in robust cybersecurity infrastructure and implementing comprehensive risk mitigation strategies are imperative for safeguarding both patient data and a healthcare organization's financial stability.

In summary, the health industry continues to face intensifying pressure as government budgets stretch, reimbursements decrease, healthcare costs continue to rise, workforce competition increases, and new threats emerge. These challenges lead to an increased need for effective operational leaders and creative financial managers who can successfully navigate today's health industry.

**FIGURE 11.2.** Healthcare data breaches of 500+ records (2009–2023).

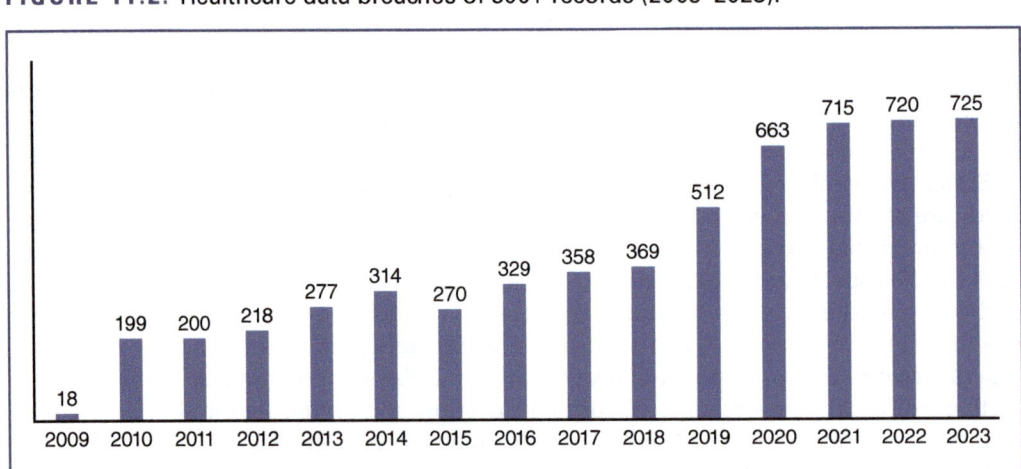

*Source:* Data from Adler, S. (2024). Security breaches in healthcare in 2023. *The HIPAA Journal.* https://www.hipaajournal.com/security-breaches-in-healthcare/.

# FINANCIAL MANAGEMENT

The business discipline of financial management involves the short-term and long-term financial decision-making processes. Long-term decision-making involves funding strategic initiatives that expand the scale or scope of an organization's mission. Examples include constructing a new hospital, purchasing new technology, expanding into new markets, or acquiring other companies. Financial managers will assess the financial costs and benefits of these initiatives (called "capital projects") to determine if they provide financial returns necessary to pay investors an adequate rate of return and to also provide residual financial benefit to the organization. Once the projects are identified and assessed as being financially viable, they must be funded for implementation.

Optimally, companies hope to be profitable enough to be able to fund new initiatives out of its retained profits. However, most companies do not have the level of sustained profitability that facilitates financial resources being readily available to make such large investment decisions. When this is the case, organizations must seek outside **investment capital** by entering the capital markets to take on debt from lenders and/or to seek equity from potential new owners. The mix of debt and equity that a company uses is referred to as its "capital structure."

Smaller health industry organizations often rely on loans (debt) from local or regional banks, or they have to seek out new ownership partners (equity) to help fund expansions of their organization. The largest health industry organizations often rely on the formal capital markets that sell structured financial assets (such as stocks and bonds), thereby enabling organizations to reach a much deeper pool of investment capital. Examples of formal stock markets that provide equity capital include the New York Stock Exchange (NYSE) and the Nasdaq Stock Exchange. An example of a formal bond market that provides debt capital is the NYSE Bonds Market. This newly acquired investment capital is then used to fund capital projects that organizations hope will expand the scale or scope of operations.

Managers typically assess capital projects for financial viability using a set of financial metrics. These metrics include payback period, discounted payback period, net present value (NPV), internal rate of return (IRR), modified internal rate of return (MIRR), and profitability index. Each of these metrics can be used individually or they can be used collectively. These metrics assess different characteristics of the project, each of which may be useful to key executives making strategic decisions. Table 11.1 lists these metrics and provides some of the strengths and weaknesses of each.

### TABLE 11.1. FINANCIAL METRICS FOR CAPITAL PROJECTS

| METRIC | VALUE | STRENGTH | WEAKNESS |
|---|---|---|---|
| Payback period | Time | Indicates when the project will break even | Does not consider the time value of money; ignores cash flows after payback |
| Discounted payback period | Time | Indicates when the project will break even | Ignores cash flows after payback |
| NPV | $ | Shows the dollar value a project will add to the company's bottom line | May bias key leaders toward larger projects |
| IRR | % | Shows a percentage return relative to investment | Redundant to NPV; flawed reinvestment rate assumption |
| MIRR | % | Shows a percentage return relative to investment; more conservative than IRR | More difficult to calculate and less intuitive than IRR |
| Profitability Index | Ratio | Indicates dollar return relative to dollar investment; useful for capital rationing | None |

IRR, internal rate of return; MIRR, modified internal rate of return; NPV, net present value.

## CASE STUDY 11.1: LONG-TERM CAPITAL INVESTMENTS

Mountainside Hospital has experienced rapid growth in its four operating rooms (ORs) and single cardiac cath lab utilization in the 3 years since it opened a new hospital after moving from its old location and aging infrastructure. Revenue has leveled off since opening, and the Mountainside System Corporate Office is looking for new ways to increase revenue at this location and across the system. Mountainside has access to space located next door in a medical office building owned by the system. They also have purchased space for a second cath lab and the possible expansion of two additional ORs. Furthermore, an area on the hospital's third floor is unused after labor and delivery services moved to a sister hospital.

The hospital's highest demand services include the cardiac cath lab, with interventional cardiologists fighting for time on the schedule, given the demographics and cardiovascular disease incidence in the local population. The COO developed a capital project that requires building out the second cath lab, creating a new cardiology office in the medical office building, and converting unused inpatient space into a five-bed cardiovascular unit in order to provide both outpatient and inpatient services. This project requires a $4.3 million capital investment in facilities and equipment. However, the Chief Medical Officer prefers an option with less capital investment in equipment for the ORs and a procedure room that costs only $1.1 million. What factors should the hospital CEO consider when recommending capital investments to the system CEO (Table 11.2)?

### TABLE 11.2. CAPITAL INVESTMENT OPTIONS

| DESCRIPTION | START DATE | CAPITAL | | | IP ADMITS/ OP VISITS* | | | EBITDA $* | | |
|---|---|---|---|---|---|---|---|---|---|---|
| | | 15 | 16 | 17 | 15 | 16 | 17 | 15 | 16 | 17 |
| Build second cath lab (Current shelled-out space ready for build out) | Q4 | $1.9M | $0 | $0 | 36 / 60 | 119 / 198 | 186 / 310 | $326K | $1,426K | $1.7M |
| Replace aging ortho/gen surgery equipment | Q1 | $400K | $0 | $0 | 65 / 9 | 105 / 15 | 127 / 19 | $207K | $346K | $425K |
| Purchase OR equipment to support incremental growth | Q1 | $400K | $0 | $0 | 12 / 42 | 22 / 77 | 27 / 102 | $138K | $286K | $380K |
| Purchase C-arm for procedure room and build out new five-bed ICU (Convert old L&D, C-section, NICU space) | Q1 | $300K | $900K | $0 | 0 / 0 | 20 | 125 / 40 | $0 | $282K | $755K |
| Complete site infrastructure preparations for second MOB | Q1 | $1.5M | $0 | $0 | 0 / 0 | 40 / 33 | 90 / 65 | $0 | $165K | $537K |

*Denotes documented, coded encounter for which data are available.
EBITDA, earnings before interest, taxes, depreciation, and amortization; L&D, labor and delivery; NICU, neonatal intensive care unit; MOB, medical office building; OR, operating rooms.

Short-term decision-making focuses on financial decisions within a 1-year time horizon. Examples include cash flow forecasting and management, revenue cycle management, and supply chain management. Cash flow forecasting and management refers to the process of estimating how cash will flow into and out of the organization throughout the year and then putting measures in place to ensure that the organization's bills are paid in a timely manner. When cash inflows exceed outflows, cash reserves will increase. When cash outflows exceed inflows, cash reserves will be drawn down. Financial managers must ensure that adequate cash is available to pay bills on time, but too much cash being available is problematic for investors because the excess cash could be put to better use investing in projects that bring in a higher return. When cash flows are positive (inflows exceed outflows), financial managers will place the excess cash into accounts or marketable securities that draw a higher rate of return (cash earns no interest). When cash flows are negative, financial managers will draw down those accounts or sell off marketable securities to free up cash to pay bills as they come due. Examples could be payments to suppliers, payroll for its employees, and interest payments on existing debt.

Revenue cycle management refers to the timeline between delivering healthcare and being paid for that healthcare. Healthcare organizations typically see a patient and provide care, then document that care and generate invoices (claims) to submit to payers such as insurance companies, Medicare, or Medicaid. Payers will process these claims to determine if the healthcare services are covered under the insurance policy. If so, the payer will generate a payment to the organization. Healthcare organizations want this length of time between provision of care and payment for care to be minimized. Revenue cycle management involves all the steps from initially seeing the patient, validating the patient has a means for paying for care (a health insurance policy or the ability to pay for care directly), documenting all of the care provided, generating a valid invoice backed up by that documentation, submitting the invoice to the payer, receiving payment, and depositing the money into the organization's accounts. In many organizations, revenue cycle management falls under the purview of the CFO.

Supply chain management, from a financial perspective, focuses on the timing of payments to suppliers. Healthcare organizations often purchase routine supplies and equipment through credit extended by their vendors. Many vendors provide incentives for early payment and penalties for late payment. Financial managers must assess if the incentives for early payment or if the penalties for late payment are strong enough to justify an early or late release of cash to pay bills as they come due. For example, if a vendor offers a large enough discount for early payment, an organization may be willing to forgo lower returns on their cash management accounts or marketable securities to receive a higher rate of return through the discount. Similarly, a low penalty for late payment may be worth incurring if their cash management accounts or marketable securities draw a higher rate of return during that late payment period. While the returns on individual supply chain transactions may be minimal, the returns are magnified when these transactions are aggregated across the entire organization.

Financial managers must balance short-term financial needs that keep an organization viable on a daily basis with long-term financial needs that ensure the organization is able to grow and remain profitable well into the future. In smaller organizations, financial managers may be involved in both types of decisions. In larger organizations, the CFO normally has separate staff who focus on either short-term or long-term financial decision-making but not both.

## FINANCIAL ACCOUNTING

Financial accounting involves the recording and reporting of an organization's financial information using a standardized set of guidelines known as GAAP. The standardized guidelines enable external reviewers to interpret the financial health of an organization. These external reviewers are often current or potential lenders. Current lenders use the financial information to determine if organizations are abiding by the terms of their loans. Potential lenders use the information to assess the riskiness of lending to the company and compare it with similar organizations to make lending decisions. Likewise, financial accounting information is useful to the organization's management team in that it helps ensure proper stewardship on behalf of the organization's ownership, as well as helping ensure that the organization is fulfilling the terms of previous borrowing from its current lenders.

Organizations use the financial accounting process to develop financial statements that provide great detail on the financial health of the organization. Financial statements are produced annually, but many larger firms are required to also produce them quarterly. The financial statements include five primary components: a letter from the top management team, a letter from the auditors, a balance sheet, an income statement, and a statement of cash flows. The letter from the top management team provides a narrative on the financial health and relevant operational insight for the period covered within the financial statements (quarterly or annual). The letter from the auditors indicates whether the financial statements have been produced using GAAP and accurately reflect the financial health of the organization. The balance sheet is a snapshot in time that shows all the assets owned by an organization, all debts owed by the organization, and the net position on all those assets after accounting for debt (referred to as "stockholders equity" in for-profit organizations and "net assets" for not-for-profit organizations). The income statement shows the revenue and expenses over a period of time covered within the financial statements (again, quarterly or annual). The statement of cash flows quantifies how cash is flowing into and out of the organization broken down along three lines: operating activities, investing activities, and financing activities.

The two most useful components are the balance sheet and the income statement. From a personal finance perspective, the balance sheet shows all the items you own (house, car, money in checking and savings accounts, etc.). The balance sheet also shows the debt you owe (a mortgage, a car loan, credit card debt, etc.). The difference between the two indicates your net wealth, which is comparable to the terms stockholders equity or net assets. Likewise, the income statement from a personal finance perspective would show all the money you earn and all the money you spend, with the difference being how much you saved throughout the year. Managers and investors use this financial accounting information to assess the ongoing financial health of the organization and its earning potential well into the future.

### CASE STUDY 11.2: ASSESSING FINANCIAL HEALTH

Sarah is a recent healthcare administration graduate of a prestigious university and has landed a coveted associate administrator position at an urban hospital within a national for-profit healthcare organization. Since she has some academic financial expertise and practical management experience, the COO assigned her to assess the business process and operational impacts on the financial health of the hospital since it has been without a CFO for over a year.

In her first meeting with the COO, Sarah was asked to look at the hospital income statement and make some recommendations on what areas the hospital could improve cost controls, while also projecting impacts and risks to operations and revenue. She wanted to make a good impression with this first project, so she dove in using what she learned about financial operations and cost analysis to tackle the challenge.

She saw that net patient revenue was growing at a healthy rate, although bad debt was also rising; however, the net operating revenue was holding steady at around 5% for the past 2 years. More concerning, total hospital expenses were rising year over year, primarily due to salaries, wages, and benefits (SW&B). These expenses had been weighing on the hospital's earnings (shown as earnings before interest, taxes, depreciation, and amortization or EBITDA), thus reducing the earnings growth rate. After studying the income statement (Table 11.3), Sarah recommended that the hospital leadership begin more detailed management reviews of operational costs, starting with salaries. What are some key things Sarah should also look for if she reviews the hospital statement of cash flows and balance sheet?

### TABLE 11.3. CONSOLIDATED INCOME STATEMENT

| (IN '000s) | 2020 | 2021 | | 2022 | | 2023 | |
|---|---|---|---|---|---|---|---|
| P&L Summary | | | Fav (Unfav) % | | Fav (Unfav) % | | Fav (Unfav) % |
| Net Patient Revenue | $143,967 | $150,249 | 4.4% | $159,430 | 6.1% | $168,784 | 5.9% |
| Bad Debt | 40,395 | 42,643 | (5.6%) | 46,288 | (8.5%) | 49,903 | (7.8%) |
| Other Revenue | 914 | 1,053 | 15.2% | 1,064 | 1.0% | 1,074 | 0.9% |
| **Adjusted Net Operating Revenue** | 104,486 | 108,659 | 4.0% | 114,206 | 5.1% | 119,955 | 5.0% |
| SW&B | $42,961 | $44,527 | (3.6%) | $46,091 | (3.5%) | $47,997 | (4.1%) |
| Supplies | 19,586 | 20,046 | (2.3%) | 20,848 | (4.0%) | 21,682 | (4.0%) |
| Other Operating Expenses | 23,989 | 23,881 | 0.5% | 24,398 | (2.2%) | 24,920 | (2.1%) |
| E.H.R. Incentive | (250) | 0 | 0.0% | 0 | 0.0% | 0 | 0.0% |
| **Total Hospital Expenses** | 86,286 | 88,454 | (2.5%) | 91,337 | (3.3%) | 94,599 | (3.6%) |
| Hospital EBITDA | $18,200 | $20,205 | 11.0% | $22,869 | 13.2% | $25,356 | 10.9% |
| EBITDA Margin | 17.4% | 18.6% | 1.2% | 20.0% | 1.4% | 21.1% | 1.1% |

EBITDA, earnings before interest, taxes, depreciation, and amortization; SW&B, salaries, wages, and benefits.

## MANAGERIAL ACCOUNTING

Managerial accounting involves the measurement, analysis, and interpretation of accounting information necessary for managers to make optimal leadership decisions. Managerial accounting does not involve a standardized set of guidelines, so managerial accounting techniques can be customized to the organization's unique needs to facilitate management decisions.

**Cost accounting** is a managerial accounting tool that helps organizations determine the cost of providing a good or service. In healthcare delivery, how does an organization determine how much an outpatient visit or an inpatient stay costs? While it can be quite easy to quantify the costs of goods and supplies consumed directly in the provision of care for an individual patient, leaders find it much more difficult to account for overhead costs associated with the top management team, functional area staff, facility upkeep, nursing staff who provide care to many patients, equipment used to provide care for multiple patients, and a host of other costs that cannot be directly attributed in whole to a specific patient encounter. Cost accounting is a process of taking all these overhead costs that occur above the point of patient care delivery and allocating them down to that patient encounter to analyze costing trends and to feed into pricing models.

Another component of managerial accounting is the **budgeting** process. The development of budgets is part of the financial planning process, but the assessment of the execution of budgets is part of the management control process. When organizations develop an overall budget, they frequently develop subordinate budgets for all the components that make up the larger enterprise. When an organization moves into a new fiscal year, budgets are allocated to all subordinate components (for instance, a hospital budget will consist of service line budgets for all services that a hospital provides to its community). As the organization moves throughout the year, the management control process results in a budget review to determine budget execution for early detection of potential problems where management can intervene and make directions to avoid larger problems that will affect the financial health of the organization.

In addition to simply determining who is over and who is under their budget execution, leaders must also understand its payer mix to determine if being over budget is good or bad. For example, an organization that provides care and is paid for every patient encounter may be over budget if their workload increases above what was expected. In this example, having spent more than the budgeted amount early in the year may not be problematic because the additional encounters will lead to additional invoices for payment, thereby bringing in additional revenue to offset being over budget. However, if the organization is prepaid for patient encounters, as in a managed care model, the additional workload will not result in additional invoices for payment. As a result, no additional revenue will be flowing into the organization to offset the additional expenditures. Therefore, a simple analysis of whether an organization has spent more or less money than forecasted in the budget must also consider what is happening on the revenue side to determine appropriate management actions.

### CASE STUDY 11.3: MANAGEMENT CONTROL PROCESS

The hospital COO was pleased with Sarah's work on highlighting areas from the income statement for more detailed reviews. She asked Sarah to build a monthly review to focus on better management control throughout the year before annual reports are completed. Sarah realized it was important to look at year-to-date (YTD) data as well as monthly comparisons, so she built the following charts (Figure 11.3).

**FIGURE 11.3.** Year-to-date and monthly comparisons.

| Southwest Hospital Expenses | | | | | |
|---|---|---|---|---|---|
| (All $ in thousands) | Current month | Budget | % Var | Prior year | % Var |
| Staff | 555 | 547 | −1.5% | 605 | 8.3% |
| Salaries | 3,022 | 3,082 | 1.9% | 3,198 | 5.5% |
| Benefits | 563 | 525 | −7.2% | 644 | 12.6% |
| Supplies | 2,078 | 1,663 | −25.0% | 1,740 | −19.4% |
| Other controllable expenses | 1,760 | 1,779 | 1.1% | 1,578 | −11.5% |
| Noncontrollable expenses | 427 | 396 | −7.8% | 486 | 12.1% |
| Total operating expense | 7,850 | 7,445 | −5.4% | 7,646 | −2.7% |

| Southwest Hospital Expenses | | | | | |
|---|---|---|---|---|---|
| (All $ in thousands) | Year to date | Budget | % Var | Prior year | % Var |
| Staff | 552 | 558 | 1.1% | 594 | 7.1% |
| Salaries | 20,262 | 21,336 | 5.0% | 21,027 | 3.6% |
| Benefits | 4,046 | 3,778 | −7.1% | 3,426 | −18.1% |
| Supplies | 11,693 | 11,433 | −2.3% | 11,172 | −4.7% |
| Other controllable expenses | 11,513 | 12,356 | 6.8% | 10,454 | −10.1% |
| Noncontrollable expenses | 2,097 | 2,913 | 28.% | 2,958 | 29.1% |
| Total operating expense | 49,611 | 51,815 | 4.3% | 48,788 | −1.7% |
| | | ≥0% | <0%–5% | <−5% | |

She made the following for the first performance review:

- Total operating expense is over budget for the month but favorable YTD.
- Southwest has improved cost controls in the total number of staff compared to the prior year.
- Salaries are within budget and are less than the prior year for both the month and YTD.
- Benefits are costing more for the month and YTD. This is an area for more research.
- Supply expenses were way over budget for the month and are now weighing on YTD performance. Recommend a detailed analysis of supply expenses compared to cases and patient days.
- Controllable expenses are within budget for the month and YTD.

What other comments or observations can you make from Sarah's initial monthly review?

## CONCLUSION

This chapter provides a broad overview of healthcare financial management. We discussed the role of the CFO and provided societal and health industry context involving the major challenges shaping the domain of healthcare finance. We aim to help expose future operational managers to some of the concepts that will help them make better financial decisions as they progress through their careers toward becoming key executives. We also aim to summarize some of the tools and concepts that will be employed by financial experts in advising key executives on the strategic decisions they will make. We provided insight into financial decision-making (financial management), recording and reporting of financial health (financial accounting), and customizable tools and techniques for effectively leading an organization (managerial accounting). The ultimate goal of the chapter is to provide foundational terminology and context covered in other chapters within this textbook, as well as in later classes that focus much more in depth on the field of healthcare finance.

## END-OF-CHAPTER RESOURCES

### CRITICAL THINKING QUESTIONS

- How might access to investment capital differ between small organizations like a physician practice and large organizations like a publicly traded integrated delivery system?
- In assessing capital projects, should financial viability be the primary (or only) consideration?
- How might the assessment of capital investment projects differ between governmental, for-profit, and not-for-profit organizations?
- Who are the primary users of financial statements, external or internal stakeholders? How might they use the information differently?
- In healthcare delivery, is cost accounting effective in helping identify the cost of patient encounters? Are all outpatient visits or inpatient stays the same, or should the cost accounting process be adjusted to account for differences in the complexity of care among patient encounters?
- How might different payment schemes influence the interpretation of budget execution data?
- When assessing budget execution, do most health industry organizations have a pure payer mix or do they have a portfolio of different types of payers? If the latter, how might this complicate the interpretation of budget execution?

### LEARNING ACTIVITIES

**CourseConnect >**

To access self-assessment questions and interactive, competency-based learning activities for this chapter, visit www.springerpub.com/courseconnect. See inside front cover and tear-out card for CourseConnect details.

### REFERENCES

Adler, S. (2024). Security breaches in healthcare in 2023. *The HIPAA Journal*. https://www.hipaajournal.com/security-breaches-in-healthcare/

Centers for Medicare & Medicaid Services. (2023a). *National Health Expenditures fact sheet*. https://www.cms.gov/data-research/statistics-trends-and-reports/national-health-expenditure-data/nhe-fact-sheet

Centers for Medicare & Medicaid Services. (2023b). *What are the value-based programs*. https://www.cms.gov/medicare/quality/value-based-programs

Hallett, E., Simeon, E., Amba, V., Howington, D., McConnell, K. J., & Zhu, J. M. (2024). Factors influencing turnover and attrition in the public behavioral health system workforce: Qualitative study. *Psychiatric Services*, 75(1), 55–63. https://doi.org/10.1176/appi.ps.20220516

Kaiser Family Foundation. (2023). *FAQs on health spending, the federal budget, and budget enforcement tools*. https://www.kff.org/medicare/issue-brief/faqs-on-health-spending-the-federal-budget-and-budget-enforcement-tools/

Markit, I. H. S. (2017). *The complexities of physician supply and demand: Projections from 2015 to 2030*. Association of American Medical Colleges.

Neprash, H. T., McGlave, C. C., Cross, D. A., Virnig, B. A., Puskarich, M. A., Huling, J. D., Rozenshtein, & Nikpay, S. S. (2022). Trends in ransomware attacks on US hospitals, clinics, and other health care delivery organizations, 2016–2021. *JAMA Health Forum* 3(12), e224873–e224873. https://doi.org/10.1001/jamahealthforum.2022.4873

Rosseter, R. (2024). Nursing shortage. *American Association of Colleges of Nursing*. https://www.aacnnursing.org/news-data/fact-sheets/nursing-shortage

CHAPTER 12

# HEALTH INSURANCE AND REIMBURSEMENT

Jason S. Turner and Angela L. Perri

## LEARNING OBJECTIVES

- Describe the primary function of insurance and the relationship of risk to insurance premiums.
- Explain how the origins of health insurance in the United States have influenced the current healthcare environment.
- Define health status risk, medical care risk, and loading factors and determine how changes in those risks will influence insurance premiums and cost-sharing arrangements.
- Distinguish between the incentives associated with prospective payments and fee-for-service payments.
- Summarize value-based payments and how they are designed to mitigate the incentives associated with prospective payment and fee-for-service payment models.

## KEY TERMS

- Actuarily fair premium
- Beneficiary
- Coinsurance
- Community rating
- Community rating by class
- Copayment
- Deductible
- Employer-sponsored insurance
- Experience rating
- Health status risk
- Loading factors
- Managed care organization (MCO)

- Medicaid
- Medical care risk
- Medicare
- Out-of-pocket maximum
- Patient Protection and Affordable Care Act (ACA)
- Premium
- Value-based healthcare

## INTRODUCTION

In 2022, the United States spent 17.3% of the gross domestic product or $4.45 trillion on healthcare. Most of those expenses are related to hospital care, professional services, and prescription drugs (Table 12.1). While $471 billion is paid for out-of-pocket individuals, many health expenditures are paid by private and governmental health insurance products like **Medicare** and **Medicaid**. Despite being spread out across a handful of for-profit and not-for-profit insurance providers, as a category, private insurance accounts for the bulk of expenditures in the United States. Medicare is the largest single health insurance payor and is followed by Medicaid, the joint federal-state plans (Centers for Medicare & Medicaid Services, 2024).

## WHAT IS HEALTH INSURANCE?

Health insurance is an arrangement that transforms unpredictable and unbudgetable events into budgetable and predictable events by pooling risks and resources. It protects individuals from unexpected, high-cost medical expenses that can be difficult to foresee. More specifically, health insurance is a risk mitigation tool that transfers the uncertainty of falling ill (**health status risk**) and the associated costs of care (**medical care risk**) from an individual to another entity for a predetermined fee. This fee is typically referred to as a **premium**, is set in advance, and is prepaid monthly.

Health insurance plans require the **beneficiary** (the individual being covered by insurance) or their proxy to pay a premium unless the beneficiary is eligible for Medicaid or is enrolled in the federal-state Children's Health Insurance Program (CHIP). In addition to the monthly premium, health insurance plans often have a deductible, a copayment, and

**TABLE 12.1. NATIONAL HEALTH EXPENDITURES BY PAYOR 2022 (AMOUNT IN BILLIONS OF U.S. DOLLARS)**

| | | |
|---|---|---|
| Out-of-pocket expenses | $471.4 | 11% |
| Private health insurance | $1,289.8 | 29% |
| Medicare | $944.3 | 21% |
| Medicaid | $805.7 | 18% |
| Other insurance programs | $171.6 | 4% |
| Public health and similar programs | $564.0 | 13% |
| Nonconsumption-related expenses | $217.8 | 5% |
| Totals | $4,464.6 | 100% |

*Source:* National Health Expenditure Accounts from CMS.gov.

some form of coinsurance. A **deductible** is the annual amount due for medical services before an insurance company begins paying for its costs A **copayment** or *copay* is the out-of-pocket amount that is due at the time of medical service. The percentage of the total amount owed after medical services are rendered that the health insurance company will cover once the annual deductible is met is referred to as the **coinsurance** rate. Plans may also provide members with an **out-of-pocket maximum**. The out-of-pocket maximum is the most money that an individual will pay for covered medical services each year. The out-of-pocket maximum includes the deductible, copays, and coinsurance but does not include monthly premiums. Once one reaches the out-of-pocket maximum for the year, the health insurer will pay 100% of the covered and essential costs for the remainder of the year.

Several underwriting mechanisms can be used to predict premiums, but the primary goal of the insurer is to set a premium that covers the expected medical costs (**actuarially fair premium**), as well as the administrative costs and requisite profit (**loading factors**). If priced correctly, the expected benefit from purchasing the insurance outweighs the cost and generates value for the insured.

## CASE STUDY 12.1: HEALTH INSURANCE FOR A 55-YEAR-OLD FEMALE

Bernice, a 55-year-old female, purchased an insurance product with an 80/20 coinsurance rate, a $50 emergency room (ER) copay, and a $2,000 deductible. Bernice was recently hospitalized in conjunction with an ER visit and was billed $7,500 for the 3-day stay. Bernice had not had any medical expenses prior to her hospitalization.

*Deductible*: The selected health insurance plan has a deductible of $2,000. When the healthcare costs reach $2,000 for the year, the health insurer will step in and begin paying for its share of costs above the $2,000 threshold.

*Copayment*: Visiting an ER requires a copayment of $50 for each visit and is independent of the cost of services provided. Copayments are commonly credited against the patients' coinsurance and deductible responsibilities.

*Coinsurance*: The insurer offers a $2,000 deductible with an 80/20 coinsurance product. Once the $2,000 deductible amount is met, the health insurer will pay 80% of every medical bill and the patient will be responsible for paying the remaining 20% until the out-of-pocket maximum is met.

| | |
|---|---|
| Amount billed | $7,500 |
| Deductible | $2,000 (inclusive of copay) |
| 80% of balance paid by insurer | $4,400 ($5,500 × .8) |
| 20% of balance paid by Bernice | $1,100 ($5,500 × .2) |
| Total from Bernice | $3,100 |
| Total from insurer | $4,400 |

Expected medical costs are calculated by estimating the probability of falling ill and seeking care and multiplying that by the cost of care if the encounter occurs. If only the prior utilization and costs of the individual or a single group are considered, the insurance firm will use **experience ratings** to set premiums. The prior experience of the individual or group is used to predict the future actuarially fair premium of the group. If, however, groups and individuals are clustered into a larger pool and the predicted medical costs are based on the aggregated experiences of everyone in the pool, the insurer is using a **community rating** methodology. High-cost groups and individuals are subsidized by lower cost groups because everyone is sharing equally in the cost. The third commonly used model to price insurance is referred to as **community rating by class** and is a mixture of experience and community rating methodologies. Community rating by class aggregates everyone into the same large pool but then creates subcategories like age, smoking status, or gender. The insurance firm then creates estimates for each subcategory and then applies the subcategory estimates to the group or individual being insured based on how they fit into the respective categories. This methodology is currently being used on the state insurance exchanges where the subcategories include gender, age, zip code, and depending on the state, smoking status.

## COMMON TYPES OF HEALTH INSURANCE COVERAGE

There are several health insurance coverage options available. They range from federal and state programs with restrictive eligibility criteria to less restrictive commercial or private insurance products open to a much larger population. Based on 2022 census reports, approximately two thirds of Americans were covered through private health insurance (65.6%), whereas only one third of Americans were covered through public health insurance (36.1%; Keisler-Starkey, 2023).

### PRIVATE HEALTH INSURANCE COVERAGE

Private health insurance is paid entirely or partially by the person receiving coverage or their employer. These plans tend to be more expensive because they do not receive governmental subsidies, nor do they have the same cost containment or negotiation leverage as state and federal plans. The two main types of private health insurance are employer-sponsored and individual plans, which can be purchased through the state marketplaces. **Employer-sponsored insurance** is purchased by employers as a condition of employment for eligible employees and their families. For those who do not have access to employer-sponsored insurance, state marketplaces (e.g., Pennie in Pennsylvania or Covered California in California) and the federal marketplace (healthcare.gov) offer both individual and family plans. In certain instances, subsidies are provided to those with lower incomes who seek insurance through the marketplaces.

### PUBLIC HEALTH INSURANCE COVERAGE

Public health insurance is subsidized or fully paid for by the government. Although these plans tend to be offered at no or subsidized costs, eligibility is generally more restrictive than private plans. The main types of public health insurance options include Medicare, Medicaid, and CHIP. Medicare is a federal health insurance program for individuals aged 65 and over, along with individuals under 65 who have end-stage renal disease, black lung disease, or a significant disability. It is funded through general tax revenue, payroll taxes, and premiums paid by eligible enrollees. Medical Assistance (MA) program, otherwise known as Medicaid, is a jointly funded federal-state program that provides health insurance coverage to low-income or disabled individuals. The federal government determines the baseline eligibility and services coverage, but states can expand eligibility and services beyond the minimums set by the federal government. CHIP is also a jointly funded federal-state program that provides coverage to children under 19 who do not qualify for Medicaid. CHIP offers free, low-cost, and full-cost plans based on income.

### MANAGED CARE ORGANIZATIONS

In addition to the public and private funding distinctions, there are variations in how health insurance firms organize themselves and form relationships with facilities, clinicians, pharmaceutical entities, laboratories, and providers of durable medical equipment. A **managed care organization** (MCO) is a group of physicians, hospitals, and other providers who work collaboratively with each other and an insurer to provide necessary care for members. Types of MCOs include health maintenance organizations (HMOs), preferred provider organizations (PPOs), point of service (POS) plans, and accountable care organizations (ACOs).

An *HMO* is a plan where members have predetermined primary care physicians referring them to specialized care. Care is generally restricted to in-network entities or to providers who are contracted with the MCO. These plans tend to have lower monthly premiums and out-of-pocket costs for the beneficiary. The insurer secures more favorable payment rates from a narrower network of providers and facilities in exchange for directing more patients to those providers and facilities—lower provider/facility margin but greater throughput.

A *PPO* does not require members to select a primary care provider, and members do not require a referral to see a specialist. Individuals within PPO plans have a much broader network. Although cost-sharing expenses are higher than in-network care, PPOs also cover out-of-network services. The greater flexibility and choice of providers and facilities translates to higher costs for patients and members. Insurers cannot extract the same HMO discounts from providers because the insurer cannot guarantee the associated increase in volume.

*POS* are like HMOs in that members must select a primary care provider. However, unlike HMOs, POS beneficiaries can opt out of the network, and a portion of those out-of-network and emergency services are covered. To keep premiums lower, members have a strong financial incentive to remain in the network where volume discounts have been secured.

With all these variants, there tends to be a trade-off between the choice of facilities and providers and the cost of care. The greater the flexibility and choice, the higher the associated premium. As networks narrow and utilization management tools become more pervasive, the expected medical costs decrease and the associated premium becomes lower than high-choice, greater flexibility options. In more recent years, as costs faced by consumers, employers, and state and federal governments have continued to increase, there has been much greater acceptance of narrow networks, referral requirements, more cost sharing, and higher deductibles by the consuming public.

## HISTORY OF HEALTH INSURANCE

Property and casualty insurance has been in the United States since 1752, when Benjamin Franklin established an insurer to cover structural fires. However, health insurance is a much more recent phenomenon. Although there are predecessors that include sick funds in the Middle Ages and mutual aid societies that insured against catastrophic events or disabilities, modern health insurance did not start in the United States until shortly after the turn of the 20th century with the Progressive Era reforms of President Theodore Roosevelt. As part of the era's efforts to implement a shorter workweek, limit child labor, and improve workers' rights, states began enacting workers' compensation laws to shift the cost of injuries from the employee to the employer. While there was initial support from the American Federation of Labor and the American Medical Association for widespread, universal healthcare insurance, the experience providers had with workers' compensation led to strong opposition to the expansion of health insurance products (Starr, 1978).

That sentiment remained, and the expansion of health insurance stalled until Baylor Hospital experienced a steep decline in revenues per patient between 1920 and 1930. Investigation revealed that local schoolteachers were hospitalized but could not pay for care. As a result, Baylor Hospital offered the 1,250 schoolteachers a 50¢ per teacher per month premium that would cover the first 21 days of hospital coverage (excluding professional and physician charges). The Baylor experiment expanded to other facilities under the moniker of hospital service plans. These plans were required to be not for profit, designed to improve the public welfare, and covered hospital charges only. They did not impede the free choice of physicians.

By 1933, the hospital service plans were determined to be insured by regulators. As a result, the plans prevailed upon state legislators to exempt them from traditional reserve requirements that mandated the entity set aside significant financial resources to pay future hospital expenses. These exempt insurance organizations required enabling legislation and became known as Blue Cross plans. Blue Shield followed the Blue Cross/hospital service plans and covered the physician-related expenses. Starting in 1939, the Blue Shield products required the free choice of physicians and were an indemnity arrangement where consumers paid the physicians directly and submitted a bill for partial or full reimbursement. Growth of the private insurance market remained relatively slow until the beginning of World War II (WWII).

As the United States entered WWII, the available workforce was significantly impacted. To combat firms' competition for labor using pricing mechanisms, the federal government passed the 1942 Stabilization Act, which limited prices, wages, and salaries to September 1942 levels. As a result of the limitations, corporations began using fringe benefits as a tool to attract and retain their workforce. Health insurance became one of those benefits and with the 1947 Taft-Hartley Bill, health insurance was made a condition of employment that was subject to collective bargaining. Coupled with subsequent and favorable Internal Revenue Service (IRS) rulings that allowed health insurance to be purchased with pretax income, the growth of private insurance ballooned over the next 20 years (Reilly, 1960; Fronstin, 2006).

Although initially proposed under President Harry Truman in 1945 during this period of rapid health insurance growth, Medicare and Medicaid were not signed into law until 1965 by President Lyndon Johnson. Largely limited to those over 65 with some additional coverage for a limited number of diseases and modeled on Blue Cross and Hospital Service Plans, Medicare Part A covers facility-related expenses. Provider-related charges are covered under Medicare Part B and were modeled on Blue Shield plans. A managed care (Part C) option similar to an HMO or PPO and a drug option (Part D) were subsequently added in 1982 and 2003, respectively.

Medicaid was signed at the same time as Medicare Parts A and B and is a joint federal-state insurance product that covers needy individuals or those from a limited number of protected categories. The federal government bears most Medicaid costs. However, the states have varying levels of financial responsibility depending upon their per capita income. Richer states receive less support from the federal government than the less rich states.

HMOs were not well integrated into Medicare, Medicaid, or employer-based health insurance plans until the early 1970s. Signed into law by President Richard Nixon, the federal HMO Act of 1973 set the stage for the development and expansion of health maintenance organizations. The act not only amended prior legislation (Public Health Service Act of 1944) that restricted the role of for-profit insurers to allow for-profit insurers to contract with providers and facilities but also required eligible employers to offer health insurance options that included at least one federally qualified HMO. It also provided money for development and accelerated the proliferation of HMOs (Conover & Wiechers, 2006).

## REGULATION

The federal government does not regulate health insurance. Individual states are responsible for regulating the rate and form of the insurance products offered within their state. Codified with the McCarran-Ferguson Act in 1945, states determine reserve requirements, benefit packages and design, payment timeliness, service mandates, and premium taxation levels. While repealing the act is often considered to allow for more active federal intervention, the act does provide some protection from antitrust litigation associated with the sharing of information related to historical losses. Repeal of the McCarran-Ferguson would likely result in insurers becoming "unwilling to engage in efficiency-enhancing cooperative activities" and would result in an even greater concentration of the health insurance market (Danzon, 1992).

The federal government has been able to move forward with two notable exceptions to the McCarron-Ferguson Act. The first is the *Employment Retirement Income Security (ERISA) Act* of 1974 and the **Patient Protection and Affordable Care Act (ACA)**. The ERISA Act was established in response to the failure of the Studebaker-Packard Corporation (Wooten, 2001). Studebaker, the automobile manufacturer, shuttered its last plant in South Bend, Indiana, and did not have adequate funds to pay promised pensions and medical insurance to the 4,000 affected employees. The federal government intervened and established a code of conduct, transparency, and reporting requirements. In the same legislation, the federal government allowed nongovernmental organizations to self-insure the health insurance offered to their employees. Rather than transitioning risk to a third party for a fee, the employer could enter an *administrative service-only* (ASO) contract with an insurance firm. The insurance firm becomes responsible for the operations of insurance-related activities, but all of the claims are paid for by the sponsoring employer. The insurer bears no risk in the self-insured arrangements. Again, greater transparency, reporting, and reserve requirements were set forth. However, in exchange for the increased regulation, the self-insured products were no longer subject to state oversight, taxation, or benefit mandates. Self-insured products may include or exclude services, providers, and facilities at their discretion. Self-insured products now account for 65% of all employer-based insurance products in the United States. The percentage of self-insured employers grows as firms get larger—82% of firms with 1,000 to 4,999 employees and 91% of firms with 5,000 or more workers are self-insured (Kaiser Family Foundation, 2022).

The Patient Protection and Affordable Care Act, or ACA, is a comprehensive healthcare reform law allowing various improvements to our healthcare system. Enacted in March of 2010, the ACA had three primary goals:

- Offer more affordable health insurance options to an increased number of consumers,
- Expand the Medicaid program to include adults with incomes below 138% of the federal poverty line, and
- Lower healthcare costs through innovative medical care delivery efforts (U.S. Department of Health and Human Services, 2022).

The ACA realized several of the initial goals. Prior to implementation, approximately 45 million of the nonelderly population were uninsured. In 2014, the rate dropped to 35.9 million, and in 2022, it was at 25.6 million individuals (Tolbert & Damico, 2023). Contributing to that drop is that most states did expand Medicaid eligibility. However, after passage, legal challenges left Medicaid expansion up to individual states. Forty-one states and districts pursued expanded eligibility, but there are holdouts in Texas, Wyoming, Kansas, Wisconsin, Tennessee, Mississippi, Alabama, Georgia, South Carolina, and Florida. A survey conducted by the Commonwealth Fund found that the percentage of people in poverty without insurance dropped from 28% to 17% within states that expanded Medicaid. However, the uninsured rates for the same group stayed stagnant within states that did not expand Medicaid, thereby showing the significant impact of this initiative (Ellison, 2014).

The same legislation required states to establish a marketplace (or use the federal option), allowing individuals or small groups to purchase insurance over the internet. The marketplaces had to offer standard benefit packages with standardized, tiered cost-sharing and premium levels. The ACA reduced purchasing barriers for health insurance; increased overall insurance coverage; and is generally perceived favorably, with 59% of adults having a favorable opinion of the legislation (Kirzinger et al., 2022). Of those who were newly insured through purchasing coverage on the federal exchange, 70% said they bought insurance because of the ACA (Ellison, 2014). What is unclear is the impact on cost and whether it has been an effective cost-containment tool. With that being said, the state-based exchanges allow for price control for consumers in cases where financial assistance is needed. All ACA plans limit out-of-pocket costs for the member, and the IRS updates the maximum out-of-pocket cost for each year's plans. Individuals with lower incomes can receive federal and state assistance through two mechanisms: advanced premium tax credits (APTC) or cost-sharing reductions (CSR). An individual can receive an APTC if their income is between 100% and 400% of the federal poverty line, and they can opt for tax refunds or premium payments directly from the insurance company. A CSR is only offered for specific plans and can occur for individuals with an income between 100% and 250% of the federal poverty line. A CSR can lower out-of-pocket costs.

One of the most important aspects of the ACA concerning individual and small-group health plans was its implementation of essential benefits. Prior to the enactment of the ACA, the scope of coverage among insurance companies varied widely. To ensure that consumers were receiving the necessary benefits, the ACA introduced 10 essential health benefits (EHBs) that must be covered (Norris, 2023; Box 12.1):

- Ambulatory services (Includes visits to doctors' offices in addition to care provided in a hospital outpatient setting)
- Emergency services (Includes all emergency services regardless of network provider [extends to ambulance transport and air ambulance])
- Hospitalization (Includes all inpatient care with any laboratory or pharmacy services and surgical care)
- Pregnancy, maternity, and newborn care (Includes all care administered ranging from maternity to newborn care)
- Mental health and substance use disorder services, including behavioral health treatment (Includes inpatient and outpatient services)
- Prescription drugs
- Rehabilitative and habilitative services and devices (Includes therapy and devices [limits on the number of visits per year can apply])
- Laboratory services (Includes any laboratory work that is classified as preventative care)
- Preventive and wellness services and chronic disease management (Includes no cost-sharing coverage for preventative care [if on the defined list])
- Pediatric services, including oral and vision care (Important to note there are no requirements that health plans cover dental or vision care for adults)

## INSURANCE REIMBURSEMENT

Healthcare expenditures have grown dramatically over the last 62 years. The National Health Expenditure (NHE) was $28 billion in 1960. By 2022, the expenses had grown to $25.74 trillion, indicating an 8.5% annual growth rate. The rate of health expenditure

## BOX 12.1: ACA ESSENTIAL SERVICES

- Ambulatory patient services
- Emergency services
- Hospitalization
- Pregnancy, maternity, and newborn care (both before and after birth)
- Mental health and substance use disorder services, including behavioral health treatment (including counseling and psychotherapy)
- Prescription drugs
- Rehabilitative and habilitative services and devices
- Laboratory services
- Preventive and wellness services and chronic disease management
- Pediatric services, including oral and vision care (excluding adult dental and vision coverage)

ACA, Patient Protection and Affordable Care Act.

growth has significantly outstripped the inflation rate (3.76%) over the same period (U.S. Bureau of Labor Statistics, 2024). The significant increases are due to the increase in prices associated with healthcare delivery, the intensity of utilization by individuals, and population growth. That said, even after controlling population growth, expenditures have grown from $146 per person to $13,493 per person over the same time frame. The growth must be largely attributed to changes in the individual intensity of utilization and increase in the price of the basket of healthcare goods and services (Figure 12.1).

It is not surprising that the basket of healthcare goods has become more expensive; less effective drugs are replaced by more effective drugs, clinicians receive more specialized education, and general technological improvements replace fewer effective technologies in medicine. The rapid progression of medicine often means that the basket of healthcare goods changes and progresses faster than other commodities. The intensity of individual utilization has also changed over the last 62 years. Some of the utilization changes may be a natural response to how facilities and providers are paid and their associated incentives.

*Fee-for-service* (FFS) is a common payment system in which a provider charges a specific price for each identifiable and distinct unit of service rendered in the course of treatment. In an FFS environment, clinicians and facilities do not generate any revenue until they provide a good or service. The more services they provide, the more revenue they generate, and as long there is a positive contribution margin, the revenues will eventually reach the break-even point where they offset the fixed and variable expenses. Once this break-even point is reached, all additional services generate profit. The natural

**FIGURE 12.1.** National health expenditures.

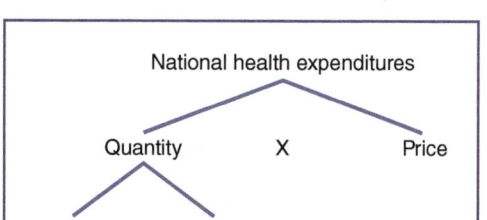

incentive in an FFS environment is to provide as many services beyond the break-even point as possible to maximize profitability. There is little to no accountability for patient outcomes. Historically, most high-cost specialty clinicians have been paid on an FFS basis and have been incented to provide as many services as possible to generate profits (Figure 12.2).

The *prospective payment system* (PPS) is at the other end of the payment spectrum and pays providers and facilities a fixed fee that is negotiated in advance for an individual and for a specified period or per a contractually defined episode of treatment. In the PPS environment, additional services and goods result in additional costs but no additional revenues. Revenue remains fixed. The natural incentive is to limit the services provided as a means of maximizing profit. Per diem rates, composite rates, capitation, and hospital diagnosis-related groups (DRGs) are all examples of prospective payment models. Low-cost primary care providers are the typical examples of providers incented, using their capitation, to limit services and potentially refer patients to higher cost specialists as a means of protecting their margins (Figure 12.3).

**FIGURE 12.2.** Fee-for-service system.

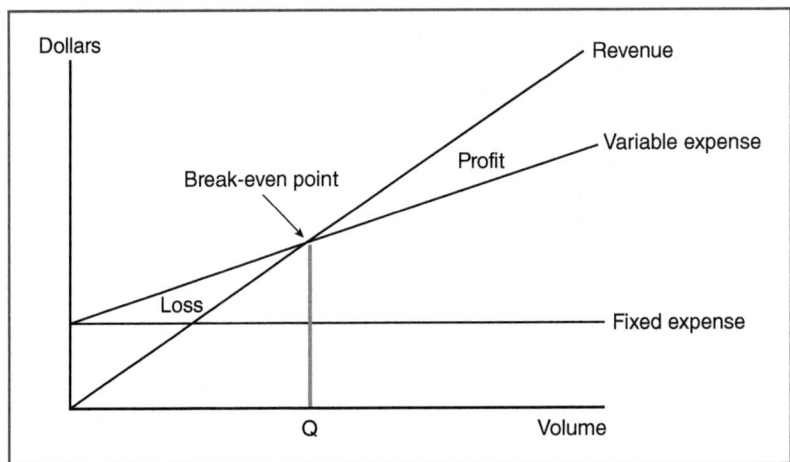

**FIGURE 12.3.** Prospective payment system.

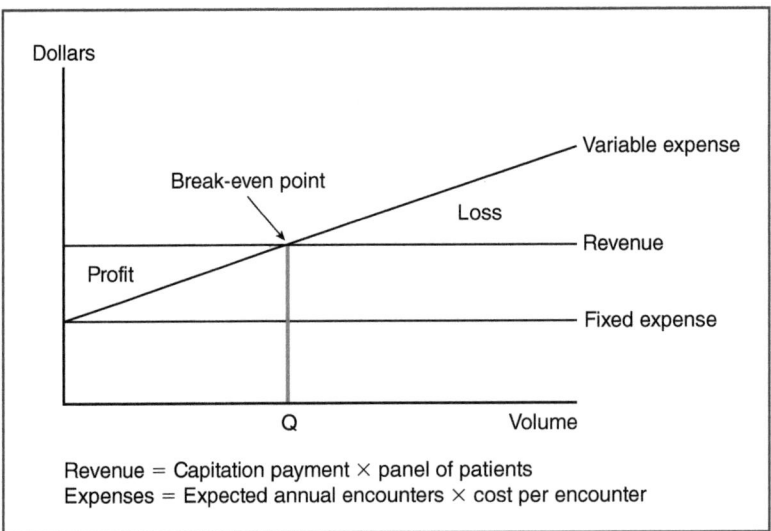

Our healthcare system has been on an unsustainable trajectory of high medical spending, and efforts must be made to combat this. Since 1970, our country has seen a continual increase in spending with no end in sight. As of 2022, U.S. healthcare spending reached $4.5 trillion. Additionally, our population is increasingly aging, with a projection of one out of every six people will be over 65 by 2050 (McPhillips, 2019). This trend presents significant challenges as older age tends to bring on more costly chronic conditions, which will only add to our increasing healthcare expenditures (Figures 12.4 and 12.5).

**FIGURE 12.4.** Total national health expenditures.

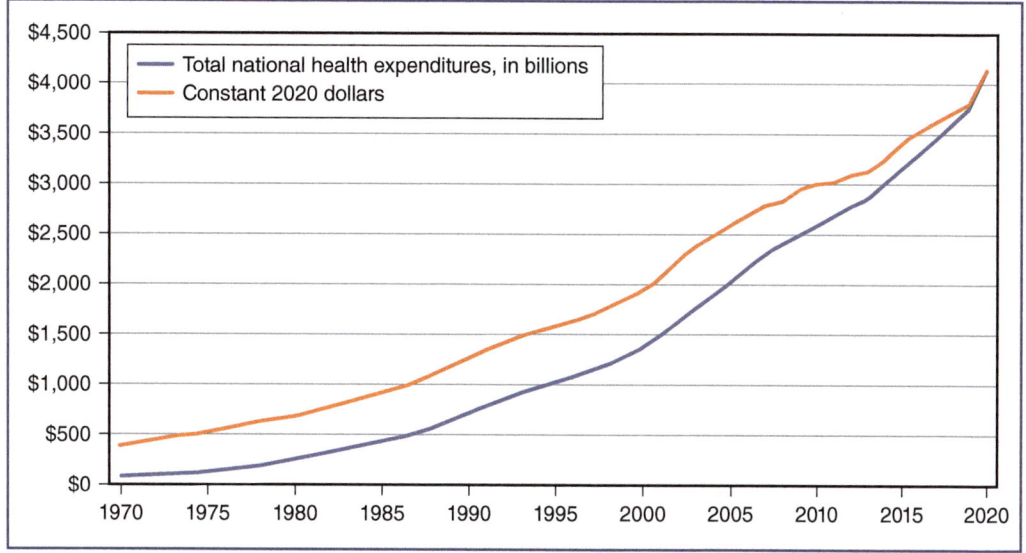

*Note:* A constant dollar is an inflation-adjusted value used to compare dollar values from one period to another.
*Source:* Data from KFF analysis of National Health Expenditure (NHE).

**FIGURE 12.5.** U.S. population predictions for senior and children.

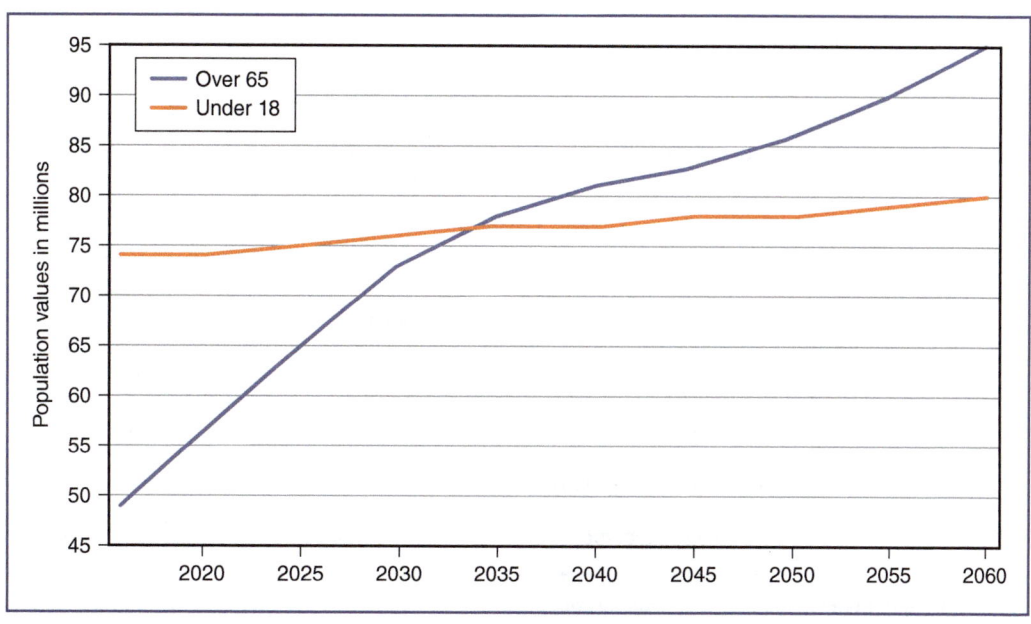

Lastly, the revenue mix seen by hospitals is continuing to shift from more reimbursement coming from governmental payers as opposed to commercial payers, leading to decreasing reimbursement rates. On average, private insurers pay nearly double the rate of Medicare payments for all hospital services (Lopez et al., 2020; Figures 12.6 and 12.7).

Recognizing the disadvantages of remaining in a fee-for-service payment system in an environment faced with increasing healthcare expenditures, an aging population, and decreasing reimbursement rates, payers (federal, state, and private) are moving to a new model of care called *value-based care*. Value-based care is a major effort that can potentially decrease medical care costs as it focuses on preventative care and ensures that patients receive holistic care from an integrated care team instead of duplicative services provided by fragmented teams. To achieve the goals of the Institute for Healthcare Improvement's Triple Aim, value-based care pairs payments to quality-of-care metrics, satisfaction, and expense per patient benchmarks. Ultimately, this improved model of care is continuously

**FIGURE 12.6.** Hospital reimbursement by payer type.

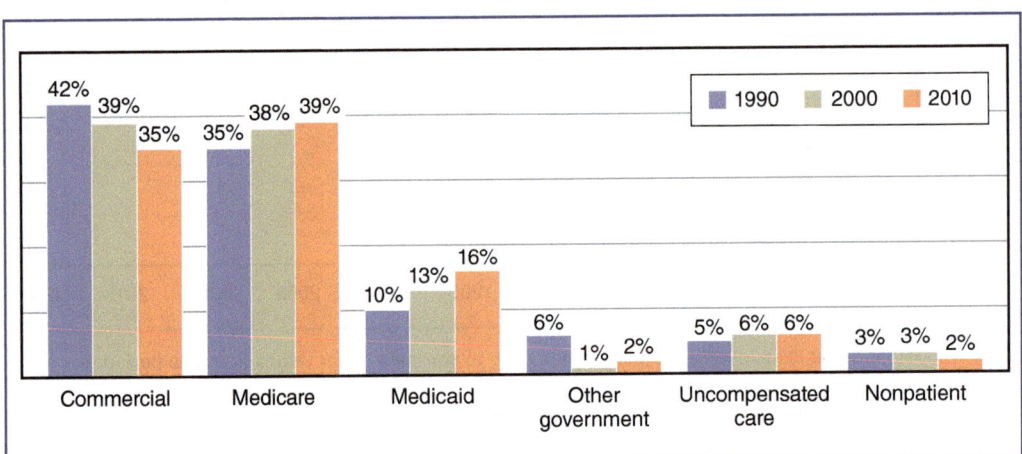

**FIGURE 12.7.** Private payment rates are higher than Medicare rates for hospital and physician services.

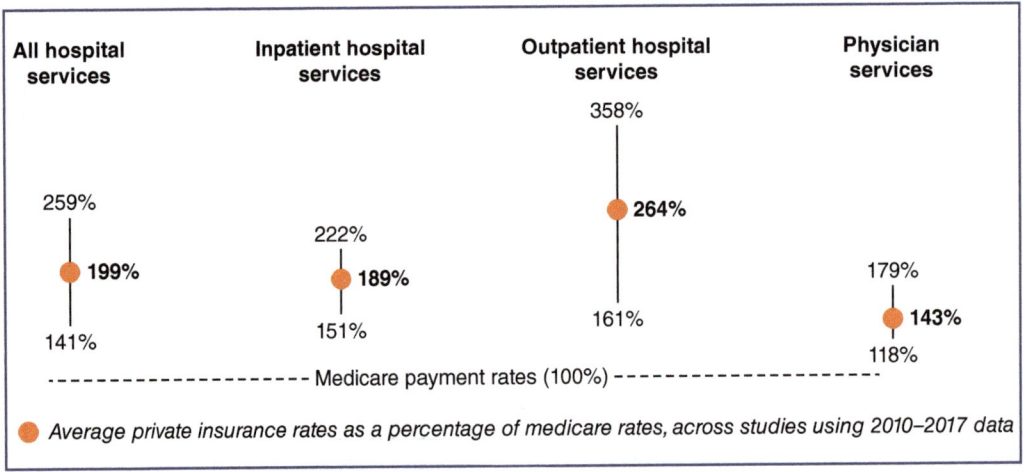

*Source:* Data from KFF; Henry J. Kaiser Family Foundation.

working to improve patient experience, enhance health outcomes, and lower healthcare costs. Patient experience, in addition to clinician experience, has become a more prevalent topic within healthcare. With higher patient satisfaction comes increased trust not only in providers but also within the entire healthcare system.

The value-based model of care shifts health status and medical care risk, which were initially borne by payors in an FFS environment, onto the providers and facilities that deliver care. Because of this, providers are incentivized to work as a team to provide care to patients as they are being held accountable for the health outcomes of various populations. The significant impact of value-based care may be the mindset shift that comes from no longer viewing patients as sources of revenue. The FFS model incentivized volume as opposed to value, leading to a diminished focus on the actual health of the patient and a focus on financials. While the value-based care model is likely to remain, the impact of the changes is decidedly mixed. Initial reports indicate some cost savings but poorer outcome measures for higher risk, vulnerable populations (Humbyrd, 2018; Lin et al., 2022).

## END-OF-CHAPTER RESOURCES

### CRITICAL THINKING QUESTIONS

- How have the historical provider and facility payment methodologies contributed to the rapid growth in healthcare expenditures?
- How do preexisting conditions impact the expected medical costs?
  - How would those impacts be reflected in premiums?
- As the population ages and NHEs grow as a percentage of the U.S. economy, are there potential impacts on other sectors of the economy?
  - How might various populations experience those impacts?
- Why might **value-based healthcare** have a negative impact on high-risk and vulnerable populations?

### LEARNING ACTIVITIES

**CourseConnect >**

To access self-assessment questions and interactive, competency-based learning activities for this chapter, visit www.springerpub.com/courseconnect. See inside front cover and tear-out card for CourseConnect details.

### REFERENCES

Centers for Medicare & Medicaid Services. (2024). *Historical national health expenditure accounts (NHEA)*. Retrieved January 17, 2024, from https://www.cms.gov/data-research/statistics-trends-and-reports/national-health-expenditure-data/historical

Conover, C. J., & Wiechers, I. R. (2006). *HMO Act of 1973*. Duke University Cost of Health Services Regulation Working Paper Series.

Danzon, P. M. (1992). *The McCarran-Ferguson Act: Anticompetitive or procompetitive?* The Cato Review of Business & Government. http://www.cato.org/pubs/regulation/reg15n2b.html

Ellison, A. (2014, July 16). *PPACA's effect on the uninsured rate: 5 things to know*. Becker's Hospital Review. https://www.beckershospitalreview.com/finance/ppaca-s-effect-on-the-uninsured-rate-5-things-to-know.html

Fronstin, P. (2006). *The tax treatment of health insurance and employment-based health benefits*. EBRI Issue Brief, 294. https://ssrn.com/abstract=910252

Humbyrd, C. J. (2018). The ethics of bundled payments in total joint replacement: "Cherry picking" and "lemon dropping". *The Journal of Clinical Ethics, 29*(1), 62–68. https://doi.org/10.1086/jce2018291062

Kaiser Family Foundation. (2022). *Section 10: Plan funding. 2022 Employer health benefits survey*. Retrieved January 17, 2024, from https://www.kff.org/report-section/ehbs-2022-section-10-plan-funding/

Keisler-Starkey, B., & Lindstrom, M. (2023). *Health insurance coverage in the United States: 2022*. U.S. Census Bureau, Current Population Reports, P60-281, U.S. Government Publishing Office.

Kirzinger, M., Hamel, L., & Brodie, M. (2022). *5 Charts about public opinion on the Affordable Care Act*. Kaiser Family Foundation.

Lin, E., Bozic, K. J., Ibrahim, S., O'Connor, M. I., & Nelson, C. L. (2022). Does value-based care threaten joint arthroplasty access for vulnerable patient populations?: AOA critical issues. *Journal of Bone and Joint Surgery, 104*(21), e92. https://doi.org/10.2106/JBJS.21.01332

Lopez, E., Neuman, T., Jacobson, G., & Levitt, L. (2020, April 15). *How much more than Medicare do private insurers pay? A review of the literature*. Kaiser Family Foundation. https://www.kff.org/medicare/issue-brief/how-much-more-than-medicare-do-private-insurers-pay-a-review-of-the-literature/

McPhillips, D. (2019, September 30). *Aging in America, in 5 charts*. U.S. News & World Report. https://www.usnews.com/news/best-states/articles/2019-09-30/aging-in-america-in-5-charts

Norris, L. (2023, September 17). *10 essential health benefits under the ACA*. Verywell Health. https://www.verywellhealth.com/what-is-covered-under-obamacare-4083032

Reilly, G. D. (1960). Legislative history of the Taft-Hartley Act. *George Washington Law Review, 29*, 285.

Starr, P. (1978). *The social transformation of American medicine*. Harvard University Press.

Tolbert, D., & Damico, A. (2023). *Key facts about the uninsured population*. Kaiser Family Foundation.

U.S. Bureau of Labor Statistics. (2024). *Databases, tables & calculators (1962-022)*. Bureau of Labor Statistics.

U.S. Department of Health and Human Services. (2022). *About the Affordable Care Act*. Retrieved January 17, 2024, from https://www.hhs.gov/healthcare/about-the-aca/index.html

Wooten, J. A. (2001). "The most glorious story of failure in business": The Studebaker-Packard Corporation and the origins of ERISA. *Buffalo Law Review, 49*, 683.

CHAPTER 13

# HUMAN RESOURCES MANAGEMENT

Dae Hyun "Daniel" Kim and William "Marty" M. Keith

## LEARNING OBJECTIVES

- Comprehend the fundamental principles of effective recruitment and selection practices.
- Grasp the legal and ethical considerations in the employment process.
- Analyze strategies for talent identification and acquisition.
- Evaluate the significance of diversity and inclusion in creating a dynamic and high-performing workforce.
- Understand the impact of social and cultural factors on hiring decisions.
- Identify best practices for creating a positive candidate experience.

## KEY TERMS

- Compensation
- Employee engagement
- Employee relations
- Employment law
- Human capital
- Human resource leadership
- Legal compliance
- Management strategy
- Recruitment
- Retention
- Selection
- Succession planning
- Talent management
- Training and development/organizational development
- Workforce planning

## INTRODUCTION

Whether you are entering a healthcare leadership position for the first time or being promoted into one, there are many aspects of human resource (HR) management that you should be aware of. The HR leader often becomes a vital ally, guiding you through the intricate challenges of healthcare leadership operations (Northouse, 2018).

One aspect of leadership revolves around the periodic evaluation of the organization's leadership competencies. As a high-ranking executive, discerning the most effective leadership styles and identifying what defines success within your organization are paramount, especially when devising talent management and succession strategies (Bolden et al., 2003). On the topic of talent management, understanding the regional healthcare job market is crucial because various questions can arise: Is your talent reservoir extensive or limited? What are the principal channels for job referrals? Does your recruitment rely on passive applications or involve proactive recruiters who actively seek out potential candidates? Beyond recruitment, the leadership must possess robust interview skills, both for accurate talent discernment and legal compliance (Collings et al., 2015).

Being equipped with a foundational knowledge of employment regulations is critical. While it is pivotal for you to be aware of national laws, one must also be cognizant of local and state-specific laws. A good grasp of employment laws will help you navigate potential issues throughout your career. Again, this is something that you will lean on your HR leader for expertise on. The basic **employment laws** you should be familiar with include Title VII of the Civil Rights Act of 1964. There are protective characteristics that should never be considered when making employment decisions. Another vital employment law is the Americans with Disabilities Act (ADA). This law has been modified over the years and requires organizations to make reasonable accommodations for employees with disabilities (Mitchell et al., 2014). The Family Medical Leave Act (FMLA) allows individuals with certain conditions to have protected time away from work. Your HR leader will guide you as you work through these. Although many employee-employer disputes play out in our court systems, the Equal Opportunity Employment Commission (EEOC) also oversees employee rights. They can and will intervene on the employee's behalf at times.

However, not all conflicts necessitate external interventions. Majority gets resolved internally, which underlines the importance of a leadership team skilled in conflict resolution and management techniques (Thomas, 2008). Collaborating with HR can assist you in finding leadership development programs tailored to your institution, ensuring leaders are equipped to handle conflicts and, more broadly, manage the invaluable asset of human capital. Financial decisions, like reducing management training budgets, may appear cost-effective initially but can have long-term repercussions if leaders are not adequately prepared (Pereira & Gomes, 2012).

Compensation strategies also play a pivotal role. Whether you aim to lead, follow, or remain competitive in the market hinges significantly on local competition (Milkovich et al., 2013). It is wise to periodically engage in market analysis, reviewing local and regional salaries, ensuring compliance with laws against collusion, and being cognizant of evolving pay transparency laws. Additionally, given the workforce's generational diversity, offering a plethora of voluntary benefits is also essential.

Lastly, effective onboarding and orientation practices lay the foundation for forging lasting employee relationships. Organizations with the infrastructure might have dedicated departments that design not just initial training and orientation but also continuous service enhancement and patient-centric competence models (Bolden et al., 2003). These departments also play crucial roles in succession planning and talent assessment for management.

# WORKFORCE DESIGN IN HEALTHCARE AND HOSPITALS

Workforce design is a strategic process that involves planning, organizing, and managing the workforce to achieve organizational goals and meet the evolving needs of patients and the healthcare system. In healthcare and hospital environments, workforce design plays a crucial role in ensuring patient care quality and safety, operational efficiency, employee engagement and retention, and financial stability.

To help ensure patient care quality and safety, there needs to be optimizing staffing levels and skill mix to meet patient needs. Additionally, staff should be trained appropriately and competently. This can be done by implementing evidence-based practices and protocols.

For operational efficiency, streamlining workflows and processes, utilizing technology to enhance productivity, and reducing unnecessary overtime and staff turnover are crucial.

To ensure employment engagement and retention are successful, there needs to be a positive and supportive work environment, and staff must have access to professional development as well as see a wide range of reward and recognition programs.

To ensure financial sustainability, labor costs must be managed effectively. Optimizing how you utilize staff will also help reduce expenses. Improving revenue generation can also be created through increased patient satisfaction.

## KEY ELEMENTS OF WORKFORCE DESIGN IN HEALTHCARE

- *Job analysis*: Identifying the tasks, responsibilities, and qualifications required for each role
- *Staffing planning*: Determining the number and types of staff needed to meet patient demand and organizational goals
- *Recruitment* and *selection*: Attracting and hiring qualified candidates who align with the organization's values and mission
- *Training and development*: Providing ongoing training to enhance staff skills and knowledge
- *Performance management*: Evaluating staff performance and providing feedback for improvement
- *Compensation and benefits*: Establishing competitive compensation and benefits packages to attract and retain top talent
- *Workforce analytics*: Using data to analyze workforce trends, identify areas for improvement, and make informed decisions

## CHALLENGES IN WORKFORCE DESIGN FOR HEALTHCARE

- *Aging population*: Increasing demand for healthcare services due to an aging population. This is true for not only the patients but also healthcare workers.
- *Technological advancements*: Rapid changes in technology and the need for staff to adapt to new systems and practices
- *Staffing shortages*: Competition for qualified healthcare professionals in certain specialties and geographic areas
- *Burnout and turnover*: High stress levels and workload can lead to staff burnout and turnover.
- *Regulatory compliance*: Adhering to complex healthcare regulations and standards

## BEST PRACTICES FOR WORKFORCE DESIGN IN HEALTHCARE

- *Involve stakeholders*: Engage physicians, nurses, administrators, and patients in the workforce design process.
- *Use data-driven decision-making*: Analyze data to identify workforce needs and trends.
- *Foster collaboration*: Promote teamwork and communication among staff members.
- *Invest in training and development*: Provide opportunities for staff to enhance their skills and knowledge.
- *Create a positive work environment*: Implement initiatives to support employee well-being and reduce burnout.
- *Monitor and evaluate*: Regularly assess the effectiveness of workforce design strategies and make adjustments as needed.

## TYPICAL METRICS AND ORGANIZATIONAL OUTCOMES MEASURED BY HUMAN RESOURCES

- Employee engagement and satisfaction:
  - Employee satisfaction surveys
  - Absenteeism and turnover rates
  - Employee recognition and rewards programs
- Workforce productivity and performance:
  - Key performance indicators aligned with organizational goals
  - Productivity metrics (e.g., output per employee, project completion rates)
  - Performance evaluations and feedback
  - Training and development participation
- Talent acquisition and retention:
  - Time to fill for open positions
  - Candidate experience and satisfaction
  - Employee turnover rates
  - Retention bonuses and incentives
- Diversity, equity, and inclusion (DEI):
  - Representation of diverse groups in the workforce
  - Employee resource groups and DEI initiatives
  - Pay equity and bias mitigation
- Compliance and risk management:
  - Compliance with employment laws and regulations
  - Harassment and discrimination prevention training
  - Employee safety and well-being programs
- Organizational culture and values:
  - Employee surveys on organizational culture and values
  - Employee recognition programs that align with company values
  - Leadership development and succession planning
- Financial metrics:
  - Labor costs as a percentage of revenue
  - Return on investment for HR programs
  - Cost per hire
  - Employee benefits costs

- Employee development and learning:
  - Training hours per employee
  - Employee development plans
  - Succession planning and leadership development programs
- Employee health and well-being:
  - Employee health screenings and wellness programs
  - Employee assistance programs (EAPs)
  - Work-life balance initiatives
- HR technology and analytics:
  - HR technology adoption and utilization
  - Data analysis to identify trends and improve HR processes
  - Employee self-service and automation

By measuring these metrics and outcomes, HR can demonstrate the value of its programs and initiatives to the organization and make data-driven decisions to improve employee engagement, productivity, and overall organizational performance.

## EMPLOYEE RECRUITMENT AND RETENTION

One constant phenomenon that the healthcare workforce has consistently been forced to navigate is change. From a global pandemic and increased workforce shortages to a growing emphasis on telehealth and digital medicine, healthcare providers are continuously expected to deliver care amid significant uncertainty and change. Unfortunately, a heightened sense of uncertainty and so many unknowns create a worsening problem: increased levels of stress and burnout among healthcare professionals. Stress and burnout affect healthcare workers at all organizational levels, including clinical and administrative employees. In the United States, burnout among healthcare employees is now recognized as a national public health issue (Terry & Matthews, 2021), and it impacts anywhere from 35% to 60% of the U.S. workforce (Melnyk et al., 2022).

All these phenomena have made employee recruitment and retention in healthcare much more complex and critical. Various studies have shown that a consistent workforce, coupled with experienced professionals, leads to continuity of care and patient safety (Jennings, 2008; Kent et al., 2020). On the other hand, rotating providers can lead to miscommunication and potential errors, leading to inconsistency in patient care.

**Recruitment** is often defined as how organizations attract qualified individuals on a timely basis and in sufficient numbers and encourage them to apply for jobs (Upenieks, 2005). In starting a recruitment process, it is imperative for organizations to provide clear information regarding the nature of the jobs and the desired qualifications. These are essential since an organization's recruitment success heavily depends on various factors, including the reputation of the job and the organization, the community in which the organization is located, the organization's work climate and culture, and workload (Albaugh, 2003). Hence, it is important for HR leaders to have various recruitment strategies in mind to be able to source the right talent for their respective organizations. HR leaders frequently utilize two main recruitment strategies: internal and external recruitment.

Internal recruitment refers to promotion or transfers from inside the organization (Gatewood et al., 2018). One distinct advantage of internal recruitment is that, from an organization's perspective, managers are already well informed about candidates' past performance and future trajectory. Furthermore, internal recruitment can show the rest of the employees that there are opportunities for advancement. From the candidates' perspective, they are already familiar with the organization, which means they do not have to spend much time on onboarding. However, there are several disadvantages to internal recruitment as well. The first disadvantage is that internal recruitment can cause a ripple effect of one individual moving into another position and an organization having to find a replacement, which can cause another role to be filled, and so on. Another negative impact is that it can promote an employee to a position that might require competencies that they might be lacking, known as Peter principle (Peter & Hull, 1969). This can have a detrimental impact on an organization because if an individual is promoted to a position that they are not apt for, other people would have to work around this person, which can lead to organizational inefficiency (Asghar, 2014).

External recruitment is defined as recruiting applicants outside the organization (Gatewood et al., 2018). The reason why HR leaders might prefer to recruit externally is because they are able to specifically target candidates with necessary skill sets and may even bring new ideas to the organization. Furthermore, external applicants might fit better in an organization with challenging work situations than those who are already working in that organization because they usually are not aware of existing office politics or tensions. There are instances where current employees refer people for positions for an organization. Employee referral is a terrific method for sourcing applicants because an employee already knows the types of individuals the company is looking for and can vouch for the people they are recommending. Hiring through employee referral can lead to new hires who attain job offers, stay longer, and perform better (Buchan, 2007).

It is important to note, however, that while recruiting the right talent is unquestionably imperative, retaining that very talent is just as important and challenging. Maintaining a stable workforce is crucial for patient safety and operational efficiency (Buerhaus et al., 2005). Turnover within an organization can also cause significant financial and training burdens. While many strategies for effective recruitment can be applied to retention, each organization needs to develop its own retention strategies because depending on the geographic location, type of facility, and type of employees, strategies would have to be tailored differently (Buerhaus et al., 2005). The following evidence-based retention strategies have proved to be effective:

- Providing adequate opportunities for internal employees to grow their careers (Zappe, 2006)
- Enhancing orientation and onboarding processes to assist employees in forming personal and professional relationships with colleagues (Gess et al., 2008)
- Creating an environment and culture where employees would continue to work by placing a strong management team (e.g., sufficient autonomy, flexible work hours and scheduling, and a work environment that incentivizes respect and collegiality; Buerhaus et al., 2005)
- Selecting the right employees during the recruitment process (Gess et al., 2008)
- Offering competitive compensation in forms of forgivable loans, signing bonuses, and bonuses during employment (Gess et al., 2008)

## EMPLOYEE RELATIONS

Employee and labor relations within healthcare settings are complex, mainly because HR professionals must be able to navigate a myriad of employment laws while also addressing the unique challenges of conflict management in a high-risk environment. However, they are still very much critical aspects of healthcare organizations because not only do they impact a positive work environment, but they also ensure compliance with both state and federal regulations (U.S. Census Bureau, 2022). It is essential to keep in mind, however, that state and federal governments are not the only governing bodies that oversee regulations. Administrative agencies such as the U.S. EEOC, a federal agency responsible for ending employment discrimination, also partake in protecting alleged victims of discrimination in the workplace (Phillips, 2016).

Under the umbrella of employment law, Title VII of the Civil Rights Act of 1964 is viewed as a cornerstone, prohibiting discrimination by employers based on race, sex, age, national origin, or religion (U.S. Census Bureau, 2022). It allowed employees in various healthcare organizations to work in an environment free from discriminatory acts. Compliance with Title VII is critical since it assists in creating an inclusive workplace environment, which is the very nature of a successful healthcare delivery system (Phillips, 2016).

Similarly, the ADA prohibits discrimination against individuals with disabilities in all aspects of employment, including job application, procedures, hiring, termination, compensation, training, and promotion (Americans with Disabilities Act Amendments Act of 2008 [ADAAA], 2008). It also provides protection to those who are deemed as having an impairment, such as individuals with disfiguring conditions due to burns (ADAAA, 2008). However, it is important to note that the ADA does not require an organization to hire someone with a disability but does not meet the requirements to conduct the job accordingly (ADAAA, 2008). Instead, the ADA notifies the employers that it is their responsibility to make reasonable accommodations on a case-by-case basis, such as providing interpreters and readers and adjusting training materials and employee's working schedules or conditions (ADAAA, 2008). See Table 13.1 and Figure 13.1 for more information.

Despite a tremendous effort from various federal, state, and legal organizations to protect healthcare employees, as shown earlier, conflicts still exist. Conflicts in healthcare organizations can be problematic since they can lead to poor quality of care provided to the patients, poorly affecting staff morale and the entire organization (Almost et al., 2016). Hence, it is critical for HR professionals to take active roles in managing and resolving conflicts effectively, which includes formulating communication and negotiation skills, understanding the dynamics of conflicts, facilitating discussions, mediating disputes, and implementing conflict resolution policies that are aligned with both best practices and legal standards in HRs (Almost et al., 2016). In other words, the intersection between employment laws and conflict management is important for HR professionals to keep track of because they are essentially the backbones of employee relations within a healthcare organization. As the healthcare landscape continues to evolve, so should strategies for managing employee relations within legal compliance and various conflict resolution methodologies.

Additionally, several laws speak specifically to labor organizing and unions. Employment laws that guide union organizations include a combination of federal and state legislation designed to protect the rights of both employees and labor unions. Some key federal laws governing union activities and labor relations in the United States include the following:

- *National Labor Relations Act (NLRA)*: Enacted in 1935, the NLRA, also known as the Wagner Act, is a foundational piece of legislation that guarantees the rights of employees to form and join labor unions, engage in collective bargaining, and participate in concerted activities for mutual aid and protection. The NLRA also establishes the National Labor Relations Board to oversee and enforce these rights.
- *Labor Management Relations Act (LMRA) or Taft-Hartley Act*: This legislation, passed in 1947, amended the NLRA and outlined regulations for union activities, addressing issues such as unfair labor practices, the rights of employers, restrictions on secondary boycotts, and the use of union dues for political purposes.
- *Civil Rights Act of 1964*: Although not specific to union organizations, this landmark legislation prohibits employment discrimination based on race, color, religion, sex, or national origin, protecting the rights of unionized workers against discrimination in the workplace.

TABLE 13.1. CHARGE STATISTICS (CHARGES FILED WITH EEOC) FY 1997 THROUGH FY 2022

| | FY 2013 | FY 2014 | FY 2015 | FY 2016 | FY 2017 | FY 2018 | FY 2019 | FY 2020 | FY 2021 | FY 2022* |
|---|---|---|---|---|---|---|---|---|---|---|
| Total Charges | 93,727 | 88,778 | 89,385 | 91,503 | 84,254 | 76,418 | 72,675 | 67,448 | 61,331 | 73,485 |
| Race | 33,068 | 31,073 | 31,027 | 32,309 | 28,528 | 24,600 | 23,976 | 22,064 | 20,908 | 20,992 |
| | 35.30% | 35.00% | 34.70% | 35.30% | 33.90% | 32.20% | 33.00% | 32.70% | 34.10% | 28.60% |
| Sex | 27,687 | 26,027 | 26,396 | 26,934 | 25,605 | 24,655 | 23,532 | 21,398 | 18,762 | 19,805 |
| | 29.50% | 29.30% | 29.50% | 29.40% | 30.40% | 32.30% | 32.40% | 31.70% | 30.60% | 27.00% |
| National Origin | 10,642 | 9,579 | 9,438 | 9,840 | 8,299 | 7,106 | 7,009 | 6,377 | 6,213 | 5,500 |
| | 11.40% | 10.80% | 10.60% | 10.80% | 9.80% | 9.30% | 9.60% | 9.50% | 10.10% | 7.50% |
| Religion | 3,721 | 3,549 | 3,502 | 3,825 | 3,436 | 2,859 | 2,725 | 2,404 | 2,111 | 13,814 |
| | 4.00% | 4.00% | 3.90% | 4.20% | 4.10% | 3.70% | 3.70% | 3.60% | 3.40% | 18.80% |
| Color | 3,146 | 2,756 | 2,833 | 3,102 | 3,240 | 3,166 | 3,415 | 3,562 | 3,516 | 4,088 |
| | 3.40% | 3.10% | 3.20% | 3.40% | 3.80% | 4.10% | 4.70% | 5.30% | 5.70% | 5.60% |
| Retaliation—All Statutes | 38,539 | 37,955 | 39,757 | 42,018 | 41,097 | 39,469 | 39,110 | 37,632 | 34,332 | 37,898 |
| | 41.10% | 42.80% | 44.50% | 45.90% | 48.80% | 51.60% | 53.80% | 55.80% | 56.00% | 51.60% |
| Retaliation—Title VII Only | 31,478 | 30,771 | 31,893 | 33,082 | 32,023 | 30,556 | 30,117 | 27,997 | 25,121 | 28,462 |
| | 33.60% | 34.70% | 35.70% | 36.20% | 38.00% | 40.00% | 41.40% | 41.50% | 41.00% | 38.70% |
| Age | 21,396 | 20,588 | 20,144 | 20,857 | 18,376 | 16,911 | 15,573 | 14,183 | 12,965 | 11,500 |
| | 22.80% | 23.20% | 22.50% | 22.80% | 21.80% | 22.10% | 21.40% | 21% | 21.10% | 15.60% |
| Disability | 25,957 | 25,369 | 26,968 | 28,073 | 26,838 | 24,605 | 24,238 | 24,324 | 22,843 | 25,004 |
| | 27.70% | 28.60% | 30.20% | 30.70% | 31.90% | 32.20% | 33.40% | 36.10% | 37.20% | 34.00% |
| Equal Pay Act | 1,019 | 938 | 973 | 1,075 | 996 | 1,066 | 1,117 | 980 | 885 | 955 |
| | 1.10% | 1.10% | 1.10% | 1.20% | 1.20% | 1.40% | 1.50% | 1.50% | 1.40% | 1.30% |
| GINA | 333 | 333 | 257 | 238 | 206 | 220 | 209 | 440 | 242 | 444 |
| | 0.40% | 0.40% | 0.30% | 0.30% | 0.20% | 0.30% | 0.30% | 0.70% | 0.40% | 0.60% |

EOEC, Equal Opportunity Employment Commission; FY, fiscal year.
*Note:* * In FY 2022, there was a significant increase in vaccine-related charges filed based on religion. As a result, FY 2022 data may vary compared to previous years.
*Source:* Data from The U.S. Equal Employment Opportunity Commission; https://www.eeoc.gov/data/enforcement-and-litigation-statistics-0

**FIGURE 13.1.** Enforcement and litigation statistics.

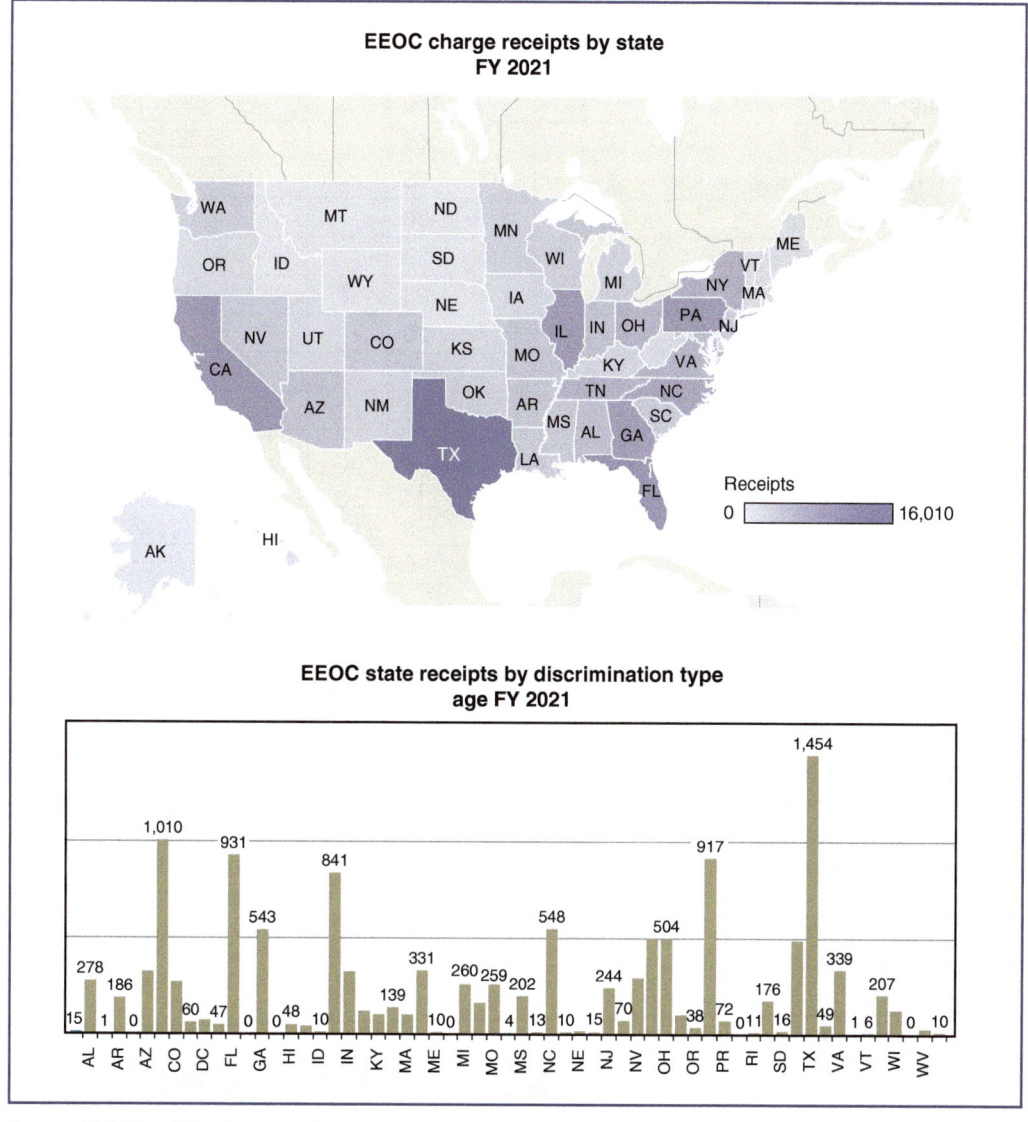

*Source:* U.S. Equal Employment Opportunity Commission. *Enforcement and litigation statistics.* https://www.eeoc.gov/data/enforcement-and-litigation-statistics-0.

- *Labor-Management Reporting and Disclosure Act (LMRDA) or Landrum-Griffin Act*: Enacted in 1959, the LMRDA is aimed at regulating the internal affairs of labor unions, ensuring democratic processes, and protecting the rights of union members through reporting and disclosure requirements for union officials and safeguards against improper union practices. In addition to federal laws, state-specific employment laws and regulations also play a significant role in governing labor relations, union activities, collective bargaining, and the rights of employees within unionized workplaces. These state laws may address issues such as public sector unionization, labor dispute procedures, and union recognition in various industries. Union organizations and employers need to stay informed about the relevant federal and state laws that govern labor relations, as well as any updates or amendments to existing legislation, to ensure compliance and fair treatment of all parties involved in the collective bargaining process and union activities.

**TABLE 13.2. RECENT WORKER STRIKES AND PROTESTS**

| TYPE OF DEMAND | WORK STOPPAGES | APPROXIMATE NUMBER OF WORKERS INVOLVED |
|---|---|---|
| Better pay | 160 | 59,730 |
| Healthcare | 65 | 33,298 |
| Health- and safety-related issues | 63 | 12,815 |
| Staffing-related issues | 39 | 9,249 |
| Improved COVID-19 protocols | 29 | 7,060 |
| Job security | 23 | 11,757 |
| Retirement benefits | 20 | 21,620 |
| Union recognition | 19 | 1,332 |
| Scheduling issues | 19 | 7,133 |
| First contract | 14 | 3,767 |
| Racial justice | 11 | 452 |
| End to sexual harassment | 9 | 528 |
| $15 minimum wage | 6 | 81 |

*Source:* Data from ILR School Labor Action Tracker. https://striketracker.ilr.cornell.edu/.

## AN INCREASE IN RECENT WORKER STRIKES AND PROTESTS

Faced with the collective voice gap described earlier, many workers are engaging in strikes and protests across the country. The new Worker Empowerment Research Network report summarizes data from the Cornell Industrial and Labor Relations School Strike Tracker, which details strikes and protests in 2021 by the type of demand workers were making. Table 13.2 demonstrates that while better pay and benefits were the most common issues leading to a strike or protest, many of the other causes or demands in 2021 reflected other issues that workers faced, including COVID-19 protections and other health and safety issues, staffing, and scheduling (https://www.ilr.cornell.edu/worker-institute/blog/publications-0/labor-action-tracker).

## ORGANIZATIONAL DEVELOPMENT

Executives and managers in various healthcare organizations generally acknowledge the importance of continuing education. However, when budgets become constrained, training initiatives are almost always the first ones to get downsized or eliminated (Frenk et al., 2022). This is because it is much more challenging to quantify the financial return on continuing education programs compared to other organizational expenses, even though managers intrinsically understand how education programs can ultimately lead to fiscal efficiency (Frenk et al., 2022). In other words, funds allocated to continuing education are often perceived as expenditures with ambiguous returns; managers can clearly see funds going out, but the benefits are slowly accruing. Consequently, especially in the current healthcare environment, while the emphasis on training and development is undeniable, it occasionally gets overshadowed by the executives.

However, this phenomenon can ultimately backfire because studies have shown that organizational development and training are crucial mechanisms to recruit, retain, and engage the organization's best talents (Frenk et al., 2022; Szilvassy & Sirok, 2022). This is mainly the case since majority of the employees get motivated by the nature of their work, specifically the opportunity to do exciting and challenging work and the opportunity to learn and grow (Harrison & Kessels, 2004). Unfortunately, this also means that if excelling employees are not in a stimulating work environment, they are potentially at risk of leaving. This goes to show the importance of persistent education and development programs, and one avenue to show the employees the investment that the organization is putting forth to these initiatives is through orientation.

Typically, new employees are provided with orientation sessions addressing common matters within an organization they will be working for. Typically prepared by the HR team, an organization's orientation provides information such as the organization's structure and leadership, mission, vision, and values, performance review processes, employee benefits, EAPs, employee work policy, and other universal precautions (Chen et al., 2004).

On a similar note, it is imperative for healthcare organizations to hold orientations sessions within each department as well because departmental orientation provides new employees an opportunity to meet colleagues that they will directly be working with (Chen et al., 2004). They are also likely to be provided with departmental processes and policies, along with on-the-job guidance so the learning curve for an individual that was hired to do a specific job can be as minimal as possible. Having new employees start working without formal training can be detrimental for both the employee and the employer. Regardless of their educational level or experience, new employees need some sort of direction and guidance that is unique to the department or the job. They should also be able to seek clarification about their new responsibilities, which is what departmental orientation is for. Incorporation of a mentor into an onboarding process, whether it be organizational or departmental, can be beneficial as well. Not only will this mentor-mentee program assist new employees by providing personalized orientation experience and navigational support for the initial days or weeks of employment, but it will also offer mentors an opportunity to enhance their own personal growth and expand their horizons in leadership and mentoring skills.

## CONCLUSION

The significance of HR management has grown exponentially due to organizations and employees both having to navigate the complexities of healthcare. This chapter has provided a deep dive into the multifaceted world of HR management within healthcare, shedding light on its multifaceted dimensions, hurdles, and methodologies. As we conclude exploring the maze of HR management, it is essential to reflect on the key takeaways and envision the path forward.

First, it is important to comprehend that HR management in healthcare is not confined to being an administrative task but is inherently strategic. In a sector where patient outcomes depend on various factors such as competence, commitment, and well-being of healthcare professionals, HR is a cornerstone of ensuring the delivery of high-quality care to patients. One overarching theme that emerges in this chapter is the importance of adaptability. Healthcare is an industry that is constantly evolving and changing, driven by shifting patient demographics, evolving regulatory landscapes, and technological advances. Hence, it is paramount for HR professionals to be agile, poised for change, and mindful of integrating new talent management strategies into the healthcare ecosystem. HR leadership theories can serve as helpful guidance for HR professionals to maximize organizational effectiveness and efficiency, ultimately benefiting patients, healthcare providers and staff members, and the entire healthcare system.

Recruitment and retention strategies stand at the forefront of HR initiatives in healthcare. The perennial shortage of skilled healthcare professionals necessitates innovative approaches to recruit and retain top talent. From targeted recruitment strategies to fostering a culture of continuous learning and development, HR professionals must be adept at creating a workplace that not only attracts but also retains the best and the brightest people.

However, this chapter also underlines the significance of compliance with the complexities of regulations managing healthcare HR management. It is imperative to pay close attention to legal frameworks such as Title VII, ADA, FMLA, and agencies like the EEOC. Not only are HR professionals operators of the workforce, but they also serve as protectors who ensure that every employee is getting an equal opportunity to excel in the healthcare organization.

In conclusion, healthcare HR management is a dynamic field that continuously evolves to meet the challenges of a complex and rapidly changing healthcare environment. The success of healthcare organizations is intricately tied to their ability to attract, develop, and retain the right talent while ensuring compliance with legal regulations. As the healthcare field continues to evolve, HR management will continue to be at the forefront of shaping healthcare delivery. The dedicated professionals in the healthcare field are the driving force that allows this field to meet the demands of today while also envisioning and preparing for tomorrow's healthcare challenges. In doing so, they are safeguarding the health and well-being of communities and paving the way for a brighter, more sustainable healthcare future.

## CASE STUDY 13.1: ENHANCING RECRUITMENT AND RETENTION STRATEGIES IN A HEALTHCARE SETTING

### ABSTRACT

This case study explores the challenges and strategies related to recruitment and retention in a healthcare setting. It aims to identify effective approaches that can attract and retain high-quality healthcare professionals while considering the unique dynamics of the healthcare industry.

### INTRODUCTION

- Provide an overview of the importance of recruitment and retention in healthcare organizations.
- Highlight the impact of workforce shortages and the need for proactive strategies.

### CASE DESCRIPTION

- Select a healthcare organization, such as a hospital or healthcare system, facing recruitment and retention challenges.
- Describe the organization's size, structure, and location.
- Identify the specific roles or departments affected by recruitment and retention issues.

### RECRUITMENT CHALLENGES

- Discuss the specific recruitment challenges faced by the organization.
- Examine factors such as a competitive job market, limited candidate pool, or difficulty in attracting top talent.
- Identify any internal or external factors that may contribute to recruitment hurdles.

## RETENTION CHALLENGES

- Explore the retention challenges experienced by the organization.
- Examine factors such as high turnover rates, burnout, lack of career development opportunities, or unsatisfactory work-life balance.
- Identify any common reasons for employee attrition within the healthcare industry.

## DATA COLLECTION AND ANALYSIS

- Conduct interviews or surveys with HR personnel, managers, and current employees.
- Gather data on recruitment metrics, such as time-to-fill positions and quality of hires.
- Evaluate turnover rates, employee satisfaction surveys, and feedback mechanisms.
- Analyze the collected data using appropriate tools and techniques.

## STRATEGIES AND IMPLEMENTATION

- Examine successful recruitment and retention strategies implemented by other healthcare organizations.
- Develop tailored strategies based on the specific challenges identified in the case study organization.
- Discuss approaches such as targeted advertising, partnering with educational institutions, or offering competitive compensation packages.
- Consider strategies for improving employee satisfaction, engagement, and career progression opportunities.

## IMPLEMENTATION AND EVALUATION

- Develop an implementation plan for the identified strategies.
- Discuss potential barriers and considerations during implementation.
- Monitor and evaluate the effectiveness of the strategies over a defined period.
- Measure improvements in recruitment metrics, turnover rates, and employee satisfaction.

## DISCUSSION

- Interpret the findings and discuss their implications for the healthcare organization.
- Highlight successful strategies and their impact on recruitment and retention efforts.
- Discuss potential challenges and limitations associated with implementing the strategies.
- Explore opportunities for continuous improvement and future research.

## CONCLUSION

- Summarize the key findings and recommendations from the case study.
- Emphasize the significance of effective recruitment and retention strategies in healthcare organizations.
- Propose strategies for sustained recruitment and retention efforts and suggest areas for further research.

*Note:* This case study can be customized based on the specific recruitment and retention challenges faced by healthcare organizations, such as rural healthcare facilities, specialized departments, or specific healthcare professions.

## END-OF-CHAPTER RESOURCES

### CRITICAL THINKING QUESTIONS

- How does healthcare HR differ from HR in other industries, and what are the unique challenges and considerations in managing healthcare personnel?
- What are the key factors influencing employee retention and turnover in the healthcare industry, and what strategies can HR professionals implement to address these issues?
- What are the ethical considerations and challenges specific to healthcare HR, such as patient privacy, confidentiality, and compliance with healthcare regulations?
- How can healthcare HR contribute to creating a diverse and inclusive work environment, and why is diversity important in the healthcare industry?
- What are the current trends and emerging issues in healthcare HR, such as the growing demand for healthcare professionals, changes in labor laws, and advancements in healthcare technology?
- How can HR professionals in healthcare organizations effectively recruit and retain top talent in a competitive labor market, and what role does employer branding play in this process?
- What are the regulatory compliance challenges specific to healthcare HR, and how can HR departments ensure adherence to labor laws, healthcare regulations, and accreditation requirements?
- In what ways can healthcare HR support employee well-being and mental health in a high-stress environment, and what programs or initiatives can be implemented to promote staff wellness?
- What are the strategies for developing effective leadership and management skills among healthcare professionals, and how can HR contribute to leadership development programs within healthcare organizations?
- How can healthcare HR departments align workforce planning with organizational strategic goals, such as providing high-quality patient care, improving efficiency, and driving innovation in healthcare delivery?

### LEARNING ACTIVITIES

**CourseConnect**

To access self-assessment questions and interactive, competency-based learning activities for this chapter, visit www.springerpub.com/courseconnect. See inside front cover and tear-out card for CourseConnect details.

### REFERENCES

Albaugh, J. (2003). Keeping nurses in nursing: The profession's challenge for today. *Urologic Nursing*, 23(3), 193–199.

Almost, J., Wolff, A. C., Stewart-Pyne, S., McCormick, L. G., Strachan, D., & D'Souza, C. (2016). Managing and mitigating conflict in healthcare teams: An integrative review. *Journal of Advanced Nursing*, 72(7), 1490–1505. https://doi.org/10.1111/jan.12903

Americans with Disabilities Act Amendments Act of 2008. (2008). H. R. 3195—ADA Amendments Act of 2008. 110th congress (2007–2008). www.congress.gov/bill/110th-congress/house-bill/3195/text

Asghar, R. (2014, August 14). Incompetence rains, er, reigns: What the Peter principle means today. *Forbes*. https://www.forbes.com/sites/robasghar/2014/08/14/incompetence-rains-er-reigns-what-the-peter-principle-means-today

Bolden, R., Gosling, J., Marturano, A., & Dennison, P. (2003). A review of leadership theory and competency frameworks. *Centre for leadership studies*, 1–44.

Buchan, J. (2007). International recruitment of nurses: Policy and practice in the United Kingdom. *Health Services Research*, 42(3), 1321–1335. https://doi.org/10.1111/j.1475-6773.2007.00710.x

Buerhaus, P. I., Donelan, K., Ulrich, B. T., Norman, L., Williams, M., & Dittus, R. (2005). Hospital RNs' and CNOs' perceptions of the impact of the nursing shortage on the quality of care. *Nursing Economics*, 23(5), 214–221.

Chen, L., Evans, T., Anand, S., Boufford, J. I., Brown, H., Chowdhury, M., Cueto, M., Dare, L., Dussault, G., Elzinga, G., Fee, E., Habte, D., Hanvoravongchai, P., Jacobs, M., Kurowski, C., Michael, S., Pablos-Mendez, A., Sewankambo, N., Solimano, G., ... Wibulpolprasert, S. (2004). Human resources for health: Overcoming the crisis. *Lancet*, 364(9449), 1984–1990. https://doi.org/10.1016/s0140-6736(04)17482-5

Collings, D. G., Scullion, H., & Vaiman, V. (2015). Talent management decision making. *Management Decision*, 50(5), 925–941. https://psycnet.apa.org/doi/10.1108/00251741211227663

Frenk, J., Chen, L. C., Chandran, L., Groff, E. H., King, R., Meleis, A., & Fineberg, H. V. (2022). Challenges and opportunities for educating health professionals after the COVID-19 pandemic. *Lancet*, 400(10362), 1539–1556. https://doi.org/10.1016/S0140-6736(22)02092-X

Gatewood, R. D., Barrick, M. R., & Feild, H. S. (2018). *Human resource selection* (9th ed.) Wessex.

Gess, E., Manojlovic, M., & Warner, S. (2008). An evidence-based protocol for nurse retention. *Journal of Nursing Administration*, 38(10), 441–447. https://doi.org/10.1097/01.nna.0000338152.17977.ca

Harrison, R., & Kessels, J. W. M. (2004). *Human resource development in a knowledge economy: An organizational view*. Palgrave Macmillan.

Jennings, B. M. (2008). Work stress and burnout among nurses: Role of the work environment and working conditions. In Hughes, R. G. (Ed.) *Patient safety and quality: An evidence-based handbook for nurses* (2nd ed., 137–148). Agency for Healthcare Research and Quality.

Kent, J. M., Thornton, M., Fong, A., Hall, E., Fitzgibbons, S., & Sava, J. (2020). Acute provider stress in high stakes medical care: Implications for trauma surgeons. *Journal of Trauma and Acute Care Surgery*, 88(3), 440–445. https://doi.org/10.1097/ta.0000000000002565

Manzoor, F., Wei, L., & Asif, M. (2021). Intrinsic rewards and employee's performance with the mediating mechanism of employee's motivation. *Frontiers in Psychology*, 12, 563070. https://doi.org/10.3389/fpsyg.2021.563070

Melnyk, B. M., Hsieh, A. P., Tan, A., Teall, A. M., Weberg, D., Jun, J., Gawlik, K., & Hoyinh, J. (2022). Associations among nurses' mental/physical health, lifestyle behaviors, shift length, and workplace wellness support during COVID-19. *Nursing Administration Quarterly*, 46(1), 5–18. https://doi.org/10.1097/naq.0000000000000499

Milkovich, G. T., Newman, J. M., & Gerhart, B. (2013). *Compensation*. McGraw-Hill Education.

Mitchell, M. S., Koen, C. M., Jr. & Darden, S. M. (2014). Dress codes and appearance policies: Challenges under federal legislation, part 2: Title VII of the civil rights act and gender. *Health Care Manager*, 33(1), 20–29. https://doi.org/10.1097/01.hcm.0000440617.09020.d3

Northouse, P. G. (2018). *Leadership: Theory and practice*. Sage Publications.

Pereira, C. M., & Gomes, J. F. (2012). The strength of human resource practices and transformational leadership: Impact on organisational performance. *The International Journal of Human Resource Management*, 23(20), 4301–4318. https://doi.org/10.1080/09585192.2012.667434

Peter, L. J., & Hull, R. (1969). *The Peter Principle*. Morrow.

Phillips, J. P. (2016). Workplace violence against health care workers in the United States. *New England Journal of Medicine*, 374(17), 1661–1669. https://doi.org/10.1056/nejmra1501998

Szilvassy, P., & Sirok, K. (2022). Importance of work engagement in primary healthcare. *BMC Health Services Research*, 22, 1044. https://doi.org/10.1186/s12913-022-08402-7

Terry, D., & Matthews, D. P. (2021). Technology-assisted supplemental work among rural medical providers: Impact on burnout, stress, and job satisfaction. *Journal of Healthcare Management*, 66(6), 451–458. https://doi.org/10.1097/jhm-d-21-00256

Thomas, K. W. (2008). Conflict and conflict management: Reflections and update. *Journal of Organizational Behavior, 13*(3), 265–274. https://www.jstor.org/stable/2488472

Upenieks, V. (2005). Recruitment and retention strategies: a Magnet hospital prevention model. *Academy of Medical-Surgical Nurses, Suppl*, 21–27.

U.S. Census Bureau. (2022). *American Community Survey (ACS)*. Revised September 29. www.census.gov/programs-surveys/acs

Zappe, J. (2006, March 3). The state of recruitment & staffing be aggressive, or be gone. *Workforce Management.* https://workforce.com/news/the-state-of-recruitment-staffing-be-aggressive-or-be-gone

# CHAPTER 14

# QUALITY AND PERFORMANCE IMPROVEMENT IN HEALTHCARE

Jill Suzanne Fennimore and Diane Denny

## LEARNING OBJECTIVES

- Develop a foundational knowledge of how quality is defined within the context of healthcare.
- Understand the multifaceted lens through which quality is measured.
- Explain how principles associated with high reliability and a culture of psychological safety are central to providing quality care.
- Describe the value of disciplined methodologies used for improvement, including the basics of **P**lan-**D**o-**C**heck-**A**ct (PDCA), Lean, Six Sigma, and change management.
- Identify core tools used in efforts intended to improve the healthcare delivery system to make it safer, more effective, and more person centered.
- Identify factors most often contributing to the success and sustainability of improvements.

## KEY TERMS

- Change management
- High reliability
- Institute of Medicine (IOM)
- Lean
- Measures/metrics/indicators of quality (structure, process, outcome)
- Patient experience
- Patient safety
- **P**lan-**D**o-**C**heck-**A**ct (PDCA)
- Quality
- Six Sigma/DMAIC

## INTRODUCTION

What does it mean to provide quality care? Some would suggest they know it when they see it, or better yet, they know it when they do not receive it. But what is "it"? In healthcare, unique challenges exist where incentives differ between what is valued by the key stakeholders—clinicians, providers, payers, and ultimately, the patient—who hold no agreed-upon definition. Quality healthcare can and often does mean different things to different people. The definition of quality and the need to improve "it" has been the focus of discussion for some time. To advance our conversation, we must begin with some definitions.

## STARTING WITH THE HISTORICAL ROOTS

Quality as a business imperative has been a widely studied topic such that we can turn to four quality giants of this past century who studied organizations and their commitment to exceeding the needs of their customers. In Table 14.1, we highlight these notable pioneers along with their principles of quality management. Walter A. Shewhart, whose work dates back to the 1920s, is often cited as the first to define quality scientifically. Best known for his fitness of use definition, Joseph Juran spoke to the importance of total quality management

### TABLE 14.1. PIONEERS IN DEFINING QUALITY FROM A BUSINESS LENS

| | SHEWHART | JURAN | DEMING | CROSBY |
|---|---|---|---|---|
| **PRINCIPLES** | Stated that the two sides of quality exist: objective and subjective.<br><br>Must focus upon the objective; define quality scientifically.<br><br>Quality standards must be expressed in quantitatively measurable product or service characteristics so that statistics may be used to determine the degree to which wants are satisfied.<br><br>Acknowledged that an important dimension of quality is value received for the price paid. | Defined quality as "fitness of use" recognizing the human dimension of quality, in addition to the technical (or freedom from defects).<br><br>Best known for the Quality Trilogy.<br><br>1. Quality **planning:** steps taken to understand and meet desired (external and internal) customer needs.<br>2. Quality **control:** actions to maintain desired capacity including measuring performance to identify gaps.<br>3. Quality ***improvement:*** activities pursued to elevate capacity to meet demand. | Emphasized quality is about people, not products.<br><br>Brought forth "14 Points" which stressed the role of management and the continuous development of people as central to organizational effectiveness.<br><br>Best known for the Deming cycle of PDCA.<br>• **Pl**an: For a change/improvement.<br>• **Do**: Carry out of the plan.<br>• **Check**: Examine the results.<br>• **Act**: Adopt the change, abandon it, or modify it to begin the cycle again. | Defined quality as "conformance of requirements".<br><br>Emphasized requirements must be clearly stated so that measurements can be continually taken to determine conformance to those requirements.<br><br>Nonconformance found is the absence of quality.<br><br>Coined the statement that quality is free. Doing things right the first time adds nothing to cost, doing things wrong does. |

PDCA, Plan-Do-Check-Act.

**FIGURE 14.1.** The Deming cycle of PDCA traditionally used in healthcare coupled with probing questions.

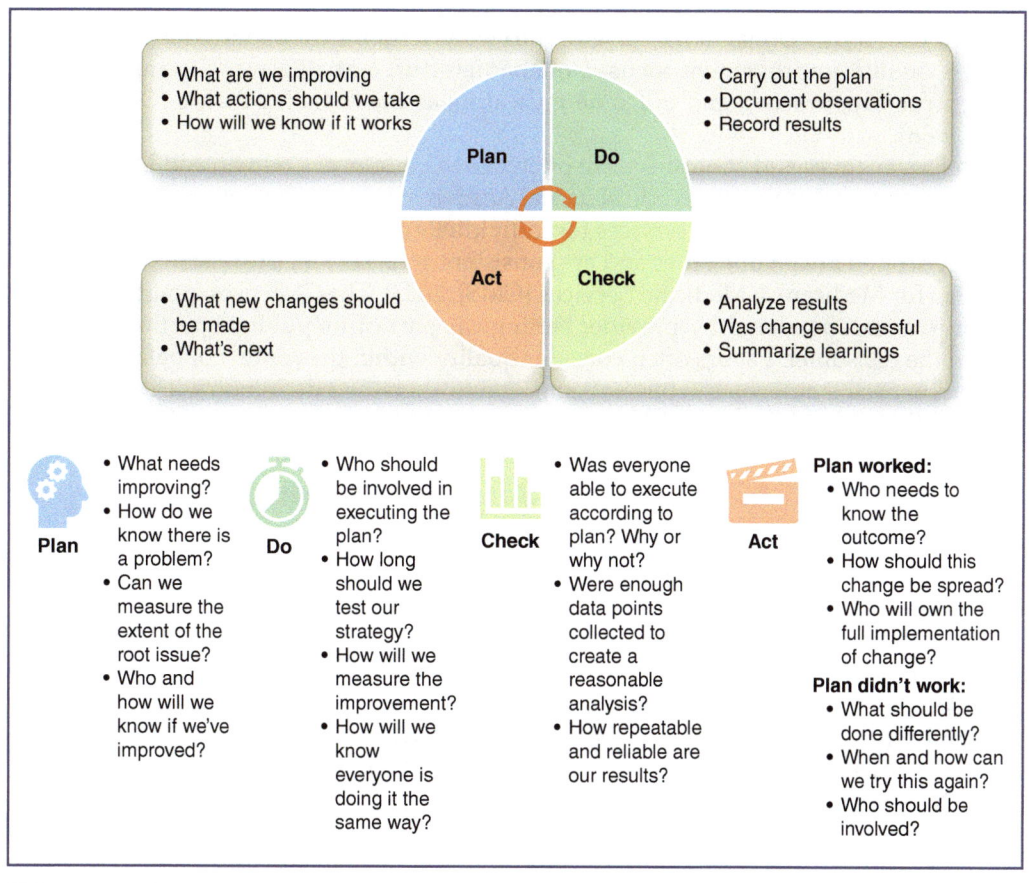

PDCA, Plan-Do-Check-Act.

and advanced the discussion from one focused upon numbers to viewing quality as interconnected to human relationships. His approach, referred to as the Juran Trilogy, is comprised of quality planning, control, and improvement as a cycle in which continuous positive change exists (Juran, 2005). Joining Juran and further championing the work of Shewhart, W. Edward Deming is most famous for his 14 Points for Management, in which he theorizes that organizations can positively impact quality while addressing costs. Credited for the **Plan-Do-Check-Act** (PDCA) cycle, Deming's method for improvement remains a widely accepted staple of many organization's quality assessment frameworks (Figure 14.1). Philip Crosby asserted that there is no such thing as a quality problem, stating that quality is free. His unique thinking affirmed that it is the systems, individuals, processes, or departments that cause the problems, necessitating rework (Crosby, 1979; Hoyer et al., 2001).

## PLACING THE DEFINITION OF QUALITY WITHIN THE CONTEXT OF HEALTHCARE

As we look to adapt such definitions to healthcare, a study of some of the great leaders of the quality movement is incomplete without mentioning two additional practitioners. In 1914, a surgeon named Ernest Codman was credited for being the first to challenge physicians and hospitals to take responsibility for patient outcomes. Compiling data on procedures by practitioners, his efforts were pivotal to the notion that standardization can lead to improved outcomes. It was not until the 1960s that the work of Dr. Avedis Donabedian gave root to what remains the foundation for much of today's quality improvement focus. Donabedian differentiated ways to measure care using structure, process, and outcome indicators as the basis for dialog (Donabedian, 1980, 1988).

While academics and clinicians alike often cite the works of Codman and Donabedian, more conventional language by the National Academy of Medicine defines quality of care as the degree to which health services for individuals and populations increase the likelihood of desired health outcomes and are consistent with current professional knowledge (Centers for Medicare & Medicaid Services [CMS], 2023). The CMS uses quality measures to compare care rendered by provider settings as part of its public reporting efforts to inform the consumer. Payors often consider quality within the context of balancing costs with the expected outcomes, while patients tend to align their definition with the care that achieves the optimal quality of life.

## MEASUREMENT AS THE IMPETUS TO IMPROVEMENT

It is hard to debate the adage in management that asserts, "You can't manage what you don't measure." The value in establishing quality measures is in their ability to reflect the characteristics of an attribute of interest along with a framework for judgment. Turning data derived from measurement into information and information into knowledge so that problem-solving may take place is the basis of all quality improvement efforts. As providers, policymakers, and payers continuously debate what constitutes quality, all understand central to any equation is the desire to improve outcome, process, and structure indicators of care at the provider, organization, and patient population levels (Evans et al., 2001; Donabedian, 2005).

Consistent with Donabedian's model for evaluation, quality is often assessed using aspects of care (or processes and structures) with a proven relationship to desirable outcomes (Box 14.1). This assessment requires our ability to capture data intended to describe the characteristics of care through each element of performance (Donabedian, 1988). Focusing on one singular metric or even a set of metrics can result in losing sight of the broader picture. Process informs outcome. Outcome informs structure. Structure informs process (Evans, 2001).

Although some outcomes are easy to measure, others are not as clearly defined. These outcomes include patient attitudes, social restoration, and physical disability. In examining the care processes, measures may appear to be more plentiful and easily understood. This is not necessarily the case, given a more complete measurement of quality requires us to evaluate the processes of care in relation to outcomes and the environment in which care takes place. Quality measures thereby become the tools by

---

**BOX 14.1: KEY CONCEPTS IN DONABEDIAN'S MODEL FOR EVALUATION**

*Outcomes:* What happens or does not happen following a process of care or intervention

*Process:* Interventions performed intended to result in a desired outcome

*Structure:* Elements found within the environment that may impact outcomes and/or processes

**TABLE 14.2. EXAMPLES OF HEALTHCARE QUALITY STRUCTURE, PROCESS, AND OUTCOMES MEASURES**

|  | | STRUCTURE | PROCESS | OUTCOME |
|---|---|---|---|---|
|  | Definition | Attributes of care providers and/or the system in which care is delivered | Specific transactions associated with encounters | Desired endpoints of care |
|  | Areas of Focus | Staff skills and training<br><br>Equipment, plant operations, physical environment<br><br>Support infrastructure | Percentage adherence or compliance to an expected standard or process intended to positively correlate to a favorable outcome<br><br>Strength of the relationship may differ by indicator | Mortality and morbidity by disease state; functional status |
|  | Example of metrics | Hours of nursing care per patient<br><br>Percentage of staff who are board certified<br><br>Availability of a particular test, diagnostic/treatment piece of equipment<br><br>Rate of RN turnover | Percentage of patients assessed for the risk of developing a blood clot<br><br>Percentage of patients who receive antibiotics before surgery<br><br>Percentage of patients who returned to the operating room<br><br>Percentage of patients readmitted for congestive heart failure | Rate of falls resulting in injury<br><br>Percentage of patients with blood clots<br><br>Rate of surgical site infections<br><br>Hospital-acquired pressure ulcers<br><br>Urinary tract infection rate |
|  | Traits | Easiest to measure | Largest area of focus | Most challenging to measure |

which leaders, practitioners, payors, patients, and others with a vested interest quantify our ability to meet our customers' expectations. Table 14.2 contains examples of quality metrics by category.

# THE VOICE OF THE PATIENT

Assuming two elements of performance exist with respect to quality healthcare, a technical and an interpersonal component, technical is often defined as the right diagnosis and right treatment, delivered in a manner that is reliable, timely, and without complication. The interpersonal component requires a process through which technical care is exchanged (Donabedian, 1988). Metrics surrounding care dimensions, such as access and patient engagement in their own care, have become the standard. This holistic view of quality acknowledges the importance of care that is effective, safe, and patient valued and aligns with the Institute of Medicine's (IOM) position for defining quality by these proprieties and more (IOM, 2001; Lohr, 1990).

*Crossing the Quality Chasm*, published in 2001 by the IOM, made an urgent call for change to the American healthcare system with the patient at the center. To better align perceived competing incentives and unify the components of quality, six aims for improvement were identified:

- *Safe*: Care without injury to those it is intended to help
- *Timely*: Carefree of waits and delays for those who receive and deliver it
- *Effective*: Care provided based on evidence-based knowledge
- *Efficient*: Care that eliminates equipment, supplies, ideas, and energy waste
- *Equitable*: Care that does not vary in quality because of individual differences and personal characteristics
- *Patient centered*: Care that puts the patient in control

The assessment of performance associated with any quality metric is dependent upon whom the improvement is intended to serve. For example, if our purpose is to serve the interest of patients, this means providing insights behind quality improvement activities to enable informed decision-making. Likewise, measures become a tool for clinicians and staff seeking to improve the care being delivered, payers and regulators with whom contractual obligations exist, and boards who share in the fiduciary responsibility for performance. Attainment of quality improvement goals is not just admirable but necessary. Figure 14.2 notes the recipients of data.

## CULTURE AND HIGH RELIABILITY

An integral part of our definition of quality, a focus on patient safety, is traced to the 1999 report *To Err is Human: Building a Safer Health System, a Precursor to the Quality Chasm*. No longer was harm seen as an inevitable consequence of delivering care. It was reported as

**FIGURE 14.2.** Recipients of meaningful quality data with associated primary intent.

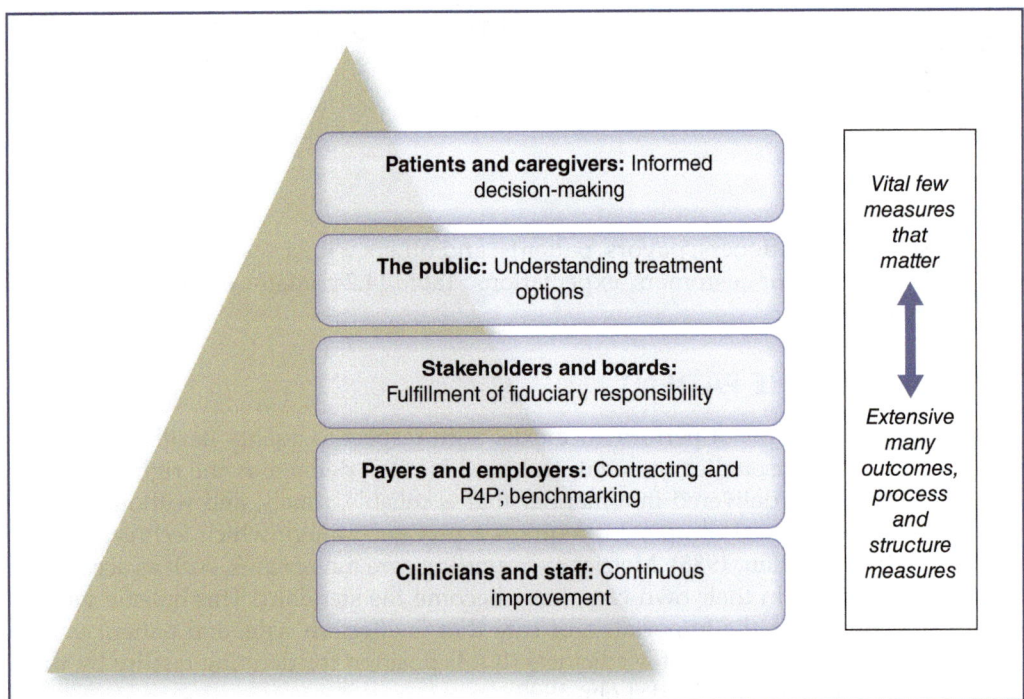

P4P, pay-for-performance.

many as 98,000 people die in any given year from medical errors that occur in hospitals. Many scholars offered an even more robust estimate of patient harm ranging from 210,000 to 400,000 preventable deaths a year, making errors a leading cause of death in the United States. While preventable medical errors have an economic cost in the billions per year, these events also result in the loss of trust in the healthcare system itself by patients and providers alike (Doll, 2010; Emanuel, et al., 2008).

Today's modern safety movement focuses upon creating an open and transparent culture, recognizing that catastrophic failures can occur in complex organizations despite the best intentions and safeguards. An organization's culture is a product of the individual and group values, attitudes, perceptions, competencies, and patterns of behavior that determine its commitment to safety.

The ability to repeatedly produce a product or service without failure in complex systems translates to **high reliability**. The challenge in healthcare is the processes that depend largely on individual interaction. People, not machines, do most of the important work. Behaviors are shaped by our environment such that reliability improves through the right mix of structure, culture, policy, technology, and workflow (Frankel et al., 2017). Successful organizations will attest that of all the environmental factors, culture is the most influential.

Traditionally, the culture within most healthcare organizations has held individuals accountable for all mishaps that transpire to patients under their care. Conversely, a just culture recognizes that individuals should not be held accountable for system flaws they have no control over. It also recognizes that errors represent often predictable interactions between humans and the systems in which they function. Competent individuals make mistakes such that a shared accountability must exist in which organizations are responsible for the systems designed and for responding fairly to the behaviors of those who work within those systems.

High-reliability organizations (HROs) design for safety and manage not only the expected but also the unexpected when stakes are high. Successful industries from which healthcare organizations are learning include nuclear power, air traffic control, and the armed services, to name a few (Polonsky, 2019; Weick & Sutcliff, 2015). Principles that enable HROs to achieve optimal performance include a preoccupation with failure, reluctance to simplify, sensitivity to operations, commitment to resilience, and deference to expertise. Marrying these principles alongside culture can easily be translated into key behavior characteristics (Table 14.3). Chassin and Loeb were among the first to explore

### TABLE 14.3. PRINCIPLES OF HIGH-RELIABILITY ORGANIZATIONS TRANSLATED TO PATIENT SAFETY

| PRINCIPLES OF HIGH RELIABILITY | IN A CULTURE OF SAFETY | BEHAVIOR CHARACTERISTICS |
| --- | --- | --- |
| Preoccupation with failure | We acknowledge that events do occur which are preventable; a continuous journey toward ZERO is the only acceptable goal. We understand the value of learning from both event and near misses. | • Individuals commit to and speak up for safety without fear.<br>• Teams are empowered with tools and techniques for error prevention with behavioral expectations defined for leaders, staff, and physicians.<br>• Leaders discuss safety issues in daily huddles, department meetings, town halls, management, and board meetings. |
| Reluctance to simplify | We improve reliability and safety through focusing upon the complete picture. We look for the nuances through our unique lens and diverse experience. We challenge the status quo. | |

*(continued)*

## TABLE 14.3. PRINCIPLES OF HIGH-RELIABILITY ORGANIZATIONS TRANSLATED TO PATIENT SAFETY (*CONTINUED*)

| PRINCIPLES OF HIGH RELIABILITY | IN A CULTURE OF SAFETY | BEHAVIOR CHARACTERISTICS |
|---|---|---|
| Sensitivity to operations | We understand that latent failures or loopholes exist in our complex systems that attempt to guard against error. We must seek these deficiencies out informed by those doing the work. | • Leaders regularly round for safety wins and concerns, encouraging a questioning attitude.<br>• Peers cross-check one another's work and hold each other accountable for safety.<br>• The organization, inclusive of its board, is committed to reporting, transparency, and learning from errors and near misses. |
| Commitment to resiliency | We bounce back; we learn from our mistakes, big and small, recognizing no system is perfect but striving to get there. We are committed to developing our skill sets and knowledge. | |
| Deference to expertise | We differentiate between normal times and high-typo times, knowing when to bend and flex. We push decision-making down and around, searching for our experts to assist in problem-solving. | |

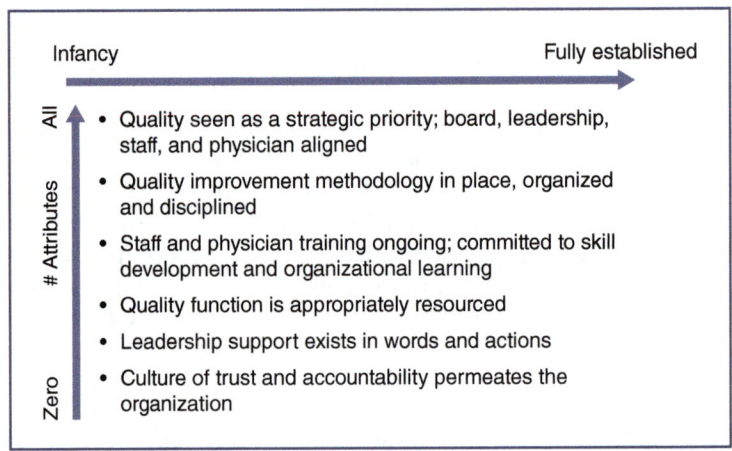

**FIGURE 14.3.** Attributes associated with quality improvement maturity.

major steps for healthcare organizations on a path toward high reliability. Central is a need to revisit approaches to improvement, citing the next generation of tools developed in industry and imported into healthcare—Lean, Six Sigma, and change management (Chassin & Loeb, 2013). The most successful organizations with a heightened quality maturity combine steadfast leadership, engaged teams, and skilled quality practitioners with a just culture and robust infrastructure (Figure 14.3; Grailey et al., 2021; Hibbert et al., 2021; Vaughn et al., 2019).

## THE RIPPLE EFFECT

A discussion of quality would not be complete without acknowledging the ripple effect or the notion that improving one characteristic of care can have both positive and negative consequences on other aspects. Even more germane is the fact that at the organizational

**FIGURE 14.4.** The ripple effect of quality, positive or negative implications.

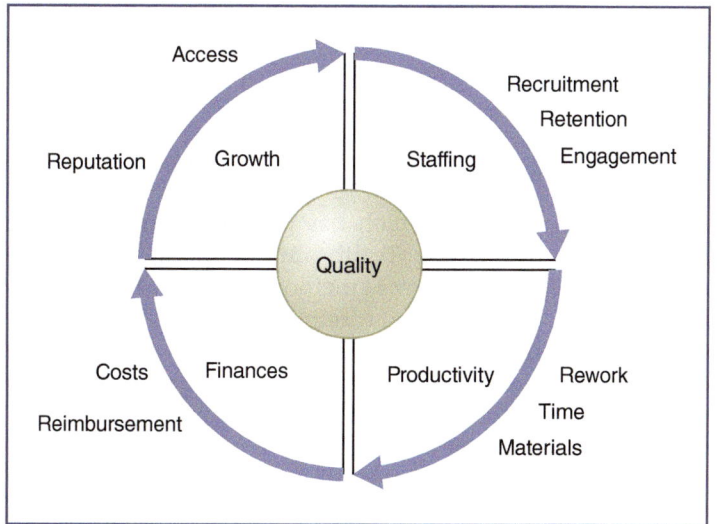

level, the cost of poor-quality care can impact other performance levers such as the ability to attract new patients; to hire, retain, and grow staff; to operate productively; and to manage finances (Figure 14.4).

Economically, ripple effects deemed substantial have been the impetus behind policymakers' and payors' attempts to incentivize quality improvement and healthcare expenditures simultaneously (Nuckols et al., 2013). Expertise from stakeholders working across sectors is needed to create a shared understanding of the opportunities to disrupt the delivery system, to change how it functions, and to ensure that quality is at the forefront of this transformation. Any change can lead to a cascading array of unplanned, nonlinear, and unexpected effects which, at first pass, may appear distant yet may, in fact, impact individual lives.

## APPLYING THE TOOLS OF THE TRADE: THE VALUE OF DISCIPLINED METHODOLOGIES FOR IMPROVEMENT

Given the complex and unpredictable landscape of the healthcare industry, safety, quality, and satisfaction problems are constant. Healthcare quality leaders are responsible for guiding their organizations in addressing these challenges with flexibility and creativity, supporting an evolution toward less complexity and improved patient and organizational outcomes (Plsek & Greenhalgh, 2001). In doing so, they will remain competitive, maintaining cost-effectiveness and efficiencies by reducing the number of defects/errors while improving quality, productivity, and customer/staff satisfaction.

### BUSINESS STRATEGY

A structured methodology for improvement must be embedded in an organization's culture to ensure its long-term viability and success. Without an intentional journey of continuous improvement, there exists an increased risk of unmet customer and employee needs and the endangerment of the organization's very existence (Achibat et al., 2023). Typically structured in today's environment at the senior leader, titles such as Chief

Quality Officer or Vice President of Process Improvement are now commonplace. This commitment to continuous improvement is a shared responsibility implemented using a variety of approaches and methodologies to analyze and solve business problems. Several approaches are further described.

## ROBUST PROCESS IMPROVEMENT OVERVIEW

Robust process improvement (RPI), which has been utilized as a pillar of The Joint Commission's Center for Transforming Healthcare since 2008, is a strategic combination of Lean, Six Sigma, and change management methodologies that provides an effective and complementary set of tools, strategies, and training programs within the healthcare space to create sustainable solutions for critical safety, quality, and satisfaction problems and to make significant improvements to faulty processes. RPI is a proven methodology for obtaining the voice of the customer to inform the areas of improvement focus and to ensure that both clinical quality and business processes are capable of consistently generating and sustaining rates of improvement (Chassin & Loeb, 2013). When applied successfully, RPI sustainably increases the efficiency of business processes, employee engagement, and empowerment, ultimately improving the quality of care.

Applying RPI to invest in employees, for example, ensuring RPI proficiency is included in staff career development, yields positive results such as improving business and clinical outcomes, moving performance to zero harm, and improving finance and operations for clinical quality and safety, inside and outside of a hospital setting (High-Reliability Training, n.d.). Figure 14.5 shows additional benefits of implementing an RPI program.

**FIGURE 14.5.** Benefits of implementing a robust process improvement program across practice areas.

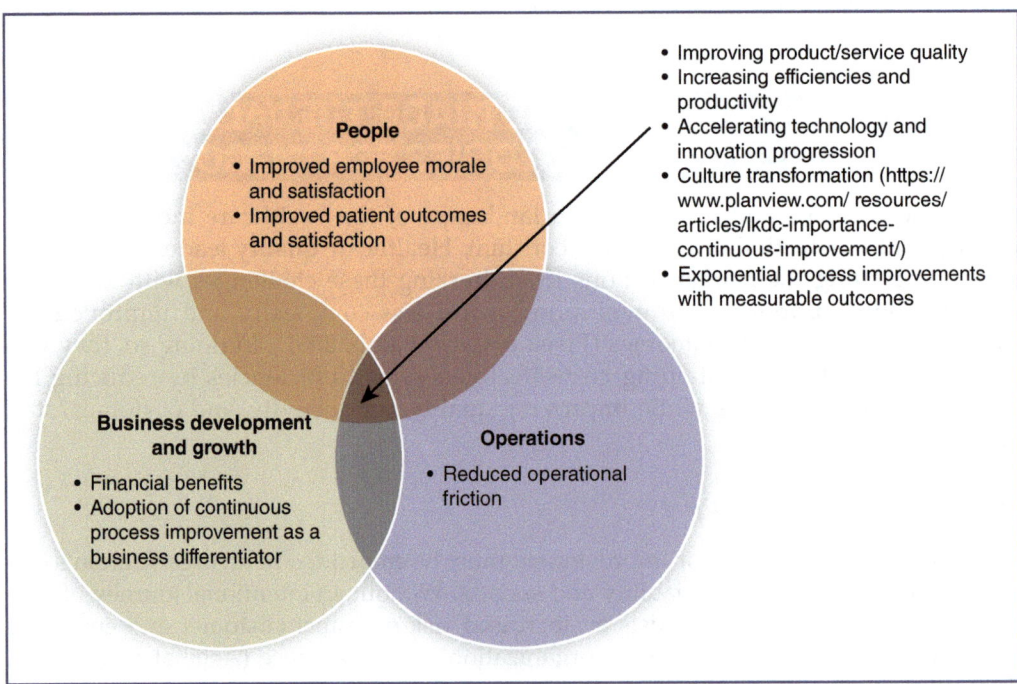

## ROBUST PROCESS IMPROVEMENT ENGAGEMENT AND A CULTURE OF KINDNESS

Research suggests that kindness yields positive business outcomes. Formulating a culture that also values kindness affords staff an environment to speak up and share ideas for improvement. Kindness promotes feelings of psychological security, thus empowering employees. Employees who work on RPI projects for themselves and/or their customers are more engaged in their work, increase their productivity and feelings of accomplishment, and tend to remain at their companies for a longer period. Furthermore, when employees receive a compliment or recognition for their efforts, their feelings of purpose, fulfillment, and self-esteem increase, and their self-evaluations improve. A culture of kindness results in employee behaviors that yield more frequent positive outcomes in all business areas (Swinand, 2023).

## HISTORY OF LEAN

A Massachusetts Institute of Technology research team, headed by James Womack, PhD, coined the term "Lean" to describe Toyota's business processes during the late 1980s (Lean Enterprise Institute, 2023). **Lean** is a way of thinking differently about optimizing flow with less waste (things the customer is not willing to pay for) to create products with more value to customers. It is a practice of continuous experimentation with the aim of achieving zero waste; included in this practice are frontline subject matter experts.

### APPLYING LEAN MANAGEMENT TO HEALTHCARE

Lean has a track record of achievement in manufacturing with tools that have been applied in the manufacturing industry more recently adopted by the healthcare industry. In both manufacturing and healthcare, communication challenges and a lack of understanding about customers' needs and wants are common root causes for problems encountered by organizational leadership and employees, as well as customers. Lean thinking and execution are about cyclical and systematic continuous learning (King, 2019).

Adding to his body of work, Deming provided a foundation for Lean management theory in his book, *Out of the Crisis* (1982), in which he presents many concepts and methodologies that can be readily applied in the healthcare setting, including the following (Simon & Canacari, 2011):

- Leading the organization
- Driving out fear
- Breaking down barriers between departments
- Transforming the organization
- Including frontline staff

### LEAN SIX SIGMA EMERGES

A continuous commitment to improving quality and enhancing productivity is cited by most as the key to improving business results and ultimately obtaining a competitive advantage. Marrying the tools, techniques, and benefits of Lean and Six Sigma produces dramatic, accelerated improvements in organizational performance. **DMAIC** (**D**efine, **M**easure, **A**nalyze, **I**mprove, and **C**ontrol) is an effective problem-solving structure that helps clarify what you are trying to achieve, making the combination of Lean and Six

Sigma techniques even more powerful when used together (Brook, 2022). The term "Lean Six Sigma (LSS)," first introduced into literature around the year 2000, has grown across industries, including healthcare (Timans et al., 2012). It has been defined by Snee (2010) as "a business strategy and methodology that increases process performance resulting in enhanced customer satisfaction and improved bottom-line results while improving quality" (Laureani & Antony, 2012). Table 14.4 provides several examples of LSS projects in healthcare and their impact.

Mount Sinai developed a multidisciplinary initiative, "Lose the Tube," focused on a Choosing Wisely recommendation to decrease catheter-associated urinary tract infection (CAUTI) rates and catheter days. Through an electronic health record catheter identification tool, daily interdisciplinary query, and clinician education, their multifaceted intervention reduced mean per-person catheter days from 3.3 to 2.9, decreased CAUTI rates from 2.85 to 0.32 per 1,000 catheter days, and reduced institutional cost by $32,245 (Cho et al., 2017).

Martin Luther King Jr. Community Hospital in Los Angeles, California, reached new heights as it became a Stage 7 facility on the Electronic Medical Record Adoption Model (EMRAM), a tool for assessing how efficiently a facility uses electronic health records. Achieved by only 6.4% of hospitals in the United States, their secret has been well documented to include LSS. Many hospital leaders were well versed in LSS methodology, including Tracy Donegan, the Chief Information and Innovation Officer. She had already been working on 15 LSS projects before attempting to reach Stage 7 recognition. One project focused on improving patient admittance flow through the hospital from the

**TABLE 14.4. THE IMPACT OF LEAN SIX SIGMA PROJECTS AT DIFFERENT HEALTH SYSTEMS**

| HEALTH SYSTEM | IMPACT |
|---|---|
| Mount Sinai (2017) | The "Lose the Tube" project reduced CAUTI rates from 2.85 to 0.32 per 1,000 catheter days. It reduced mean per-person catheter days from 3.3 to 2.9. It reduced costs by $32,245. |
| Johns Hopkins All Children's Hospital (2017) | They revamped their onboarding process and increased the number of hospital-employed providers who are active with health plans by nearly 38 percentage points. In February 2015, less than 50% of all employed providers were active with payers. By February 2016, this increased by 20 percentage points. By the end of 2016, over 77% of employed providers were active with payers, while the volume of providers continuously increased. |
| Martin Luther King Jr. Community Hospital (2018) | By improving patient admittance flow through the hospital from the emergency department project, they reduced their median time by 22%. (Original median time was 471 minutes.) |
| Legacy Salmon Creek Medical Center in Vancouver (2012) | Reduced the time it takes to secure a bed for ICU-transferred patients by 50%. Visual management boards with performance measurements. Recognition of good work by specific employees |
| Tallahassee Memorial Healthcare (2017–2019) | Improved patient outcomes and satisfaction. Improved staff efficiency and effectiveness. Minimized travel distances and turns. Separated patient and family traffic from staff to support circulation |

CAUTI, catheter-associated urinary tract infection.

emergency department. Their original median time in the emergency department was 471 minutes; after utilizing LSS strategies to analyze and adjust their process, they reduced their median time by 22%. Martin Luther King Jr. Community Hospital is a leader in process improvement using LSS (Admin, 2019).

Tallahassee Memorial Healthcare (TMH) embarked on a $157M project to build a new hospital, using LSS to streamline patient and employee processes. The project featured evidence-based design concepts to improve patient outcomes and increase patient satisfaction. As the project progressed toward completion in April 2019, TMH utilized LSS principles to improve efficiency and effectiveness by minimizing travel distances for patients and visitors and separating family and patient traffic to increase circulation.

# CHANGE MANAGEMENT

Fifty percent of organizational change initiatives fail. **Change management** frameworks and methodologies can help all stakeholders navigate the change and transitions in experience, from the initial phase of a project throughout implementation to resolution and project closing. When employees and customers are prepared for change and leaders support and manage it, a safe environment is created that helps accelerate the change (Miller, 2020).

## HISTORY OF CHANGE ACCELERATION PROCESS

The Change Acceleration Process (CAP) model, originating at General Electric, is the process of moving the current state of the process/service/product to an improved state by speeding up the transition state, which is the period from implementing a project to achieving and maintaining the sustained results. Healthcare leaders have used CAP on the people side of change by supporting the development of behaviors that will accelerate process improvement and ensure sustainable change. The CAP model includes several key elements, such as leading change, creating a shared need, shaping a vision, obtaining buy-in, making the change last, and monitoring progress. Each component comprises tools that can be used to better understand the issues at hand and develop a comprehensive plan. Fundamental, substantial change can occur when the CAP model and improvement tools are used together (Dawson, 2019). Table 14.5 shows the attributes and benefits of PDCA, Lean, Six Sigma, and change management.

### TABLE 14.5. ATTRIBUTES AND BENEFITS OF PDCA, LEAN, SIX SIGMA, AND CHANGE MANAGEMENT

| PDCA | SIX SIGMA | LEAN | CHANGE MANAGEMENT |
| --- | --- | --- | --- |
| Streamline and improve a repetitive work process | Focus on reducing variation and elimination of defects | Focus on reducing waste and lead time | Focus on seven steps for the CAP model for moving from the current state through the transition state to the improved state |
| Develop a new business process | Data and metrics orientation—geared to reduce variation | Leaders and workers are included in RPI and learn by innovating their work flows, service, and/or quality concerns | Quick and systematic |

*(continued)*

**TABLE 14.5. ATTRIBUTES AND BENEFITS OF PDCA, LEAN, SIX SIGMA, AND CHANGE MANAGEMENT (*CONTINUED*)**

| PDCA | SIX SIGMA | LEAN | CHANGE MANAGEMENT |
|---|---|---|---|
| Get started with continuous improvement | Financial impact varies greatly | Financial impact varies greatly | Creates a shared need and shaping a common vision to support organizational and process improvement change |
| Rapidly iterate on change and see immediate results | Focus on the bottom line—less focus on "across the board" | Supports "across the board" continuous improvement and learning | Provides alignment and acceleration of process changes and the business functions |
| Minimize errors and maximize outcomes | Best practiced by individuals and teams with Six Sigma skills | Best practiced by those that do the work | Promotes teamwork and the people (behavioral) side of change |
| Test multiple solutions quickly | Views variation as waste | Views non-value add as waste | |
| Ongoing feedback loop for iterations and process improvements. | Can take months to complete | Can achieve quick results | |
| | Uses DMAIC tollgates for report outs | Can use an A3 template to report out | |
| | ** | ** | ** |

CAP, change acceleration process; DMAIC, Define, Measure, Analyze, Improve, and Control; PDCA, Plan-Do-Check-Act; RPI, robust process improvement.
**To access additional illustrations for this table, please visit **www.springerpub.com/courseconnect**.

## TRAITS OF SUCCESS: FACTORS CONTRIBUTING TO THE SUSTAINABILITY OF SUCCESSFUL IMPROVEMENTS

To achieve the fullest potential of RPI methods and to sustain the results of PI initiatives, it is essential to take several factors into consideration. Success in sustainable improvement projects hinges on a committed leadership that not only provides a clear vision but also aligns strategies with company goals, allocating necessary resources in terms of time and personnel for project implementation. Effective communication is paramount, with messaging that elucidates initiatives, fosters a culture conducive to process improvement, and highlights the connection between improvement efforts and outcomes impacting quality, service, safety, and stakeholder experience. Additionally, leadership must support the infrastructural requirements for change, ensuring the identification of champions and sponsors and establishing a management system or council (Morfaw, 2014). A deep understanding of RPI tools and techniques is essential, coupled with ongoing training and education to enhance employee competencies. The sustainability of improvement endeavors involves refining RPI programs through policy adjustments, alignment with organizational objectives, rigorous audits, data analysis, and responsive management reviews (Morfaw, 2014). Furthermore, the selection, prioritization, and regular review of projects through DMAIC tollgates are crucial for progress. Establishing a robust reporting and tracking system facilitates accountability and transparency. Notably, addressing cultural shifts from the project's inception is imperative, as neglecting this aspect risks the initiative's eventual dissolution (Antony et al., 2017). As underscored by Antony et al. (2017), without due consideration for cultural change, the momentum of improvement efforts is at risk of waning over time.

## CASE STUDY 14.1: IMPROVEMENT IN PRACTICE

The following is a case study that illustrates efforts deployed by a community hospital in New Jersey with a goal of reducing the number of missed physical therapy visits.

**Maximizing Rehabilitation Visits (Sarah King, DPT; Pamela Randolph, DPT; Jill Anderson, MBB/PMPP; Charlene Hendrickson; and Cheryl Prall, RN)**

*Background/aim*: Rehabilitation missed visits have fluctuated between 15% and 24% over the last 3 years. Missed visits are wasted resources for any department. Reducing both no-shows and cancellations can improve productivity, positively affect the financial bottom line, and ultimately improve patient outcomes and satisfaction.

*Objective*: To reduce the number of missed visits of rehabilitation patients from 24% to 17% (the national standard) or below

*Methods*: The 2015 baseline analysis of the hospital revealed an outpatient rehabilitation missed visit rate of up to 24%. The department identified and presented this opportunity to the Lean Steering Committee, which approved a Lean Team. The Lean Leader utilized the DMAIC model to guide the performance improvement project and associated action plan. Various tools such as a formalized team charter, data collection and analysis, process mapping of both the current and future state processes, root cause analysis, brainstorming, action planning, capturing metrics, and control plan were used throughout the Lean project. The Lean Leader guided frontline staff throughout the DMAIC process. As a result, the team collaboratively arrived at a future state with key drivers, which included the following:

- Assignment of lead roles to players in the department
- Call reminders
- Patient education handouts on policy change
- The use of shared case notes
- Discharge communication between staff members to remove future appointments

This new process flow was rolled out through in-service, small groups, and staff meetings. Expectations were set and communicated.

*Results*: The baseline data for 2015 Q1 missed visit was 24%. The Lean project started in June 2015. With the new process fully implemented in Q3, a significant improvement was noted, with a 16% missed visit rate (Figure 14.6). With a rise in missed visits in November and December in Q4 due to winter variables, the year-end result was 18%. Noticing this trend, leadership regrouped the team, educated new employees, and refocused staff on the common goal. The 2016 Q1 rate was 14%, a significant change from the prior year, irrespective of winter weather challenges. As of December 2017, the missed visit rate was 13.8%. By assigning ownership, involving frontline staff members, and including them in the design of the future state, the project saw sustained success. Further, by clearly defining each team player's role, the staff held one another accountable. This quality goal was added to the staff's departmental goals, as a means of continuously motivating all key players to carry out the improved processes consistently and ensure consistent physical therapy services for patients.

**FIGURE 14.6.** Number of missed physical therapy visits.

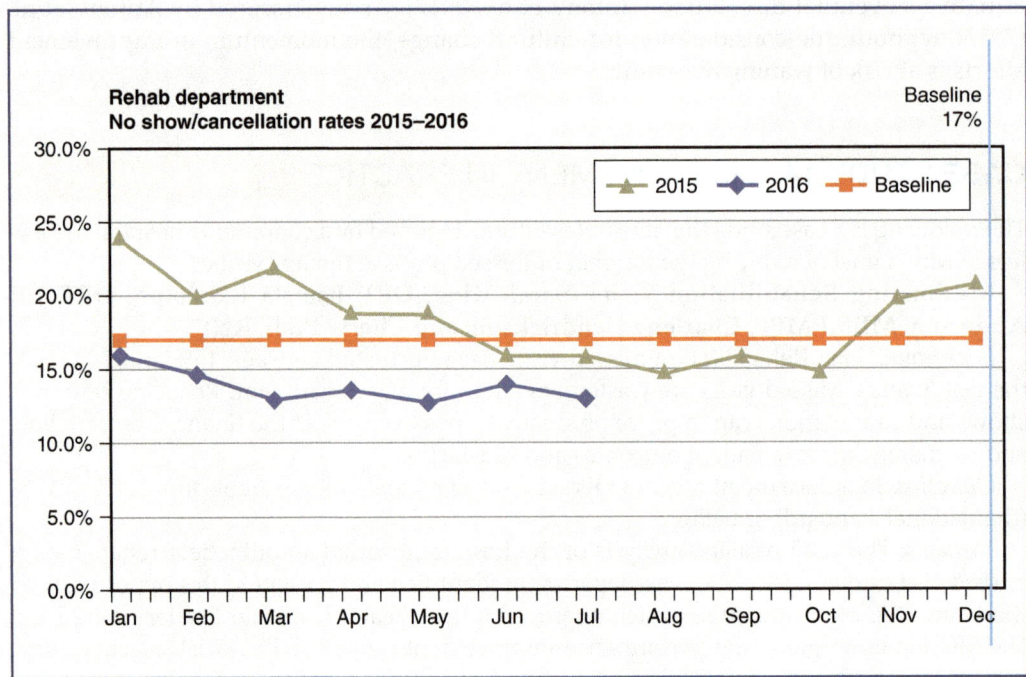

*Conclusions*: Processes put in place from this initiative resulted in a decrease in missed physical therapy visits. This project was budget neutral and resulted in additional revenue capture. The success of this project had the potential to be duplicated across service lines.

## COMMON TOOLS WITHIN THE ROBUST PROCESS IMPROVEMENT TOOLBOX

In addition to the tools identified in the case study, there are many tools to provide structure and standardization while making the delivery of healthcare safer, more effective, and person centered. See Table 14.6 for commonly used tools for problem identification, improvement, and analysis and Table 14.7 for commonly used tools for data analysis and presentation.

## TABLE 14.6. COMMONLY USED TOOLS FOR PROBLEM IDENTIFICATION, IMPROVEMENT, AND ANALYSIS

| TOOL NAME | DEFINITION | EXAMPLE | CITATION | NOTES |
|---|---|---|---|---|
| Kaizen | A Japanese word that translates loosely to "change for the better," an improvement tool with the purpose of eliminating waste and creating value for the customer. Commonly referred to as continuous improvement. | ** | The Council for Six Sigma Certification. (2018). *Six sigma green belt certification: Training manual.* Harmony Living, LLC. | Focuses on small incremental improvements. Follows the PDCA cycle. |
| Workouts | Improvement tool designed to engage and motivate all team members. | ** | Global Six Sigma. (2017). Work-out: the most effective tool for process improvement. 6sigma. https://6sigma.com/work-effective-tool-process-improvement/ | Fulfill roles and assign responsibilities. Design the event. Conduct the event. Implement decisions. |
| FMEA | A tool that can be applied during any phase to help identify risk priorities for various inputs and errors within a process. | ** | The Council for Six Sigma Certification. (2018). *Six sigma green belt certification: Training manual.* Harmony Living, LLC. | |
| RCA | Used to identify root causes or problems or defects when a team has reached the analyze phase without a clear idea of primary causation. | In addition to the fishbone, asking "why" five times is another tool to obtain the root cause(s) of an issue. | The Council for Six Sigma Certification. (2018). *Six sigma green belt certification: Training manual.* Harmony Living, LLC. | |
| Fishbone | A diagram that allows brainstorming of possible problem causes; organizes them in a logical way; and lets teams visualize priorities, trends, and relationships between the ideas. | ** | The Council for Six Sigma Certification. (2018). *Six sigma green belt certification: Training manual.* Harmony Living, LLC. | |

*(continued)*

## TABLE 14.6. COMMONLY USED TOOLS FOR PROBLEM IDENTIFICATION, IMPROVEMENT, AND ANALYSIS (CONTINUED)

| TOOL NAME | DEFINITION | EXAMPLE | CITATION | NOTES |
|---|---|---|---|---|
| Process Map | A visual diagram that uses standard shapes and connections to create a map of a process that can be understood by most employees/team members. | ** | The Council for Six Sigma Certification. (2018). *Six sigma green belt certification: Training manual.* Harmony Living, LLC. | |
| SWI | Ensures consistency, timing, and repetition of a process. The best method for producing a product or providing a service. | ** | https://www.learnleansigma.com/template/swi-template-excel/ | Takt time, work sequence, standard inventory. |
| 5S Plus Safety | A Japanese approach to organizing a workspace; relies on visual cues and a clean work area to enhance efficiencies | ** | The Council for Six Sigma Certification. (2018). *Six sigma green belt certification: Training Manual.* Harmony Living, LLC. | Sort: Remove trip hazards; Set: Straighten up to make work more accessible and easy to store; Shine: Everything is clean and working properly Standardize: Develop ongoing procedures for sort, set, and shine; Sustain: Create a culture that follows these steps each day; Safety: Modify and remove hazards for an accident-free workplace |
| Types of Waste | *Muda* is a Japanese word that translates to waste; eight types | ** | healthcare version** | DOWNTIME |
| Gemba (including Gemba walks) | A Japanese term for actual place; any place where value-creating work occurs | ** | https://citoolkit.com/templates/gemba-walk-template/; Lean Enterprise Institute. (2022, May 19). *Gemba—What does it mean?* https://www.lean.org/lexicon-terms/gemba/#:~:text=Gemba%20(%E7%8F%8F%BE%E5%A0%B4)%20is%20the%20Japanese,It%20is%20also%20spelled%20genba., | Gemba walk: Going to the site to gauge the situation through direct observation |

FMEA, failures mode and effects analysis; PDCA, Plan-Do-Check-Act; RCA, root cause analysis; SWI, standard work instructions.
**To access additional illustrations for this table, please visit www.springerpub.com/courseconnect.

## TABLE 14.7. COMMONLY USED TOOLS FOR DATA ANALYSIS AND PRESENTATION

| | TOOL | BENEFITS/USAGE | THUMBNAILS FROM QI MACROS |
|---|---|---|---|
| 1 | Descriptive Statistical: Normality | • Anderson-Darling statistic determines if data is normal.<br>• If *p*-value is >.05 data is *not* normal. (Null hypothesis, $H_0$, states that data is normal.)<br>• Most of the standard hypothesis testing tools in QI Macros work with data that is close to normal. | ** |
| 2 | Bar chart | • Compares different categories of data<br>• Visually simple, familiar, and easy to understand<br>• Does not provide statistical insights or analysis<br>• Histograms and Pareto charts are more sophisticated types of bar chart used for data analysis. | ** |
| 3 | Pie chart | • Shows the relationship of parts to a whole<br>• Visually simple, familiar, and easy to understand<br>• Difficult to interpret if too many data categories<br>• Does not provide statistical insights or analysis | ** |
| 4 | Histograms | • Show the range, shape, and spread of variable data<br>• Compare the data to the customer's requirements (specification limits)<br>• QI Macros will draw a bell curve onto the histogram and calculate the Cp, CpK, Pp, and PpK, which show how well the process is meeting customer requirements. | ** |
| 5 | Pareto | • The Pareto principle, or 80/20 rule, states that 80% of consequences result from 20% of causes.<br>• Plots causes as bars on the x-axis ranked by frequency, from most frequent on the left to least frequent on the right<br>• Line chart showing cumulative percentage is superimposed over bar chart. | ** |
| 6 | Dot plot | • Type of frequency histogram that shows distribution of data points<br>• Each data point is shown as a dot along the x-axis. Dots stack to show relative frequency.<br>• Useful if number of discrete values is limited.<br>• Difficult to interpret if too many discrete values | ** |
| 7 | Box plot | • Box plots compare data variation within and between different data sets.<br>• They contain a lot of information about the median, range, and distribution of the data in a visually simple, yet meaningful, way.<br>• The box shows the range from the 1st to 3rd quartile (IQR that contains 50% of the data), with a horizontal line showing the median (midpoint, or boundary between 2nd and 3rd quartiles).<br>• The whiskers show the highest and lowest values in the range, up to a limit of 1.5 4 IQR. Data points outside of the limit, "outliers," are shown by an "x." | ** |

*(continued)*

## TABLE 14.7. COMMONLY USED TOOLS FOR DATA ANALYSIS AND PRESENTATION (*CONTINUED*)

| | TOOL | BENEFITS/USAGE | THUMBNAILS FROM QI MACROS |
|---|---|---|---|
| 8 | Scatterplot | • Used to evaluate correlation between *x* and *y* variables<br>• Option in Excel to add a trendline that visualizes whether the correlation is negative (sloping down to the right) or positive (sloping up to the right) and how close the data points are to the trendline (indicating the strength of the correlation)<br>• QI Macros calculates the correlation coefficient *r* (slope of the line) and coefficient of determination $r^2$ (strength of the correlation).<br>• Correlation does not prove causation. | ** |
| 9 | Time series plot | • Type of line chart that plots time on the *x*-axis to show changes in *y* over time<br>• Simple and easy to understand but does not show statistical data for analysis<br>• Run charts and control charts are more sophisticated versions of time series charts used for statistical analysis of process data. | ** |
| 10 | Run chart | • A run chart is a time series plot that includes a line to indicate the midpoint of the data (choose mean/average or median).<br>• "Sigma lines" can be added to indicate 1, 2, and 3 standard deviations on either side of the midpoint.<br>• Standard deviations can be calculated (and Sigma lines added) manually in Excel or automatically in QI Macros. | ** |
| 11 | Control chart | • Type of run chart that shows the upper and lower control limits for a process.<br>• Control limits are ±3 standard deviations from the mean.<br>• For a process to be "in control," 99.7% of the data should fall within the upper and lower control limits.<br>• For a process to be "stable," there are additional rules about how the data is distributed within zones created by the Sigma lines.<br>• Stability analysis differentiates between "common cause variation" (expected variation within the control limits for the process) and special cause variation (due to an error, defect, or unforeseen circumstances). | ** |
| 12 | Hypothesis testing | • Determines whether two sets of data are the same or different, statistically<br>• Null hypothesis $H_0$ states that the two data sets are the same. Alternative hypothesis $H_a$ states that the data sets are different.<br>• If the *p* is low, the $H_0$ must go. | ** |

(*continued*)

### TABLE 14.7. COMMONLY USED TOOLS FOR DATA ANALYSIS AND PRESENTATION (*CONTINUED*)

| | TOOL | BENEFITS/USAGE | THUMBNAILS FROM QI MACROS |
|---|---|---|---|
| 12a | ANOVA | • Compares the means of more than two sets of data ($H_0$: data sets are the same)<br>• If $p > .05$ the data sets have a >95% chance of having the same mean (i.e., there is no significant difference) and if $p > .05$ the opposite is true and data sets are statistically different.<br>• Useful for determining if processes are stable under different conditions or at different times | ** |
| 12b | T-test: one sample | • Compares the mean of one data sample to a target mean ($H_0$: sample mean is equal to target mean)<br>• Use for smaller samples or samples with a known standard deviation<br>• Useful for determining if a process is meeting customer requirements | ** |
| 12c | Correlation | • Linear association between two variables, used to determine if the variation in $y$ is proportional to the variation in $x$<br>• Correlation coefficient ($r$) will always be between $-1$ and $1$.<br>• Negative correlation means that as $x$ increases, $y$ decreases; positive correlation means that as $x$ increases, $y$ also increases; zero correlation means that $x$ and $y$ are not correlated.<br>• The numerical value (i.e., closer to $-1/+1$ or closer to 0) indicates the strength of the correlation.<br>• Correlation does not prove causation. | ** |
| 12d | Regression | • Used to evaluate effects of one or more independent variables ($x_1, x_2$) on a single dependent variable ($y$)<br>• Uses coefficient of determination ($r^2$, "R squared") to establish the strength of the linear relationship between two variables. The value of $r^2$ will always be between 0 and 1.<br>• Useful for analyzing possible causes of variation in the output of a process (analyze phase of DMAIC) and/or optimal input values for a process to achieve desired output (control phase of DMAIC)<br>• Strong regression does not prove causation. | ** |
| 13 | Ishikawa fishbone diagram (under improvement tools) | • Used (along with five "whys") for root cause analysis<br>• Problem statement goes in the "head" and causes in the "bones."<br>• Main bones are categories of causes (e.g., environment, materials, personnel, equipment, policy, patients). | ** |

ANOVA, analysis of variance; DMAIC, **D**efine, **M**easure, **A**nalyze, **I**mprove, and **C**ontrol; IQR, interquartile range.
**To access additional illustrations for this table, please visit **www.springerpub.com/courseconnect**.
*Source:* Created by Zoe McInally, MBBS, MHA Rutgers University Student, CLSSGB.

## CONCLUSION

Defining quality in healthcare is a nuanced task and one that is essential for ensuring optimal patient outcomes. Healthcare organizations have a responsibility to the patients they serve to continuously strive to provide care that is safer, more effective, and more person centered. They have an obligation to focus upon quality at multiple levels in a delivery system that is considered fragmented and poorly organized and in need of transformation.

Achieving major gains in outcome, process, and structure metrics that define quality, regardless of our lack of a universal definition, would undoubtedly result in patients experiencing care that is more reliable, responsive, integrated, and widely available and move us further along the continuum to a more patient-centric (or customer-centric) model (IOM, 2001). Yet, true improvement in healthcare requires change to occur not only at the individual level in which patients experience care but also at the microsystem or provider level in which care is delivered by the team; the organizational level in which supporting functions exist in aggregate; and the external environment level which includes payment mechanisms, policy, and regulatory factors.

Our ability to measure and ultimately demonstrate quality requires us to focus upon those approaches to improvement that provide our greatest opportunity. This translates to the adoption and use of various proven strategies, tools, and techniques; the establishment of an infrastructure with committed resources; and a strong resolve by the leadership responsible. The methodologies of Lean, Six Sigma, and change management hold this tremendous promise as the backdrop for continued improvement.

## END-OF-CHAPTER RESOURCES

### CRITICAL THINKING QUESTIONS

- How does the lack of a standard definition of quality contribute to the complexity of measuring and improving the provision of care and services in healthcare?
- How do principles associated with high reliability contribute to the pressing need for organizations to focus upon all dimensions within the IOM's framework in which safety is a central requirement?
- Given that the various methodologies for quality improvement (whether using Lean, Six Sigma, or change management) offer new and compelling ways to break down organizational silos and support a culture of continuous assessment, what barriers exist to their adoption?
- Considering the various tools in existence for planning, data collection, analysis and problem-solving, and process control, what techniques and approaches offer the most significant potential for team engagement and success?
- Change is not with its challenges. Propose ways in which you would address those resistant to change. How does leadership set the tone for a culture that values continuous improvement, defining quality as a strategic priority?

### LEARNING ACTIVITIES

**CourseConnect ▸**

To access self-assessment questions and interactive, competency-based learning activities for this chapter, visit www.springerpub.com/courseconnect. See inside front cover and tear-out card for CourseConnect details.

### REFERENCES

12 critical success factors for Six Sigma effectiveness. (2002). *Measuring Business Excellence*, 6(3). https://doi.org/10.1108/mbe.2002.26706cab.007

Achibat, F. E., Lebkiri, A., Aouane, E. M., Lougraimzi, H., Berrid, N., & Maqboul, A. (2023). Analysis of the impact of six sigma and lean manufacturing on the performance of companies. *Management Systems in Production Engineering*, 31(2), 191–196. https://doi.org/10.2478/mspe-2023-0020

Admin. (2019, March 12). California Hospital's success shows possibilities of health IT, Lean Six Sigma. *Six Sigma Daily*. https://www.sixsigmadaily.com/hospital-success-health-it-lean-six-sigma/

Antony, J., Snee, R. D., & Hoerl, R. W. (2017). Lean Six Sigma: Yesterday, today and tomorrow. *International Journal of Quality & Reliability Management*, 34(7), 1073–1093. https://doi.org/10.1108/ijqrm-03-2016-0035

Brook, Q. (2022). *Lean Six Sigma and Minitab: The complete toolbox guide for business improvement*. OPEX Resources.

Centers for Medicare and Medicaid Services. 2023. *Quality measures.* Accessed September 24, 2023/ update. https://www.cms.gov/Medicare/QualityInitiatives-Patient-Assessment-Instruments/QualityMeasures

Chassin, M. R., & Loeb, J. M. (2013). High-reliability health care: Getting there from here. *The Milbank Quarterly*, 91(3), 459–490. https://doi.org/10.1111/1468-0009.12023

Cho, H. J., Khalil, S., Poeran, J., Mazumdar, M., Bravo, N. G., Wallach, F., Markoff, B., Lee, N., & Dunn, A. (2017). "Lose the tube": A choosing Wisely initiative to reduce catheter-associated urinary tract infections in hospitalist-led inpatient units. *American Journal of Infection Control*, 45(3), 333–335. https://doi.org/10.1016/j.ajic.2016.10.023

Crosby, P. B. (1979). *Quality is free: The art of making quality certain*. McGraw-Hill Book.

Dawson, A. (2019). A Practical Guide to performance improvement: change acceleration process and Techniques to maintain improvements. *AORN Journal*, 111(1), 97–102. https://doi.org/10.1002/aorn.12895

Doll, M. C. (2010). Apathy toward patient safety: Has 10 years made a difference? *Journal of American Association of Physician Assistants*, 23(2), 26–30. https://doi.org/10.1097/01720610-201002000-00005

Donabedian, A. (1980). *The definition of quality and approaches to its assessment*. Health Administration Press.

Donabedian, A. (1988). The quality of care: How can it be assessed? *JAMA*, 260(12), 1743–1748. https://doi.org/10.1001/jama.260.12.1743

Donabedian, A. (2005). Evaluating the quality of medical care. *The Milbank Quarterly*, 83(4), 691–729. https://doi.org/10.1111/j.1468-0009.2005.00397.x

Elboq, R., Hlyal, M., & Alami, J. E. (2020). Lean manufacturing and Six Sigma critical success factors -A case study of the Moroccan Aeronautic Industry. *International Journal of Supply Chain Management*, 9(4), 24–35. https://doi.org/10.59160/ijscm.v9i4.3777

Emanuel, L., Berwick, D., Conway, J., Combes, J., Hatlie, M., Leape, L., Reason, J., Schyve, P., Vincent, C., & Walton, M. (2008). What exactly is patient safety? In K. Henriksen, James B. Battles, Margaret A. Keyes, Mary L. Grady (Eds.), *Advances in patient safety: New directions and alternative approaches* (Vol. 1: Assessment). Agency for Healthcare Research and Quality.

Evans, D. B., Edejer, T. T., Lauer, J., Frenk, J., & Murray, C. J. (2001). Measuring quality: From the system to the provider. *International Society for Quality in Health Care*, 13(6), 439–446. https://doi.org/10.1093/intqhc/13.6.439

Feldman, K. (2023, August 5). How CAP can revolutionize your organization's change management. *isixsigma.com*. https://www.isixsigma.com/dictionary/change-acceleration-process-cap/

Frankel, A, Haraden., C., Federico, F., & Lenoci-Edwards, J. (2017) *A framework for safe, reliable, and effective care*. Institute for Healthcare Improvement and Safe & Reliable Healthcare White Paper.

Grailey, K. E., Murray, E., Reader, T., & Brett, S. J. (2021). The presence and potential impact of psychological safety in the healthcare setting: An evidence synthesis. *BMC Health Services Research*, 21(1), 773. https://doi.org/10.1186/s12913-021-06740-6

Hibbert, P. D., Basedow, M., Braithwaite, J., Wiles, L. K., Clay-Williams, R., & Padbury, R. (2021). How to sustainably build capacity in quality improvement within a healthcare organisation: A deep-dive, focused qualitative analysis. *BMC Health Services Research*, 21(1), 588. https://doi.org/10.1186/s12913-021-06598-8

Institute of Medicine (US) Committee on Quality of Health Care in America. (2001). *Crossing the quality chasm: A new health system for the 21st century*. National Academies Press (US).

Joint Commission International. (n.d.). High reliability training. https://www.jointcommissioninternational.org/what-we-offer/high-reliability/high-reliability-training/robust-process-improvement/

Juran, J. M. (2005). The quality trilogy. In John C. Wood and Michael C. Wood (Eds.), *Joseph M. Juran: Critical Evaluations in Business and Management* (Vol. 19, p. 54). Routledge.

King, P. L. (2019). *Lean for the process industries: Dealing with complexity* (2nd ed.) Productivity Press.

Lean Enterprise Institute. (2023, January 27). *What is lean?—Lean thinking*. Lean Enterprise Institute. https://www.lean.org/explore-lean/what-is-lean/

Lohr, K. (1990) Committee to design a strategy for quality review and assurance. In Medicare (Ed.), *Medicare: A strategy for quality assurance* (Vol. 1). National Academy Press (US).

Miller, K. (2020, March 19). 5 steps in the change management process. *HBS Online. Business Insights Blog*. https://online.hbs.edu/blog/post/change-management-process

Morfaw, J. (2014). *Fundamentals of project sustainability*. [Paper presentation] PMI® Global Congress 2014—North America, Phoenix, AZ. Newtown Square, PA. Project Management Institute.

Nuckols, T. K., Escarce, J. J., & Asch, S. M. (2013). The effects of quality of care on costs: A conceptual framework. *The Milbank Quarterly*, 91(2), 316–353. https://doi.org/10.1111/milq.12015

Pellegrini, C. A. (2015). High reliability science and surgery: The Joint Commission's Process Improvement Methodology. *The Bulletin.* https://bulletin.facs.org/2015/10/high-reliability-science-and-surgery-the-joint-commissions-robust-process-improvement-methodology/

Plsek, P. E., & Greenhalgh, T. (2001). Complexity science: The challenge of complexity in health care. *BMJ, 323*(7313), 625–628. https://doi.org/10.1136/bmj.323.7313.625

Polonsky, M. S. (2019). High-reliability organizations: The next frontier in healthcare quality and safety. *Journal of Healthcare Management/American College of Healthcare Executives, 64*(4), 213–221. https://doi.org/10.1097/JHM-D-19-00098

Simon, R. W., & Canacari, E. (2011). A practical guide to applying lean tools and management principles to health care improvement projects. *AORN Journal, 95*(1), 85–103. https://doi.org/10.1016/j.aorn.2011.05.021

Swinand, A. (2023). Why kindness at work pays off. *Harvard Business Review.* https://hbr.org/2023/07/why-kindness-at-work-pays-off?

Timans, W., Antony, J., Ahaus, K., & Van Solingen, R. (2012). Implementation of Lean Six Sigma in small- and medium-sized manufacturing enterprises in the Netherlands. *Journal of the Operational Research Society, 63*(3), 339–353. https://doi.org/10.1057/jors.2011.47

Weick, K., & Sutcliff, K. (2015). *Managing the unexpected: Assuring high performance in an age of complexity* (3rd ed.). Jossey-Bass.

CHAPTER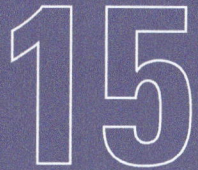

# PROJECT MANAGEMENT IN HEALTHCARE

Allen K. Solenberg, Jr. and Roie S. Rennert

## LEARNING OBJECTIVES

- Understand the importance of project management in healthcare for optimizing processes and outcomes.
- Comprehend the critical phases of healthcare project management: initiation, planning, execution, monitoring, and evaluation.
- Explore the challenges specific to healthcare projects and strategies to address them.
- Analyze real-world healthcare project cases to derive lessons and best practices.
- Apply project management tools and techniques to solve healthcare management problems.

## KEY TERMS

- Evaluation
- Execution
- Monitoring
- Planning
- Project management

## INTRODUCTION TO PROJECT MANAGEMENT IN HEALTHCARE

Initially developed for large-scale engineering projects in the early 20th century, **project management** has evolved into a distinct methodology designed to achieve specific objectives within set constraints (Meredith et al., 2017). Its principles have been adapted for various industries, including healthcare, where the complexity of medical technologies and systems necessitates structured management approaches. In healthcare, project management is critical for enhancing patient care quality, streamlining operations, and handling industrial complexities (Heldman, 2018).

This chapter comprehensively explores healthcare project management, covering its core principles, challenges, strategies, and tools. It begins by emphasizing the importance of project management in improving processes and patient outcomes through systematic methodologies. Subsequent sections detail the critical phases of healthcare project management—initiation, planning, execution, monitoring, and evaluation—focusing on strategic goal setting, resource allocation, stakeholder engagement, and alignment with overarching objectives.

Project management is applied to various healthcare projects, from small-scale improvements to major implementations like system-wide electronic health records (EHRs). Its versatility in healthcare is demonstrated through its application in grassroots enhancements and broad strategic initiatives. Real-world case studies, such as EHR implementation and hospital expansion, provide insights into successful practices and tools like Gantt charts and Agile methodologies in optimizing project outcomes.

## KEY PHASES OF HEALTHCARE PROJECT MANAGEMENT

### INITIATION PHASE

The initiation phase is the foundational step in starting a project, leading to detailed planning and execution. In this phase, project managers and teams create a business case to articulate the problem, expected benefits, and alignment with organizational goals (Singh & Williams, 2021). Key activities include defining project requirements, determining stakeholder teams, appointing a project sponsor, and outlining responsibilities. This phase also involves assembling initial documentation to help leaders decide whether to approve, modify, delay, or reject the project (Singh & Williams, 2021).

The creation of the project charter marks a critical point in this phase. This document serves as an official affirmation of the project's initiation, detailing project goals, scope, key stakeholders, and the boundaries of project activities (Singh & Williams, 2021). It ensures that all parties understand what the project will and will not cover. At the outset, the project manager sets the context by defining its background, the challenges or opportunities addressed, and an outline of expected deliverables and high-level strategies. This stage includes identifying an executive sponsor who will champion the project to senior leadership and be accountable for its success. Project timelines, budget estimates, and potential risks are also forecasted.

Furthermore, the initiation phase includes detailed planning of end-user requirements and stakeholder roles necessary for successful project completion. The project manager's authority and responsibilities are clearly defined, collaborating with stakeholders to delegate tasks. This culminates in the creation of a stakeholder register included in the project charter. A communication plan is also established, detailing meeting frequencies, preferred communication methods, and schedules for updating on project progress (Singh & Williams, 2021).

### PLANNING PHASE

The **planning** phase is critical for setting the stage for successful execution by refining the project scope, objectives, requirements, and methodologies (Singh & Williams, 2021). This phase involves several key steps, such as identifying stakeholders, detailing project requirements, defining the project scope, conducting risk assessments, creating a resource plan, establishing a project schedule, and defining metrics and key performance indicators (KPIs). It also includes drafting a detailed project management plan.

A central element of this phase is the risk/issue register, a vital tool for managing potential and current challenges in healthcare projects (Tables 15.1 and 15.2). This register tracks risks with their impacts and mitigation strategies; logs current issues with assigned responsibilities; maintains project alignment with goals; and fosters a proactive, transparent culture among stakeholders.

Stakeholder alignment is crucial; it involves gathering key participants such as clinical leaders, technology teams, administrators, and patients to ensure everyone is on board with the project's vision and objectives. Facilitated discussions help stakeholders

### TABLE 15.1. SAMPLE RISK REGISTER

| RISK ID | RISK DESCRIPTION | PROBABILITY (LOW/ MEDIUM/HIGH) | IMPACT (LOW/ MEDIUM/ HIGH) | MITIGATION STRATEGIES | OWNER |
|---|---|---|---|---|---|
| R01 | Delay in delivery of medical equipment | Medium | High | Coordinate with alternate suppliers; increase order lead time | John Doe |
| R02 | Changes in healthcare regulations affecting project scope | Low | High | Regular monitoring of regulatory updates; engage a healthcare compliance consultant | Jane Smith |
| R03 | Data migration delays due to incompatible legacy systems | High | Medium | Conduct a premigration systems assessment; plan for additional data cleansing and mapping resources | Alex Johnson |

### TABLE 15.2. SAMPLE ISSUE REGISTER

| ISSUE ID | ISSUE DESCRIPTION | DETECTED ON | IMPACT | ACTION TAKEN | RESOLUTION DEADLINE | OWNER |
|---|---|---|---|---|---|---|
| I01 | Critical software bug identified in the testing phase | 03/15/2024 | High | Deployed immediate patch; scheduled for a comprehensive fix in next update | 03/20/2024 | Chris Lee |
| I02 | Staff resistance to new EHR system implementation | 03/10/2024 | Medium | Initiated additional targeted training sessions; organized feedback sessions to address concerns | Ongoing | Morgan Taylor |
| I03 | Overrun of the project budget in the execution phase | 03/20/2024 | High | Reviewed financial allocations; identified noncritical expenditures for reduction; applied for additional funding | 04/01/2024 | Jamie Rivera |

EHR, electronic health record.

understand and agree upon the project scope and requirements, which are documented to minimize ambiguity. This clear definition helps guide all subsequent project activities, from resource allocation to timeline creation. Resource planning allocates necessary human, material, and financial resources based on project scope and objectives, adjusting as needed to address resource misalignments. This planning is essential to avoid delays and unnecessary costs. The project schedule, detailed with milestones and task dependencies, ensures efficient, coordinated progress across functional areas.

Finally, establishing metrics and KPIs allows monitoring of ongoing project performance and outcomes. KPIs are crucial for tracking efficiency and effectiveness and are directly linked to project objectives and requirements. The comprehensive project management plan that results from this phase includes governance policies, communication protocols, change management procedures, and strategies for team engagement, providing a roadmap for project execution.

## EXECUTION PHASE

The **execution** phase marks the transition of healthcare projects from planning to action, where concepts are realized through team collaboration (Singh & Williams, 2021). During this phase, project managers effectively coordinate all project components and stakeholder activities, adapting to the inherent volatility of the healthcare environment (Mansaray, 2019). This volatility often requires agile responses to scope changes and unforeseen challenges, protecting the project's objectives and requirements.

Effective change management strategies and risk mitigation plans developed during the planning phase are critical in managing adjustments. Throughout the execution phase, maintaining clear communication and structured coordination is essential. Regular status meetings, project management tools, and real-time reporting dashboards ensure that all stakeholders are informed and engaged. These gatherings align team efforts and celebrate key achievements, boosting motivation and fostering a collaborative atmosphere. The team's ability to translate planning into tangible outcomes while remaining flexible and responsive to changing circumstances is pivotal. This approach enables healthcare projects to navigate uncertainties and drive meaningful change effectively.

*Practical point:* Think of the execution phase as the time in the project when we "actually do the work."

## MONITORING PHASE

The **monitoring** phase ensures that the healthcare project remains aligned with its objectives as execution unfolds (Singh & Williams, 2021). This phase utilizes the metrics and KPIs established during the planning phase to assess project health and monitor progress. It embodies the principle of "measure twice, cut once," maintaining rigorous oversight over the project's execution.

This phase enables comprehensive monitoring through a variety of tools and protocols. Project management platforms provide real-time updates on task status, milestone completion, and schedule adherence. Automated reports offer insights into budget and resource utilization (Figure 15.1), while dashboards visualize KPIs for quick evaluation. Regular meetings focus on reviewing progress, discussing deviations, and making necessary adjustments.

This vigilant oversight allows the team to detect early signs of deviation from planned paths, enabling timely interventions to prevent more significant issues. Adjustments made during this phase help realign the project with its intended schedule, resources, scope, and quality objectives. The Monitoring Phase is crucial in securing successful outcomes for healthcare projects by fostering continuous vigilance, adaptation, and data-driven decision-making.

**FIGURE 15.1.** Pie chart showcasing the allocation of resources in a medical equipment procurement project.

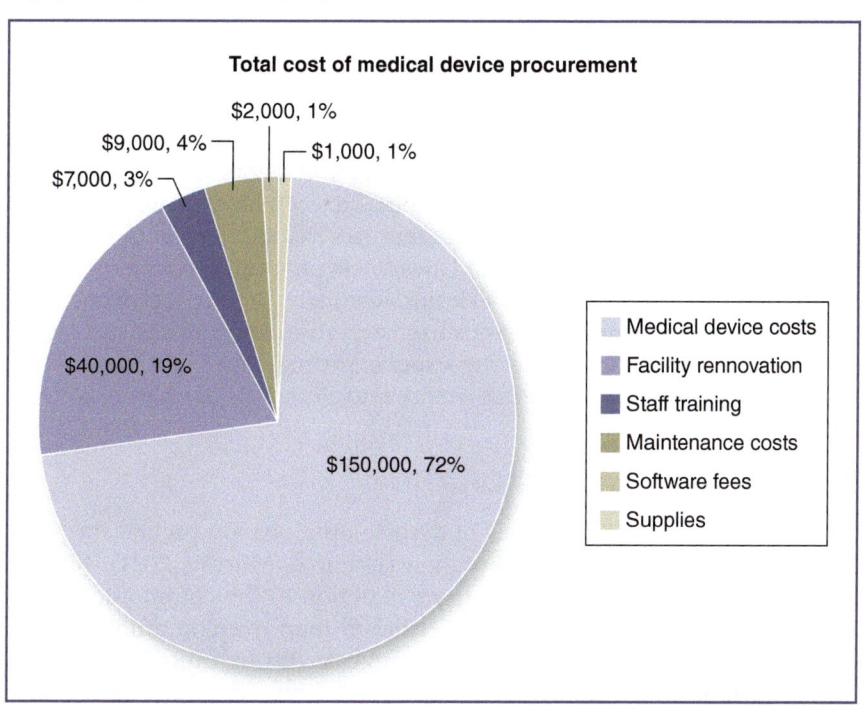

## EVALUATION PHASE

Following project execution, the **evaluation** phase allows for a reflective assessment to learn and improve for future projects (Singh & Williams, 2021). This phase focuses on analyzing what worked well, what did not, and how the project's outcomes align with the initially set objectives and requirements. Through this evaluation, the team can identify whether goals were met or exceeded or if there were any shortfalls, using metrics data to pinpoint effective strategies (Aburayya et al., 2020).

Feedback from stakeholders, including patients, clinicians, administrators, and team members, adds a subjective layer to the evaluation, offering diverse perspectives on their satisfaction with the project results and processes. This feedback provides essential context and highlights areas for improvement. The evaluation phase is crucial for extracting lessons learned, reflecting on challenges, and examining changes and team dynamics. These insights are instrumental in refining future project management practices, contributing to a cycle of continuous improvement. By systematically evaluating project results and stakeholder experiences, healthcare organizations can enhance project outcomes and raise overall performance standards over time.

## CHALLENGES IN HEALTHCARE PROJECT MANAGEMENT AND STRATEGIES

### REGULATORY AND COMPLIANCE

Healthcare operates in a complex regulatory environment which poses significant project management challenges (Scoleze Ferrer et al., 2020). Rather than having deep regulatory expertise, successful project managers assemble and engage specialized experts to ensure compliance. A robust compliance team provides legal and regulatory knowledge to identify issues and requirements related to laws like the Health Insurance Portability and Accountability Act (HIPAA) and the Health Information Technology for Economic and Clinical Health Act (HITECH; Miller & Payne, 2016). Project managers must integrate experts into planning to assess risks and shape mitigation strategies. Ongoing engagement ensures protocols adhere to regulations.

Comprehensive documentation also provides evidence of compliance across project phases. Detailed audit trails, transparent reporting, and rigorous recordkeeping demonstrate adherence if scrutinized by oversight bodies. Project managers institute processes for thorough documentation. Continual training reinforces a culture of compliance from leadership to frontline staff. Routine education and awareness programs on regulatory needs make compliance a collective responsibility at all levels. Regulatory and compliance challenges demand a collaborative effort combining specialized expertise, comprehensive documentation, and organizational education. By enabling experts, maintaining vigilance, and promoting awareness, project managers integrate adherence into all aspects of project execution.

## INTERDISCIPLINARY COLLABORATION

Effective communication and synthesis of diverse opinions are pivotal for project managers to foster interdisciplinary collaboration (Urton & Murray, 2021). Recent studies indicate leaders frequently need to pay more attention to the communication required; undercommunicating risks 10 times more criticism than overcommunicating (Flynn & Lide, 2022). Project managers must overcommunicate through regular meetings, status reports, and collaborative platforms. Tailored messaging resonates with each group's priorities—whether clinicians, administrators, or patients. Iterative feedback loops ensure continued engagement to surface concerns. Change impacts are transparently conveyed. Furthermore, synthesizing varied viewpoints into unifying project goals requires perspective-taking, empathy, conflict resolution, and finding compromises to align relevant stakeholders. Through compassionate leadership and clear communication, project managers enable interdisciplinary collaboration.

*Practical point:* The amount of materials, tools, and responsibilities under the project manager's purview can appear overwhelming. Fundamentally, a project manager is an information synthesizer and expert communicator who seeks to create situational awareness for teammates and senior leaders and, through that communication, drive the project forward. The project manager is the "quarterback" who provides the information necessary for their teammates to succeed.

## RESOURCE CONSTRAINTS

Healthcare projects often have budget limitations, equipment shortages, overloaded personnel, and other constraints (Bacelar-Silva et al., 2022). Judiciously managing scarce resources poses a significant challenge. Project managers must collaborate closely with department leaders to negotiate resourcing trade-offs and prioritization. Open communication about constraints sparks creative problem-solving, like cross-department equipment sharing.

Resource optimization techniques distribute limited assets strategically across critical activities. Accurate task and workload estimation informs realistic plans within constraints, and schedule refinements can distribute demands over time. Taking a system-wide view beyond departmental silos enables better collective resource planning. For instance, centralized asset management systems provide visibility into project equipment availability. A portfolio lens highlights redundancies and facilitates coordinated allocations. Resource constraints necessitate interdepartmental collaboration and alignment of priorities to execute projects strategically. Open dialogue, creative resourcing, workload balancing, and systems thinking optimize allocations to achieve objectives despite limitations.

*Practical point:* Commonly, projects must abide by the "iron triangle" rules, which manage project scope, budget, and schedule. Another way of thinking about this is managing how much of the project we can complete versus how fast we can complete the project versus how expensive it will be to complete the project.

## PATIENT-CENTERED APPROACH

Adopting a patient-centered approach presents significant opportunities and complex challenges (Blount, 2019). At the heart of this approach is ensuring that patient needs, preferences, and well-being are integral to project outcomes, which requires carefully balancing diverse priorities. Key to this balance is integrating patient perspectives into project requirements and planning. Methods such as surveys, focus groups, and advisory councils are instrumental in capturing patient insights to shape project objectives.

It is crucial to minimize care disruptions during project transitions. Effective change management strategies—like staggered rollouts, scheduling during off-peak hours, contingency planning, and robust communication—help mitigate impacts while maintaining patient safety and continuity of care. Implementing patient-centered solutions, though challenging, significantly enhances project value. For example, implementing an EHR should improve patient access to and exchange of medical information. Authentic patient engagement involves shared decision-making, coordinated care, and ensuring responsive access, all reflecting patient priorities.

Success in patient-centric projects demands collaboration among users, clinicians, project teams, and patients. Continuous patient feedback during project execution fosters ongoing improvements. Embracing a spirit of compassion and partnership positions patients as active participants in shaping their care experiences. A genuinely patient-centered approach requires that healthcare projects be designed collaboratively, keeping patient interests at the core. This focus aligns projects with their intended goals and values and serves as the guiding principle or "north star" for project endeavors. Moreover, understanding the challenges and pitfalls common in projects is vital for project managers, preparing them to navigate complexities effectively (Table 15.3).

### TABLE 15.3. REASONS FOR PROJECT FAILURE AND COMMON MITIGATION TECHNIQUES

| REASON FOR FAILURE | MITIGATION TECHNIQUE |
| --- | --- |
| Lack of clear objectives and vision | Establish and communicate well-defined, achievable goals that align with organizational strategies. |
| Inadequate stakeholder engagement | Involve key stakeholders early and frequently in the planning and decision-making processes to ensure alignment and buy-in. |
| Poor communication | Implement structured communication plans specifying frequency, channels, and updated content to keep all stakeholders informed and engaged. |
| Insufficient planning and resource allocation | Conduct detailed planning sessions to estimate resource needs accurately and build contingency plans for potential challenges. |
| Lack of flexibility | Remain open to changes and agile in responding to new information or external pressures, adjusting project plans as necessary. |
| Ineffective risk management | Identify potential risks early, assess their impact, and develop strategic mitigation or contingency plans. Continuously monitor for new risks throughout the project. |

## CASE STUDY 15.1: ELECTRONIC HEALTH RECORDS IMPLEMENTATION

Boston Medical Center: EHR Implementation Case Study: https://www.ncbi.nlm.nih.gov/pmc/articles/PMC6102772/.

*Challenge:* Transitioning from paper-based to digital records requires overcoming technical hurdles, changing resistance from staff accustomed to traditional methods, and ensuring data security and patient privacy amid the digital landscape (Starren et al., 2021).

*Example:* The Boston Medical Center (BMC) implemented the Epic EHR system in 2012. At the time, BMC was the largest safety-net hospital in the United States, with over 400,000 yearly patient visits. The implementation process was complex and challenging, but BMC overcame the obstacles and successfully transitioned to an EHR system.

*Strategy:* BMC's EHR implementation team employed various strategies to tackle its challenges. To surmount technical barriers, the team invested in extensive training and support for staff. In combating resistance to change, the team highlighted the benefits of the EHR system to staff and actively involved them in the decision-making process. To safeguard data security and patient privacy, the team instituted stringent security protocols and conducted training on HIPAA compliance.

*Success:* BMC's EHR implementation has been a success. The system has improved patient care by streamlining data access, enabling clinicians to make informed decisions more quickly. It has also enhanced care coordination and reduced the risk of medical errors. BMC has also seen improvements in operational efficiency, with reduced paperwork and streamlined billing and coding.

*Lessons learned:* One critical lesson from BMC's EHR implementation is the importance of thorough staff training. BMC also learned that it is essential to address resistance to change through clear communication and engagement strategies. Additionally, involving clinical staff in designing and customizing EHR interfaces ensures that systems align with their workflow, fostering smoother adoption.

Table 15.4 provides a detailed overview of the roles and responsibilities that contributed to BMC's successful implementation of the EHR system.

**TABLE 15.4. SAMPLE ROLES AND RESPONSIBILITIES IN BMC'S EHR IMPLEMENTATION PROJECT**

| ROLE | RESPONSIBILITIES |
|---|---|
| Executive Sponsor (CIO) | Provide project oversight, secure funding, and ensure alignment with the hospital's strategic goals |
| Project Manager | Coordinate the project initiation, develop the project charter, and assemble the project team |
| IT Department Leaders | Oversee technical planning, including system architecture, hardware requirements, and data migration strategies |
| Clinical Leads | Work alongside IT to tailor the EHR system to clinical needs, ensuring usability and effectiveness for healthcare providers |
| Training Coordinator | Develop and execute a comprehensive training program for all end users, including physicians, nurses, and administrative staff |
| Implementation Teams | Comprised of IT specialists, clinical staff, and vendor representatives; responsible for system setup, customization, and testing |
| Change Management Specialists | Address resistance and facilitate adaptation among staff to the new EHR system |

*(continued)*

**TABLE 15.4. SAMPLE ROLES AND RESPONSIBILITIES IN BMC'S EHR IMPLEMENTATION PROJECT** (*CONTINUED*)

| ROLE | RESPONSIBILITIES |
|---|---|
| Quality Assurance Teams | Monitor the EHR system's performance post-implementation, identifying issues and implementing fixes |
| Data Analysts | Monitor system usage and performance metrics to provide insights for ongoing improvements |
| Project Evaluation Team | Assess the project's overall success against objectives post-implementation, including impact on patient care and operational efficiency |
| Feedback Coordinators | Gather and analyze end-user feedback to identify areas for improvement and lessons learned for future projects |

BMC, Boston Medical Center; CIO, chief information officer; EHR, electronic health records; IT, information technology.

## CASE STUDY 15.2: STAFF AUGMENTATION AND VIRTUALIZATION

PRISM Vision Group (PVG) is a vertically integrated company with 150+ eyecare specialists and over 100 locations in the Mid-Atlantic United States. PVG includes optometrists, ophthalmologists, and retina specialists who provide eye care services ranging from routine eye exams to cataract surgeries and retina-specific treatments.

*Challenge:* Recruitment and retention difficulties in the healthcare industry adversely affect office staffing levels and patient care (Singh et al., 2019). High clinical and nonclinical staff turnover is costly from a recruitment and training perspective and can hinder office flow and provider efficiency. Clinical staff, including physician scribes, are integral care team members who can comprehensively document patient visit details and function as nonprovider physician extenders, allowing physicians to serve more patients.

*Example:* In 2023, PVG piloted a program to "virtualize" clinical scribes for their retina specialists, providing an opportunity for clinical staff to work remotely while still serving the practice. Virtual scribes, recruited nationwide, would be linked into the practice via Zoom. The providers and virtual scribes wearing Bluetooth headsets would share their screens and communicate, updating the patient care visit in the EHR in real time. The aim was to recruit 50 virtual scribes by Q2:2023 and serve physicians in each retina care division.

*Strategy:* The virtual scribe project was agile and consisted of iterative sprints to build momentum and establish quick wins. PVG devised a plan to bring managerial oversight to the virtual scribe program and develop a specialized recruitment lane to recruit virtual scribes nationwide. The new manager was a highly trained former in-person scribe and trainer and rapidly developed a curriculum for training scribes virtually. On-site assessments identified pain points and ensured that the proper equipment and workflows were in place at offices to ensure program success.

*Success:* The program expanded the potential recruitment pool and recruited exceptionally talented former in-person scribes seeking remote work. Individuals were more engaged (as measured by company engagement scores) and had a consistent workforce (as measured by turnover) than their in-person peers. Providers extolled the program, claiming they could serve more patients and that the scribes' dictation and charting were "best in class".

*Lessons learned:* There were two critical lessons learned in the virtual scribe program. The first was that changing the work-from-home macroenvironment disadvantaged industries requiring an in-person presence. To PVG, this presented a unique strategy to allow disaffected former scribes to practice their craft from the comfort of their homes, thus increasing candidate pools and scribe retention. The second lesson spoke to the importance of assigning accountability and managerial ownership. PVG could focus on scaling the program while optimizing office workflows by appointing a dedicated manager.

*Practical point:* The issue of organizational focus on successful project outcomes cannot be understated. Often, attention, not ability, determines how quickly and well a project can be completed.

## APPLICATION OF PROJECT MANAGEMENT TOOLS AND TECHNIQUES IN HEALTHCARE

### GANTT CHARTS AND TIMELINES

Gantt charts and timelines are essential in healthcare project management, providing a visual roadmap from the beginning to the end of a project (Kerzner, 2017). These tools extend beyond mere organization; they improve resource allocation and strategic planning. Gantt charts display project milestones, tasks, subtasks, and interdependencies, which are essential for managing the complex coordination of healthcare projects (Figure 15.2). The tools act as a common reference point, aiding stakeholders in understanding task durations, overlaps, and critical path activities, which supports informed decision-making and helps avoid bottlenecks.

The strategic application of Gantt charts ensures timely project completion and efficient resource distribution. Gantt charts enable project managers to allocate resources—personnel, equipment, and facilities—optimally, effectively meeting project requirements. Additionally, Gantt charts assist in identifying potential resource conflicts, allowing managers to proactively adjust allocations or timelines to improve operational efficiency and cost-effectiveness (Heagney, 2016).

**FIGURE 15.2.** Gantt chart depicting facility expansion project.

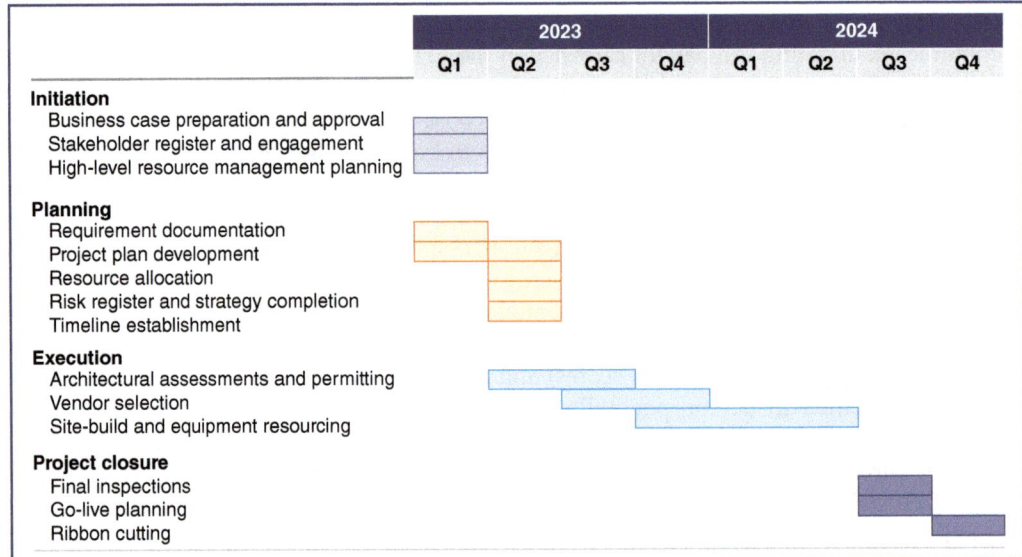

Additionally, Gantt charts promote accountability and transparency. Each milestone has an assigned responsible party, which clarifies ownership and aids in progress tracking. The visual display of task progression enables team members to evaluate their contributions and pinpoint areas needing focus. Regular updates on the Gantt chart keep all stakeholders informed, foster collaboration, and allow quick responses to project deviations.

## RISK ASSESSMENT AND MANAGEMENT

Risk assessment and management are vital in healthcare project management, guiding teams through the complex factors influencing patient safety and project success. This process is crucial for pinpointing and addressing healthcare-specific risks, including clinical errors, regulatory noncompliance, technological failures, and privacy breaches (Singh & Williams, 2021).

A thorough understanding of healthcare dynamics is necessary to pinpoint risks accurately. Healthcare projects intersect with critical areas like patient care, regulatory adherence, and data security, making them particularly vulnerable to various challenges. Identifying risks is the initial step in crafting projects that preemptively consider and counteract potential problems. Effective risk management strategies are vital to maintaining patient safety and ensuring regulatory compliance (Wang et al., 2023). Strategies involve assessing potential risks' likelihood and impact and developing preventive measures and contingency plans. This proactive approach is crucial in minimizing and managing risks efficiently.

Beyond preventing financial losses, healthcare risk management prioritizes patient well-being and care quality (Chakraborty, 2019). This might include implementing comprehensive staff training, adhering strictly to health regulations, setting up redundant systems to handle technical disruptions, and performing regular security audits to protect patient information. The strategy's effectiveness depends on seamless integration into the overall project planning and execution, establishing a vigilant, patient-focused culture within the organization.

Part of project risk assessment includes the ongoing management of known issues that appear throughout project execution. Commonly, project managers maintain an "issue log" that documents the nature of the problem encountered, the date of the issue, the steps taken to resolve the issue, the responsible party for issue resolution, and the expected resolution date (First Step for Consultancy & Training, 2022). Managing risks and issues effectively is crucial for project success. According to Wonjo (2022), there are four generally accepted strategies for handling challenges in project management:

- *Avoidance:* This strategy involves taking proactive steps to prevent an issue or risk entirely or to a significant extent. By anticipating potential problems in advance, project teams can plan to avoid them altogether.
- *Mitigation:* While some risks cannot be avoided entirely, mitigation strategies aim to reduce their impact or likelihood. This approach involves implementing measures that lessen the severity of the risk's effects should it materialize.
- *Transference:* Sometimes, the best approach is to transfer the risk or issue to a third party. This means assigning the responsibility for managing the risk to another entity that will bear the consequences and manage the resolution.
- *Acceptance:* Sometimes, the cost of mitigating a risk may outweigh the benefits, or the risk may not significantly threaten the project's overall success. In such cases, the risk is accepted as part of the project's inherent challenges.

Risk assessment and management are crucial in healthcare projects, underscoring a commitment to patient safety and care quality. These processes are integral to maintaining high standards of care by pinpointing specific risks and employing targeted mitigation strategies. Integrating risk management into project activities reinforces a healthcare organization's dedication to ethical practices, regulatory compliance, and excellence in service delivery.

## AGILE METHODOLOGIES IN HEALTHCARE PROJECTS

Integrating Agile methodologies into healthcare project management responds strategically to the dynamic nature of the healthcare sector. Agile is a cultural shift and a project management approach emphasizing continuous learning and improvement (Ciric Lalic et al., 2022). It empowers teams to handle uncertainties and enhances flexibility in executing projects. Agile requires moving away from traditional, linear "waterfall" methods to accommodate the constant advancements, evolving patient needs, and regulatory changes characteristic of healthcare (Table 15.5). Rooted initially in software development, Agile is particularly effective in healthcare due to its adaptability to change.

Agile divides projects into short, manageable phases or "sprints," promoting iterative development. This structure supports continuous feedback loops, allowing teams to learn and adapt rapidly. Unlike traditional methods that define the entire project scope upfront, Agile is flexible, adapting to new insights and changes throughout the project lifecycle. This approach is congruent with evidence-based medical practices, integrating ongoing medical insights. The inherent flexibility of Agile suits the unpredictable healthcare environment. It enables project teams to adjust objectives in response to new clinical data, patient feedback, or regulatory updates. Agile's adaptability facilitates timely adjustments, ensuring project alignment with patient needs and the broader healthcare context. Regular, collaborative interactions among multidisciplinary stakeholders enhance transparency, prevent silos, and utilize diverse expertise effectively, contributing to project success. By embracing change and promoting iterative, collaborative processes, Agile methodologies provide a robust framework for healthcare project management, aligning well with the industry's fluid nature.

### TABLE 15.5. TRADITIONAL PROJECT MANAGEMENT VERSUS AGILE METHODOLOGIES

| FACTOR | TRADITIONAL PROJECT MANAGEMENT | AGILE PROJECT MANAGEMENT |
| --- | --- | --- |
| Scope | Defined upfront, more rigid | Evolves iteratively, more flexible |
| Planning | Detailed multiphase plans created early | High-level plan with details emerging iteratively |
| Timeline | Linear phases, defined at the outset | Iterative sprints, timeline emerges |
| Change | Changes are more complex, causing delays | Embraces change within sprints |
| Team | More compartmentalized roles | Self-organizing and cross-functional |
| Communication | More formal, milestones | Daily standups, continuous |
| Documentation | Extensive documentation required | Working products prioritized over documentation |
| Customer involvement | Milestone reviews | Continuous customer feedback |
| Mindset | Follow the plan | Flexibility, adaptability |

## PROJECT MANAGEMENT INFORMATION SYSTEMS

Project management information systems (PMIS), such as Microsoft Projects, Asana, and Smartsheet, play a pivotal role in enhancing project planning, execution, and closure across various industries, including healthcare (Singh & Williams, 2021). Such systems provide structured support that proves invaluable in healthcare environments. PMIS platforms enable project managers to assign tasks effectively by matching responsibilities with team members' expertise and availability, boosting productivity and operational efficiency. Time-tracking features are critical in this sector, where the timing of task completion can significantly influence patient outcomes. This functionality helps track the duration of each task, pinpoint bottlenecks, and make timely adjustments to keep projects on track.

Resource allocation tools within PMIS platforms allow for the optimal distribution of essential resources, whether medical equipment, supplies, or human resources such as medical staff. Proper resource distribution ensures that tasks are well supported, minimizing waste and maximizing project efficiency. PMIS platforms also enhance communication and collaboration by providing centralized hubs for information sharing and updates on project progress. Beyond essential functions, PMIS offers comprehensive project reporting and robust document management capabilities. Project managers can generate detailed reports to guide decision-making and utilize secure document management features to share and store project-related documents efficiently.

## THE PROJECT PLAN

The project plan, a formal and comprehensive document, is the bedrock of any project (Singh & Williams, 2021). It meticulously outlines the project's objectives, scope, deliverables, timeline, and necessary resources. This pivotal document guides the project team and stakeholders through each phase. A well-structured project plan is indispensable in healthcare, where coordination across departments and facilities is paramount.

*Defining objectives:* Project objectives are a project's precise goals. In healthcare, objectives can range from enhancing patient outcomes to implementing an innovative health information system. Clearly defined objectives provide unwavering direction and are a touchstone for measuring the project's success.

*Scoping the project:* The scope defines boundaries, including inclusion and exclusion criteria. It acts as a shield against shifting expectations and scope creep, which refers to the unwarranted addition of tasks not initially outlined in the project plan. In healthcare, a well-defined scope ensures that all necessary tasks are encompassed while preventing mission drift.

*Deliverables and tangible outcomes:* Deliverables, tangible or intangible, are the fruits of a project's labor. These include a novel software system, a comprehensive report on patient outcomes, or a groundbreaking healthcare policy formulation. Precisely defined deliverables leave no room for ambiguity, ensuring every team member comprehends the deliverables and outcomes.

*Adhering to timelines:* Timelines offer a comprehensive overview of tasks and deadlines, serving as the project's temporal backbone. This structure maintains alignment and enables stakeholders to anticipate critical milestones. A meticulously crafted timeline in healthcare proves indispensable, as precise timing often holds lifesaving importance.

*Optimizing resources:* Resources encompass everything from personnel and equipment to materials and budget. Effective resource planning guarantees the availability of all essential resources precisely when needed, preventing delays and cost overruns.

## CONCLUSION

This chapter has highlighted the vital role of effective project management in healthcare, showing how it enhances patient care quality and operational excellence. We have covered essential project phases—initiation, planning, execution, monitoring, and evaluation—and discussed their importance in healthcare alongside the challenges of regulatory compliance, interdisciplinary collaboration, and patient-centric approaches. Using tools like Gantt charts and Agile methodologies has proven crucial for managing complex healthcare projects.

Effective project management is central to optimizing healthcare processes and outcomes. Strategies to navigate regulatory, collaborative, and patient-focused challenges have been explored, underscoring the dynamic nature of healthcare project management, which continuously adapts to technological advances, patient needs, and regulatory changes. Continuous learning and improvement are crucial for enhancing patient outcomes. Healthcare project management is an ongoing process that benefits significantly from the scientific method and clinical innovation.

The digital transformation in healthcare is introducing technologies like artificial intelligence, machine learning, and advanced data analytics, which are set to revolutionize project planning and management. Innovations like virtual/augmented reality, cloud-based project management, and blockchain enhance design collaboration, data security, and patient engagement. These tools promise to improve agility, visibility, risk management, and patient centricity while emphasizing the importance of human oversight in balancing technology with personalized care. The future of healthcare project management will focus on responsibly leveraging technology to improve patient experiences and drive innovation, maintaining a fundamental commitment to positive outcomes for all stakeholders. As the field evolves, so will the methodologies and tools at the disposal of healthcare professionals, ensuring ongoing adaptability and resilience.

## END-OF-CHAPTER RESOURCES

### CRITICAL THINKING QUESTIONS

- How does effective project management contribute to improving patient care quality in healthcare institutions?
- What are the key differences between project management in healthcare and other industries? What are the key similarities?
- How can healthcare project managers mitigate the risks associated with regulatory compliance during project execution?
- How is data used to drive project management objective setting and execution forward?
- Reflect on the role of communication in ensuring the success of healthcare projects.
- What are the key differences between the traditional (waterfall) project management methodologies and Agile methodologies? When might we use one methodology versus the other?
- What tools would one use to navigate the projects outlined in the case studies?

### LEARNING ACTIVITIES

**CourseConnect ▶**

To access self-assessment questions and interactive, competency-based learning activities for this chapter, visit www.springerpub.com/courseconnect. See inside front cover and tear-out card for CourseConnect details.

### REFERENCES

Aburayya, A., Alshurideh, M., Al Marzouqi, A., Al Diabat, O., Alfarsi, A., Suson, R., Salloum, S. A., Alawadhi, D., & Alzarouni, A. (2020). Critical success factors affecting the implementation of TQM in public hospitals: A case study in UAE hospitals. *Systematic Reviews in Pharmacy*, 11(10), 230–242. https://doi.org/10.31838/srp.2020.10.39

Bacelar-Silva, G. M., Cox III, J. F., & Rodrigues, P. P. (2022). Outcomes of managing healthcare services using the Theory of Constraints: A systematic review. *Health Systems*, 11(1), 1–16. https://doi.org/10.1080/20476965.2020.1813056

Blount, A. (2019). *Patient-centered primary care*. Springer.

Chakraborty, M. (2019). Managing risk, recovery & project management. *Recovery & Project Management*. https://doi.org/10.6084/m9.figshare.7886141.v1

Ciric Lalic, D., Lalic, B., Delić, M., Gracanin, D., & Stefanovic, D. (2022). How project management approach impact project success? From traditional to agile. *International Journal of Managing Projects in Business*, 15(3), 494–521. https://doi.org/10.1108/IJMPB-04-2021-0108

First Step for Consultancy & Training. (2022). *What is issue log? Definition with examples*. Retrieved October 22, 2022, from https://www.linkedin.com/pulse/what-issue-log-definition-examples-first-step1/

Heagney, J. (2016). *Fundamentals of project management*. AMACOM.

Heldman, K. (2018). *PMP: project management professional exam study guide*. John Wiley & Sons.

Kerzner, H. (2017). *Project management: A systems approach to planning, scheduling, and controlling*. John Wiley & Sons.

Mansaray, H. E. (2019). The role of leadership style in organisational change management: A literature review. *Journal of Human Resource Management*, 7(1), 18–31. https://doi.org/10.11648/j.jhrm.20190701.13

Meredith, J. R., Shafer, S. M., & Mantel, S. J., Jr. (2017). *Project management: A strategic managerial approach*. John Wiley & Sons.

Miller, A. S., & Payne, B. R. (2016). *Health IT security: An examination of modern challenges in maintaining HIPAA and HITECH compliance.* https://digitalcommons.kennesaw.edu/ccerp/2016/Academic/8

Scoleze Ferrer, P. S., Galvão, G. D. A., & de Carvalho, M. M. (2020). Tensions between compliance, internal controls and ethics in the domain of project governance. *International Journal of Managing Projects in Business, 13*(4), 845–865. https://doi.org/10.1108/IJMPB-07-2019-0171

Singh, H., & Williams, P. S. (2021). *A guide to the project management body of knowledge: PMBOK® guide.* Project Management Institute.

Singh, T., Kaur, M., Verma, M., & Kumar, R. (2019). Job satisfaction among health care providers: A cross-sectional study in public health facilities of Punjab, India. *Journal of Family Medicine and Primary Care, 8*(10), 3268. https://doi.org/10.4103/jfmpc.jfmpc_600_19

Starren, J. B., Tierney, W. M., Williams, M. S., Tang, P., Weir, C., Koppel, R., Payne, P., Hripcsak, G., & Detmer, D. E. (2021). A retrospective look at the predictions and recommendations from the 2009 AMIA policy meeting: Did we see EHR-related clinician burnout coming? *Journal of the American Medical Informatics Association, 28*(5), 948–954. https://doi.org/10.1093/jamia/ocaa320

Urton, D., & Murray, D. (2021). Project manager's perspectives on enhancing collaboration in multidisciplinary environmental management projects. *Project Leadership and Society, 2*, 100008. https://doi.org/10.1016/j.plas.2021.100008

Wang, Y., Wong, E. L.-Y., Nilsen, P., Chung, V. C., Tian, Y., & Yeoh, E.-K. (2023). A scoping review of implementation science theories, models, and frameworks—An appraisal of purpose, characteristics, usability, applicability, and testability. *Implementation Science, 18*(1), 43. https://doi.org/10.1186/s13012-023-01296-x

Wonjo, R. (2022). 4 Practical risk mitigation strategies for your business. *mondayblog.* Retrieved October 22, 2022, from https://monday.com/blog/project-management/risk-mitigation

# CHAPTER 16

# HEALTHCARE MARKETING

Steven W. Howard and Jacob S. Collins

## LEARNING OBJECTIVES

- Understand the fundamental marketing principles and their role in businesses related to health.
- Enumerate essential marketing tools, such as marketing research, segmentation, positioning, marketing mix analysis, data visualization, and basic analysis.
- Illustrate marketing in the digital age, including new disruptive competitors in healthcare and digital influences.
- Understand systematic marketing problem analysis in healthcare.

## KEY TERMS

- Advertising
- Buyer behavior
- Digital marketing
- Direct marketing
- Marketing mix
- Market segments
- Search engine marketing
- SMART goals
- Target marketing strategy

## INTRODUCTION TO HEALTHCARE MARKETING

This chapter builds upon the foundations laid in Chapter 10, "Strategic Planning." Just as initiatives in operations, finance, reimbursement, quality, and performance improvement cascade from the overarching organizational strategy, so the marketing efforts of the organization must be rooted in strategy. At the highest level, marketing enables the healthcare organization to meet its strategic objectives by communicating its mission and values, together with its future vision and important information about its services and products to all the stakeholders that impact its success (Howard et al., 2018). Marketing messages are also crucial for promoting the healthcare organization's services and products.

Most intuitively, this includes patients and their families who need to be aware of the organization's services and to have an accurate perception of its brand, but it also includes payers, employers, referring physicians, the broader community, and even internal audiences like employees or the board of directors. Typical goals of healthcare marketing efforts include improving brand awareness, attracting new patients, and strengthening relationships with and more actively engaging existing patients. This chapter enables the reader to better understand the meaning and purpose of marketing, the principal components of marketing in the healthcare context, the more recent and emerging aspects of marketing in the digital age, and future directions for healthcare marketing.

## MARKETING STRATEGY

Marketing strategies cascade out of the organization's overarching strategic plan and help it achieve its goals, particularly those related to its image in the market and for volumes of products or services to be provided. The process starts with setting **SMART goals** that are aligned with organizational strategies. SMART goals are goals that are **S**pecific, **M**easurable, **A**chievable, **R**ealistic, and **T**ime oriented. Examples of strategic marketing SMART goals can be statements like, "Grow our interventional cardiology service volume by 20% in the next 18 months" or "Within the next 12 months, position our cancer center brand to be in the top 2 among those over age 65 in our community." After setting objectives, the marketing team will proceed with market research to analyze the market, including competitors and demand for the product or service in question, and to better understand buyer behaviors.

## MARKETING LEADERSHIP

In most organizations, the marketing team is led by a chief marketing officer or senior vice president (SVP)/vice president (VP) of marketing, although in some organizations, they might be referred to as a chief communications officer. Irrespective of their title, the role of these leaders is to help guide the development of the marketing strategy. This role is responsible for understanding organizational priorities as determined by the executive leadership group, communicating them back to the broader marketing team, and ensuring that they are reflected in the strategies developed by the marketing team. Examples of these types of priorities are service line development and growth, expansion into new geographies, and outreach to new consumer segments.

In addition to driving marketing strategy development, many marketing leaders are responsible for strategic initiatives that create new marketing capabilities. The development of digital marketing capabilities, reputation tracking and analysis, and consumer insights and behavioral capabilities are all examples of strategic capabilities and showcase how leadership within the marketing group helps to determine the skill set of the marketing group. Typically, these senior leaders are also responsible for managing relationships with various third-party agencies such as creative development, campaign and targeting analytics, or ad placement services, which are important because they can represent a significant expense for healthcare organizations. Finally, these leaders are also responsible for building and managing effective teams that can achieve the marketing goals of their organizations.

## MARKET AND COMPETITOR ANALYSIS

The organization must define the geographic area in which the product or service under analysis will be competitive. Often, a primary *service area* will be the priority over secondary service areas (Thomas, 2020). For example, a health system with a quaternary academic medical center may define the market area for heart transplantation as a multistate area since few organizations are accredited to perform these procedures, they are infrequent, and the need for donor organs necessitates a broad catchment area. Contrast this with the same health system's orthopedic department joint replacement services, which may primarily serve only a 1-hour commuting radius from the hospital because many local community hospitals offer the same service, the same joint replacement implants are broadly available to any hospital, and patients and their families prefer not to travel long distances if they can stay nearer to home. Further, contrast these examples with the same health system's primary care services offered through its physician organization. Patients will seldom travel more than 15 to 30 minutes from home for routine services like primary care, and there are many other competitors in the area, ranging from independent physicians to multispecialty clinics to larger health systems' physician organizations.

Once the geographic service area is determined, the marketing team will analyze the *competitors* providing the same, similar, or even *substitute* services in the same market area (Berkowitz, 2021; Porter, 2008). Knowing the competitors' strengths and weaknesses vis-à-vis the marketing team's own product and service offerings is essential as we move to the later steps of marketing research and positioning.

## MARKET SEGMENTATION AND TARGET MARKETING

Once the marketing team has defined the service area and competitors, it must more clearly define categories of customers or audiences to which it will customize and deliver messages. These groupings are **market segments**. For example, market segments for joint replacement surgery could include payers (for contracting into their networks); large employers (for direct contracting); high-income seniors with Medicare; adult children of older, more frail elders; or primary care physicians who need to refer their patients for joint replacement surgery. The team must consider the size of each segment (how many people are within the area), the power or influence each has in the decision process, and the thought process each works through in deciding which joint replacement surgery center should be selected (Kotler et al., 2008). Typically, the organization does not have sufficient resources to heavily market to every conceivable market segment, so the segments must be prioritized.

This prioritization results in a **target marketing strategy**—focusing on a few audiences to whom messages and media/communication vehicles can be customized for maximum impact (Thomas, 2020). In our joint replacement example, let us assume the marketing team has chosen to target women over age 50 who are researching joint replacement for themselves, their spouses, or an elderly parent. We might also simultaneously target community physicians who refer those patients and the insurers who decide which providers are in the network and, therefore, available to the insured patients.

## BUYER BEHAVIOR

Once the marketing team understands who is making the decisions on which provider to choose and who must be the focus of its communications, the next step is to better understand that person's decision-making processes. **Buyer behavior** is one of the most important and preceding steps to marketing research. The marketing team must understand *how* customers (typically payers, patients, and their families) consider their health-related problems, how they seek out information for decision-making, and ultimately how they choose the providers from whom they will receive healthcare services or products. Buyer behavior includes more rational components, like considering the insurer's provider network, quality scores of providers, prices, schedules, wait times, and locations. However, less rational emotional aspects can be just as powerful—fear about outcomes, rumors and word-of-mouth reputations, hassles of parking, concerns about crime around the hospital, and so forth. In our joint replacement example, the marketing team may learn that the women of the household are most commonly the healthcare decision-makers and that they will invest significant time in learning about the options and choosing what they perceive to be the best joint replacement clinic for their loved ones or themselves. Note that joint replacement is generally a nonurgent, "shoppable" service that lends itself well to high-information, time-consuming shopping behaviors.

## THE MARKETING MIX: PRODUCT, PRICE, PLACE, AND PROMOTION

The **marketing mix**, comprising *product, price, place, and promotion*, also known as the "4 Ps of marketing," is a basic model for developing effective marketing strategies for any business, including healthcare organizations. After setting marketing strategy, analyzing the market and competitors, selecting the primary audiences (or targets) for the subsequent marketing campaign, and analyzing how that audience thinks about the healthcare product or service purchasing decision, the next step is working through the 4 Ps (Thomas, 2020). Overall, the marketing mix enables the healthcare organization to attract and retain patients, communicate healthcare services, and build a strong brand presence. The 4Ps are as follows:

*Product:* In healthcare, *product* can mean a physical product as we might think about it in the areas of consumer goods, electronics, automobiles, and so forth. Indeed, *products* in healthcare often include physical products like prescription or over-the-counter drugs; durable medical equipment like wheelchairs, hospital beds, and oxygen concentrators; or even surgical implantable items like hip or knee implants and related hardware. However, more often, it refers to the services, medical treatments, procedures, or even healthcare facilities being offered. That means *product* could be heart bypass surgeries at a tertiary hospital, an MRI scan at an outpatient imaging center, a sinus surgery at an outpatient ENT clinic, or a routine annual exam at a primary care office. Marketers must clearly define the features, advantages, and benefits (FAB) of their healthcare offerings and understand how they meet the needs of their target audience (they will be articulating messages to these audiences in subsequent steps). If the marketing team has done a good job of selecting the best target audiences and done a thorough job of studying their buyer behavior, they will have a good understanding of the types of *product* attributes most important to each target audience (e.g., quality, convenience, technology, effectiveness, ambiance, comforting staff).

*Price:* The term *price* is often used generally (and too casually) to represent any financial aspect of healthcare (as is also true for the term *cost*). In this chapter, *price* specifically refers to the financial, or even nonfinancial, costs the purchaser and/or consumer may pay for healthcare services or products offered. This could be as simple as a few dollars for a bottle of over-the-counter aspirin at a retail store, or as complicated as the discounted contractual payment from an insurer to a surgery center, or the fixed or percentage cost-sharing the consumer pays for that surgery.

If the payer is Medicare or Medicaid, the healthcare marketer may have no choices about price—their organization will be a price-taker, since the government names the price it will pay. If the payer is private insurance, the organization will negotiate with the insurer, but the negotiation may be more focused on conversion factors rather than individual prices for each of the hundreds of services the healthcare organization offers. Generally, the pricing needs and strategies for healthcare services only approach those of traditional consumer goods when the services in question are not covered by insurance (or not covered well), for example, dentistry, optometry, orthodontia, chiropractic, or medical spa services.

*Price* can also include nonfinancial costs like the fear of stigma for being seen at a mental health clinic or the indirect cost of taking time away from work to go to a doctor's office during the patient's workday. In fact, those are some of the aspects that make *price* in healthcare so complicated, the separation of the roles of payer and consumer and sensitive nonfinancial issues, as well as complicated insurance reimbursement models, government payers and their regulations (especially Medicare and Medicaid), and even regional variations.

*Place:* Place in marketing refers to the distribution channels and locations where customers can buy products. With physical healthcare products, this can be more straightforward and similar to traditional consumer markets. However, healthcare services are intangible, inseparable, and not inventoriable, limiting the organization's options for distribution. Typically, healthcare services use the *direct* or *zero-level* distribution model in which the service is directly provided to the patient/consumer at one location (though there may be multiple locations, like in our earlier examples for sinus surgery centers or primary care offices). Telemedicine has also enabled more options for *place* to expand in the healthcare marketing arena.

The goal of the *place* component of the marketing mix is to make healthcare services readily accessible and more convenient for the target audience. Thus having done thorough work in the market analysis, competitor analysis, and buyer behavior phases of the marketing planning is crucially important. There are multiple aspects of *place* to be considered. First, where should the healthcare organization's physical locations be placed? Often, the marketing team finds themselves needing to work with marketing existing service lines at existing locations. However, sometimes there is flexibility to plan new or changing locations. This is when the earlier analysis of demographics, epidemiology, the economics of the market area, and competitors is so important.

*Promotion:* The fourth P of the marketing mix is *promotion*. Promotion includes all the activities and communication strategies used to create awareness and encourage the target audience to choose your organization over the competition. The tools of promotion include advertising, public relations, social media marketing, content marketing, personal selling, and other promotional efforts. Crafting the message is an important first step before launching into using these specific promotional tools. If the marketing team has conducted thorough research of the market, competitors, and buyer behavior, it can then craft messages that will speak to the problems, worries, and thought processes of the target audiences. Effective messages must highlight the unique selling points of the organization's services and build trust and credibility among the target audiences. The team must also be mindful of the sensitive nature of healthcare marketing and comply with regulations and ethical considerations.

After crafting messages that will speak to the hearts, needs, and worries of the target audiences, the marketing team then must choose the most effective tools or media in the promotional mix to deliver them. Traditionally, the **promotional mix** is the array of tools in the marketer's metaphorical toolbox: advertising, personal selling, publicity and public relations, sales promotion, direct marketing, and digital marketing (Thomas, 2020).

**Advertising** is probably the most visible and common tool in the promotional mix. This includes traditional advertising media, like TV, radio, and newspaper, as well as crossing over into the digital marketing category with tools like digital display ads on healthcare websites. As is important with all aspects of the promotional mix, it is most important to match the medium with the target audience and the message being conveyed.

**Personal selling** is quite common in promoting more costly physical healthcare products, like MRI machines or orthopedic surgical implants, but is less overt for healthcare service organizations like health systems. Health systems do, however, exercise a type of personal selling when they employ provider relations personnel to develop and maintain relationships with referring physicians across the broader service area.

**Publicity and public relations** are probably the oldest forms of healthcare marketing and continue to be very important parts of the promotional mix. Publicity is indirect and unpaid, such as a news story or press release. Public relations is the broader umbrella of managing the organization's brand and relationships with the media and other community stakeholders.

**Sales promotions** are the limited-time special deals you see at the grocery store, big-box stores, online retailers, and so forth. These include special promotional offers like buy-one-get-one-free deals, coupons, special discount sales days like Black Friday, or special rebate offers. The usual objective is to get buyers to try new things and/or to buy more than the usual amount, and they are often used for entering new geographic markets or launching new product or service liens. While very common in consumer goods, they are much less common in consumer-oriented healthcare services marketing.

**Direct marketing** is directly sending messages to the potential buyer, usually at least somewhat personalized. These could take the form of direct mailings to people's homes or workplaces sent through the postal service, direct telephone telemarketing calls, cell phone text messaging, or **email marketing**. An excellent direct email list can be developed if patients are asked to sign up with the provider to receive ongoing information. This is known as opt-in marketing, and privacy laws like the Health Insurance Portability and Accountability Act (HIPAA; in the United States) and the General Data Protection Regulation (GDPR in Europe) require that patients opt in to any additional marketing efforts by the providers, other than for any ongoing communications related to their current care. Opt-in email marketing is an attractive tactic for healthcare marketers because it is inexpensive and can be highly targeted given that consumers are asked to list the types of topics that they would like to receive more information about.

## DIGITAL MARKETING

The advent of the internet and the introduction of social media have created a new array of opportunities to reach potential patients through **digital marketing**. This medium allows marketers to engage consumers in new ways, utilizing highly targeted ads based on a consumer's digital behaviors, as well as web search-based advertising that allows marketers to engage consumers who are actively searching for their services. The data-rich nature of digital marketing allows healthcare marketers with limited budgets to engage their patients and consumers in ways that can reduce wasted marketing spend and create higher conversion rates among ad recipients. The following sections detail some of the most used digital marketing tools and terminology.

Digital marketing can employ many of the traditional approaches previously described, including direct marketing, though it does so in a digital, internet-enabled fashion. Instead of billboards or newspaper ads, digital marketers use display ads and in-app or in-webpage ads. Instead of using a physician or other expert for an interview on TV or in a newspaper, digital marketers do so using social media, YouTube, or a similar digital medium. Instead of "snail mail" direct marketing, they use email, SMS text, WhatsApp, and the like. While marketers were always able to create interesting, newsworthy content, they depended upon media companies to choose whether to use it. That is no longer a limitation as digital marketers can now use **content marketing** approaches to directly publish anything the organization desires to advance its promotional messages supporting the overall brand or specific product or service lines.

While celebrity and expert endorsements have long been useful marketing tools, they have evolved significantly in the digital age. In addition to using medical experts, sports teams, and so forth to promote healthcare organizations' brands and messages, today we can better control the dissemination through YouTube and social media channels. Additionally, healthcare marketers can also pay social media influencers to endorse the organization and promote its digital content.

## DISPLAY ADVERTISING AND PAY PER CLICK

Display advertising is essentially the web-based version of traditional print media advertising and includes images, video, or audio that is shown within the content of a website. These ads can be purchased by impression, much like traditional media, but much of display advertising is what is known as pay per click (PPC) advertising. These are ads that are embedded within websites. Organizations do not pay for the ads unless a recipient clicks on the ad, which can help to reduce marketing spend. In many cases, display advertising can be targeted only to those users who entered specific key words into a search bar or who have exhibited specific online behaviors. The ability to target these ads can help improve conversion waste and reduce unnecessary marketing spend.

## SOCIAL MEDIA PLATFORM ADVERTISING

Social media platforms such as Facebook, X (formerly Twitter), Instagram, TikTok, and others have provided a rich medium for marketers to connect with healthcare consumers. Consumer engagement on these platforms is incredibly high, and users provide the various platforms with a tremendous amount of information about their demographics, preferences, desires, and needs. This wealth of information makes social media platforms an ideal space for healthcare marketers to create highly targeted ads, while the large number of consumers engaged on the platforms ensures that a high number of impressions can be garnered by purchasing advertising. Additionally, company-administered social media profiles provide an opportunity for healthcare providers to engage directly with their consumers to build up their brand, improve perceptions, and create lasting relationships with their consumers outside of the clinical space.

## SEARCH ENGINE OPTIMIZATION AND PAID SEARCH

**Search engine marketing** allows marketers to connect to consumers who are already actively seeking their services. The use of search engine marketing is one of the most effective tools for a marketer because the potential for conversion is highest among users already seeking a healthcare provider. Search engine marketing can take two forms, **search engine optimization (SEO)** and **paid search marketing**. SEO is when web designers optimize the content and tagging of their websites so that they will index well against the algorithms used by search engines to provide organic recommendations to their users (Thomas, 2020). The better that a webpage indexes against a search, the higher its position in the results returned to the end user. By optimizing the content, marketers can ensure that their website is presented near the top of the rankings, resulting in impressions and potential conversions.

The other type of search engine marketing is paid search, which can be used as a stand-alone tactic or in conjunction with SEO. Compared to SEO, paid search marketing is a quicker and less labor-intensive way to connect consumers with the providers for whom they are searching. Paid search marketing allows marketers to buy PPC ads that will be displayed ahead of the organic search terms. These purchased ads can be tied to keywords, similar to organic search results, and are denoted as ads when the search terms are presented to the consumer. The prominence of these ads within the search results, as well as the ability to tie ads to keywords without the long and labor-intensive process of SEO, is an attractive option for marketers.

# EVALUATING THE MARKETING CAMPAIGN IN THE DIGITAL AGE

## MEASUREMENT AND ANALYTICS

The increase in the use of digital marketing has driven growth in marketing analytics. The wealth of data available to marketers can be used to help improve ad targeting to make them more relevant to the recipient, to determine what campaigns are most successful, to evaluate the financial outcomes of any given campaign, and to select the creative that will most likely cause a consumer to take the desired action. The following details some of the analyses that are commonly conducted and the types of data that are used.

## DATA-DRIVEN TARGETING

Targeting has long been a tool to help reduce waste in marketing and to ensure that impressions are made on those who are most likely to *convert* to being buyers. Traditional print and TV media can be targeted via demography of the readership and viewership, respectively, and marketers have always purchased the placements that most closely aligned with their potential patients and consumers. Recently, the growth of digital marketing as a key healthcare marketing vertical has created an environment in which targeting can be taken to even greater lengths.

Within the digital space, profiles can be built on not only the broad demographics of the consumer (as they are in traditional media) but can also be tied to a more nuanced understanding of the consumer's preferences. Linking data to various third-party data sources like credit card company data and search data creates significant opportunities for highly targeted campaigns. In some cases, healthcare providers are even building predictive models that allow them to use third-party data to predict health needs, all without utilizing any of the patient's protected health information (which is highly regulated by HIPAA in the United States and GDPR in Europe). One of the questions for marketers is the appropriateness of the ways in which they are using third-party data and the care they are taking to respect the consumer's privacy.

Jeff House, Vice President for Managed Health, Payor Industry Intelligence and Insights, said of the changes, "Over the past decade, one of the major shifts in healthcare marketing analytics has been the ability to diversify segmentation across a broader range of attributes. Historically, simple demographic attributes (age, gender, and income) were the basis of primary segmentation. But that's also all marketers had to use at the time. However, with the evolution of consumer/patient research and growth in related technologies and datasets, we now have a broader scale of attributes related to behaviors, attitudes, preferences and experiences. Models, frameworks and decision tools can now factor-in more and more-sophisticated attributes to shape brand and drive behavior" (J. House, personal communication, July 28, 2023).

**CASE STUDY 16.1:** UNIVERSITY OF PITTSBURGH MEDICAL CENTER'S USE OF DATA-DRIVEN TARGETING AND DIGITAL MARKETING TO IMPROVE CARE FOR PATIENTS WITH LIVER DISEASE

University of Pittsburgh Medical Center (UPMC) has long been a source of hope for patients requiring solid organ transplant. Liver transplants, in particular, are a life-saving procedure for many patients suffering from liver disease or liver cancer. The challenge for these patients has always been the limited supply of organs for transplantation. Luckily for patients, it is now possible to transplant part of a liver from a living patient to those in need and both patients' livers will regenerate in a procedure known as a living donor liver transplant (LDLT). However, due to the newness of this procedure, patients and even physicians are not aware of this life-saving alternative.

In order to improve care for these patients and promote LDLT as an option, UPMC transplant surgeons turned to their colleagues in marketing for help identifying potential patients and reaching them in a cost-effective manner. One of the challenges for the marketing team is that there are a very small number of patients who actually require this surgery. This meant that mass media channels would potentially be wasteful, and while they were employed at the beginning of the campaign to generate *buzz*, the team knew that a highly targeted and trackable digital campaign would be the best way to reach these potential patients. These efforts would also be more trackable so that the campaign could be evaluated for effectiveness and course corrected if specific tactics were not successful.

The marketing intelligence team at UPMC was able to utilize their database of hundreds of consumer variables tracked for every individual nationwide, along with public health information about the incidence of liver disease by zip code to build a predictive model that would tier consumers based on their likelihood of needing a transplant. Using this machine learning model, the marketing team was able to create a list of potential patients without accessing any HIPAA-protected data. The consumers on this list could then be targeted across a range of digital marketing channels, including display ads, social media, and other digital channels.

These highly targeted ads were only shown to those consumers most likely to need them and were created in such a way as to be sensitive to the needs of patients with relevant conditions and not to alarm those consumers who received the ad but did not suffer from one of the conditions. The campaign generated a significant response, which was tracked via the digital marketing channels, and additional communications to the physicians likely to be managing these patients' conditions were added to increase the conversion rate. The efforts of these marketers added significant volume to the liver transplant program, and ultimately, many lives were saved as a result of these efforts and those of the transplant surgeons caring for these patients.

## CONCLUSION

When healthcare organizations know their patients and communities very well and when they understand the strengths and limitations of each part of the promotional mix, they can craft and deliver highly effective messages. This kind of impactful marketing communication helps the organization present itself to the community, differentiate itself from competitors, and persuade audiences to make the choices being promoted to advance health and healthcare in the organization's service area. Taken together, strong implementation of the marketing mix is essential for helping achieve the healthcare organization's mission and strategic goals.

## END-OF-CHAPTER RESOURCES

### CRITICAL THINKING QUESTIONS

- Design a SMART goal to promote a new initiative in your organization, using marketing strategies to gain buy-in.
- Think about *promotion* and a recent advertising campaign that you feel was very successful. Discuss the details about that campaign and the specific aspects that made it effective.
- Digital marketing methods and tools are commonly adopted by healthcare marketers today, including email, display marketing, social media, and SEO. Which of these is most effective? Most ineffective? Why, and under what circumstances?

### LEARNING ACTIVITIES

**CourseConnect ▶**

To access self-assessment questions and interactive, competency-based learning activities for this chapter, visit www.springerpub.com/courseconnect. See inside front cover and tear-out card for CourseConnect details.

### REFERENCES

Berkowitz, E. (2021). *Essentials of health care marketing* (5th ed.). Jones & Bartlett.

Howard, S., Gupta, S., Malik, M., & Ferreira, W. (2018). Strategic management and marketing. In M. Counte, B. Ramirez, B., D. West & W. Aaronson (Eds), *The global healthcare manager: Competencies, concepts, and skills.* ACHE Learn.

Kotler, P., Shalowitz, J., & Stevens, R. J. (2008). *Strategic marketing for health care organizations.* Jossey-Bass.

Porter, M. E. (2008). *On competition.* Harvard Business Press.

Thomas, R. K. (2020). *Marketing health services* (4th ed.). Health Administration Press.

CHAPTER 17

# HEALTHCARE INFORMATION TECHNOLOGY

Suzanne J. Paone and Ann Marie Evans

## LEARNING OBJECTIVES

- Understand the importance of transformative changes in healthcare that are underpinned by technological innovations.
- Identify the importance of future stakeholder expectations in healthcare services driven by advancement in other industries.
- Describe the importance of aligning technology plans with an organization's strategic planning process.
- Explain technological healthcare advancement in modular stages (MS) and the risks/rewards of an organization's migration through the stages.
- Explore the role of leadership in advancing to a transformational stage.

## KEY TERMS

- Advanced leadership skills
- Blockchain technology
- CRM (customer relationship management)
- Industry stakeholders
- Innovative technology
- Modular stages
- Stage 1
- Stage 2
- Stage 3
- Technology plans

## INTRODUCTION

Each day, digital capabilities are used in every industry to accomplish the mission and goals of all types of public, private, for-profit, and not-for-profit organizations. According to recent studies, health consumers would not think of pursuing a pathway to manage a critical health-related diagnosis without engaging systems and information (Boyce et al., 2024). The investment of core health information technology (IT) platforms across hospitals, physician offices, clinics, and long-term care, as well as other care facilities, provides a profound impact on the health of our society. One recent rigorous study, in fact, demonstrates that core technologies available to consumers and health providers today, such as mobile applications, wearable devices, electronic health records (EHRs), and telemedicine capabilities, acutely reduce the probability of engaged consumers developing type 2 diabetes (Nguyen et al., 2024). The challenge of effectively engaging healthcare consumers, healthcare providers, management staff, and communities to optimize the use of systems is an opportunity for transformational health industry leaders.

To understand the capabilities of health information today, we explore the evolution of health information platforms and systems, particularly in organizations that provide healthcare services. Whether we focus on hospitals, health systems, or health providers, the history of health IT platforms lags behind the development of core systems in other sectors of the United States economy, such as financial services, manufacturing, airlines, and hospitality. Prior to the 1980s, very few health providers invested more than 1% of their total organizational revenues on IT platforms. At that time, most technology capabilities in health provider systems involved mainframes that submitted billing claims for services to the federal government for services provided to Medicare recipients. Rudimentary human resource applications began to evolve in the 1980s and 1990s, as did the use of supply chain systems and platforms, mostly from companies selling software to organizations in other economic sectors and adapting those software systems to hospitals.

Early in the 1990s, the federal government began to challenge the effectiveness of billing claims for services submitted by hospitals. For health provider systems, this meant that reimbursement questions centered on testing services, such as laboratory tests, radiology exams, and other types of patient testing such as colonoscopies or cardiac stress exams, and pharmaceuticals prescribed in hospitals, clinics, and physician offices. The need to track the business transactions associated with testing in these service areas predicated the evolution of ancillary clinical information systems such as laboratory, pharmacy, and radiology information systems. The evolution of specialized software systems for the healthcare industry has now begun to mirror other industries based on organizational and regulatory demands.

The mid-1990s saw a plethora of software companies produce products to automate not only testing areas but also some of the high-cost areas of the health industry such as operating rooms and surgical services areas, as well as emergency room bed allocation, all problem operational departments in hospitals in the United States. By the mid-1990s, larger health systems in the United States, especially academic medical centers, implemented core software programs in these parts of the business. At the same time, these organizations, like other businesses, deployed secure, internal networks and personal computing capabilities.

Healthcare provider market consolidation began in the mid- to late 1990s, creating large and complicated healthcare delivery networks that implemented administrative solutions to address the needs of doing business as large organizations. This included the implementation of many standardized administrative systems being used in other parts of the economy, such as systems to manage the supply chain associated with acquiring goods as well as human resource information systems. In terms of the business needs specific to healthcare, this era showed the evolution of complex patient accounting systems that automated the complicated revenue cycle processes associated with scheduling customer services, coding for clinical services, using complicated medical data, and submitting billing claims not only to the federal government but also to private insurance companies using evolving digital standards.

The missing link in many of these systems and data advancements in the mid- to late 1990s was the automation of the clinical processes in complex health settings. From the standpoint of both physician offices and hospitals, software systems designed specifically to automate clinical processes and integrate patient accounting functions evolved rigorously in the late 1990s and early 2000s. This included the evolution of structured software methods to document care, place testing orders, review the results of orders, and incorporate data from platforms that were already in place in the laboratory, radiology, and pharmacy information systems. Vendor companies led the development of these clinical software platforms, which evolved from companies that sold software to automate ancillary departments and patient accounting in hospitals and physician offices.

Emphasizing the importance of health in the United States, in the early 2000s, serious concerns among the general public, constituents in the federal government, and leaders in private corporations percolated regarding the cost, quality, and perceived lack of consistency in the U.S. healthcare system. Sentinel quality works published at the time cast aspersions on the workflows and processes in the U.S. healthcare system, causing concern not only in academic circles but also in the public media. The advent of quality management programs and third-party benchmarking services placed demands on evolving U.S. healthcare systems to automate processes with an emphasis on quality and customer safety. As discussed in a recent study by Aggarwal et al. (2024), the function of both clinical and administrative knowledge workers in the health industry began to center on competencies related to the use of technology with rigorous expectations similar to those already established in other industries, such as financial services, airlines, and manufacturing.

In 2009, federal legislation ignited the implementation of advanced clinical transactional software systems referred to as EHRs. Clinical platform systems evolved from an internal medical records focus to include external health data capabilities, such as secure customer portals and capabilities of exchanging health information from organization to organization. Elements of the financial incentive program still exist today in the form of legislation that supports data exchange between disparate providers of healthcare with a focus on efficiency and safety (U.S. Department of Health and Human Services, n.d.).

As basic transactional software platforms permeated healthcare provider organizations along with advanced personal computing capabilities, secure networks, and handheld devices, health provider organizations produce tremendous amounts of information. Whether it be the way providers provide clinical care or the way they manage financial or human resources, systems and platforms evolved to include capabilities, such as mobile, computing, and the incorporation of secure internet information processing. In recent times, we see data being turned not only into meaningful management information but also into predictive patterns and algorithms that provide the capability for an organization to move along advanced models of surviving to thriving and competing in complicated health economies.

The rapid evolution of systems and data in the last 30 years in health organizations enables leaders to not only advance the mission of an organization in the most efficient manner possible but also to add new value to the complex digital health economy. While capabilities such as artificial intelligence (AI) offer tremendous potential value in both clinical and administrative areas, studies caution that leaders must first manage the quality implementation of base digital capabilities and ensure the quality of data generated by their organizations (Schulman et al., 2023). This deep understanding of the potential capabilities of technology and information as an asset differentiates organizations from those who sustain in current markets from those who transform and optimize the impact of their organizations on society.

## LEADERSHIP OPPORTUNITIES

Leaders in current-day healthcare management are at the cusp of beginning the transformative industry changes that will continue with next-generation healthcare leaders. Healthcare spending in the United States has reached a record growth of 2.7% in 2021, reaching 4.9 trillion—or $14,570 per person—and accounting for 18.3% of the nation's gross domestic product (Centers for Medicare and Medicaid Services [CMS], 2024; https://www.cms.gov/Research-Statistics-Data-and-Systems/Statistics-Trends-and-Reports/NationalHealthExpendData/nationalHealthAccountsHIstorical-).

The unsustainability of these spending levels in tandem with a chaotic and complex healthcare delivery system is not meeting the needs of the consumers the industry is there to serve. As a result, levels of competition in healthcare will continue to progress, and despite high entry barriers, new entrants into the industry are unavoidable.

The needs of the consumer are evolving and require disruptive innovation. Healthcare leaders in provider organizations are beginning to experience market changes and the healthcare consumer will leave organizations that fail or lag in innovation. Our current state healthcare system is crowded with inpatient beds, multiple-month appointment lag times, antiquated management structures, entrenched behavior, culture and politics, and a lack of consumer transparency. Supporting innovation through IT, data, and technological advancements has immense potential to propel healthcare forward, creating efficiencies and strides in the industry. Technology innovations are an underpinning of making the current state of healthcare a distant memory and improving care for the populations served.

This chapter provides an overview of the **industry stakeholder**-driven need for **innovative technology** in healthcare, reviews the various **modular stages** (MS) an organization may progress through in terms of technology, and elaborates on the leadership characteristics that enable an organization to achieve advanced modular stages.

## TRANSFORMATIVE CHANGE THROUGH TECHNOLOGICAL INNOVATION

Provider organizations that thrive proactively tune into and forecast the expectations of stakeholders such as consumers and the communities that they serve. With this focus, they innovate and deploy technology that supports the mission and transformative change. Select providers thrive using various strategies enabled by technological innovation. These strategies include differentiating themselves in existing markets, increasing market share in existing markets, creating new markets, advancing safety and quality, and reducing the unit cost of delivering products and services.

An example of an innovation-based strategy that supports aggressive differentiation in new or existing markets is the use of systems called **CRM** or **customer relationship management** systems. The legacy of using the systems to support product and service excellence comes from other industries, such as the retail, financial, and manufacturing business sectors of the economy. CRM technology is centric around managing customer data at all levels of the business relationship with its consumers. The goal is to know your customers better. The use of CRM in healthcare provides a technological basis for providers and other organizations that support providers (e.g., equipment companies, pharmacies) to connect with customers, analyze their needs, and deliver tailored services and responses to establish and increase high-value customer retention. As discussed by Baashar et al. (2020), while research on the effective use of these platforms shows ubiquitous adoption outside of healthcare, there are significant gaps in the research demonstrating consistent use of these fundamental technical and operational capabilities in healthcare.

Learning from other industries, we know that innovation-based strategies fail if the focus is exclusively technological in nature. For technology systems and platforms to provide innovative capabilities for any organization, there must be an alignment of people, processes, strategic outcome measures, and effective technology management. Like any other industry, the call to action in the healthcare sector is to align strategic plans with the thoughtful acquisition and management of cost-effective, realistic, and appropriate technology platforms and services to serve the healthcare organization. This involves aligning strategic plans with well-formulated **technology plans**.

## STRATEGIC PLANS MUST INCLUDE A FOCUSED, INTEGRATED TECHNOLOGY PLAN

Technology plans (both short and long term) are a critical part of the strategic planning process in any organization, including those delivering healthcare services. Strategic technology plans also recognize the power of data; they encompass data mining resources and the ability to turn data into strategic information. Akbarzedeh (2022) proposed improvements to IT planning using a balanced scorecard (BSC) approach with inputs related to Strengths Weaknesses Opportunities and Threats (SWOT) analysis, organizational risk, and the organization's state of maturity. Strategic algorithms like a BSC can aid in defining parameters supporting successful IT implementation by overcoming complexities within organizations.

## MODULAR STAGES OF TECHNOLOGY ADVANCEMENT

Technology advancement and data mining are related to healthcare provider organizations in three distinct modular stages:

- *Stage 1*: Day-to-day operational use (e.g., electronic medical record platforms, revenue cycle, and consumer-facing patient engagement software programs)
- *Stage 2*: Intermittent-based regulatory and competitor-based market changes (e.g., Hospital Value-Based Purchasing[VBP] Program, volume leakage, and insurer authorization requirements)
- *Stage 3*: Leading mission-based market change based on innovation (e.g., consumer access, AI, telemedicine, and other digital innovations)

Stage 1 and Stage 2 are pillars of safety and stability and an important requirement to keep the organization operating at a foundational level. However, healthcare entities that focus only on Stage 1, with occasional steps into Stage 2 for regulatory and compliance purposes, risk stagnation and, over time, will compromise the future of the organization. The key to success is a clear understanding of stability in Stages 1 and 2 as a critical bridge to operational efficiencies, sound workflows, and effective compliance protocols. Operational proficiencies, in most cases, will create the foundation of investment pipelines to fund innovative activities. In the most simplistic example, organizations with interoperability issues within their electronic medical record and other clinical systems, antiquated revenue cycle systems/processes, and manual compliance processes are not capitalizing on the opportunities in Stages 1 and 2. They are incapable of innovating in Stage 3 and may lack the resources to support innovation. It is highly likely that too many valuable resources, in the form of both human and financial capital, are caught in the former stages and wasted.

## ADVANCING THROUGH THE MODULAR STAGES

Perceptive leaders exhibit tendencies that optimize and manage Stage 1 to keep operations running at high levels while focusing on achieving the advanced stages (Stages 2 and 3). Resources are attributed to Stage 1 at optimal levels and care is taken to ensure resources remain adequate. Excess resources garnered through Stage 1 productivity are directed to the advancement of Stages 2 and 3.

The most common technology investment and what is often referred to as a costly clinical information system platform is the EHR. Stages 1 and 2 organizations optimize these high-investment platforms and align the investment in any systems or platforms they designate as the *EHR* with tangible quality metrics. The optimization of EHR technologies happens at all levels of healthcare delivery. Organizations characterized as Stage 2 (using EHRs to instantiate best practices in the organization) have demonstrated operational efficiencies by optimizing EHR investments, specifically related to documentation, ordering of testing and ancillary services, and enabling mobile clinicians to review and act on testing results more efficiently (Sieja et al., 2021). Conversely, we see some outpatient environments utilizing EHR investments at a Stage 1 level. Legacy issues with healthcare technology prevail in some markets. As an example, over 3,000 providers in New York City studied since 2007 report inconsistent workflow challenges and adoption challenges with medical and nonmedical staff. This underrepresents productivity and efficiency across multiple busy clinics with EHR platforms implemented and transacting business but not optimized (Parsons et al., 2012). It is rare to see an organization that has optimized the EHR platform to a Stage 3 level. This represents a significant transformational opportunity for the future.

Moving from optimized transactional technology platforms in Stage 2 to Stage 3 requires balanced, focused leadership on the part of healthcare organizations but it is attainable. Calculated risk-taking and change management are necessary in tandem with strong integrity, ethics, and accountability. One common thread that we see in organizations that move from Stage 2 to Stage 3 is a strong propensity toward aligning with stakeholders. The value of healthcare services is delivered from the perspective of the consumer stakeholder, whether that consumer be an individual, an employer, a community, or other representative group. Technology platforms and the data they render in this framework are merely enablers for healthcare provider organizations to establish excellence and demonstrate direct value to consumers in the marketplace.

Stage 3 healthcare organizations evolve through the implementation and cost-effective sustainment of transactional platforms, knowing an analysis of the quality of the data produced by those platforms, and a recognition that investments in technology must align with leadership-based process optimization. There is evidence in the literature that increasingly educated healthcare consumers have a willingness to receive and, in many ways, expect organizations that represent healthcare excellence to evolve through these innovation stages. In a study by Esmaeilzadeh (2020), a survey of consumers showed a willingness to accept and participate with clinicians in what they perceived to be appropriate risks of adopting AI-based clinical decision support technologies within the trust fabric of established provider-consumer relationships.

## ATTAINING MODULAR STAGE 3

The attainment of Stage 3 strategic innovation alignment is not isolated to select academic healthcare organizations. Organizations that support leaders who champion change, challenge the status quo, and accept appropriate risk have an opportunity to significantly leverage Stages 1 and 2 technology investments for the betterment of their consumer, provider, and employee communities. For example, we see significant market movement in the use of integrated consumer wearable devices in both the physical and mental health space. These reliable and innovative strategies maintain critical connections with consumers while allocating resources outside of traditional high-cost centers of care such as hospital clinics (Pardamean et al., 2020). Similarly, contemporary studies report sites where robotics initiatives, leveraging AI algorithms and verified data from transactional clinical and financial systems, are being used to engage direct benefits for geriatric populations, once again, in cost-appropriate settings of care (Sevnja et al., 2023).

## TECHNOLOGY INNOVATION IN HEALTHCARE ADMINISTRATIVE FUNCTIONS

The strategic progression of well-led healthcare organizations from Stage 2 to Stage 3 is also reflected through financial and administrative innovations. Select organizations thrive in the complicated insurance-based reimbursement models by layering AI applications within optimized revenue cycle technologies to aggressively reduce claims denials and lessen financial liabilities on community health systems as an example in the construct of social well-being (Johnson et al., 2023).

External to the workings of any healthcare organization, we see other examples of a progression from Stage 1 to 2 technology innovation. According to workforce challenges present in all industries, there is also evidence that health organizations can optimize the function of traditional human resource information system (HRIS) platforms to align with people strategies in high-performing healthcare organizations (Mauro & Borges-Andrade, 2020).

For example, analysis of **blockchain technology** capabilities in healthcare demonstrates significant organizational benefits in areas of transparency and lower cost interoperability by leveraging these technologies. The capability of multiple healthcare organizations to move toward a blockchain infrastructure for select financial and administrative frameworks assumes that these organizations have optimized their transactional financial platforms. Even given that assumption, there are significant capabilities that counterbalance security and other concerns of moving forward with blockchain-enabled healthcare models (Poquiz, 2022). Imagine a network of competitive but partnered operable healthcare organizations efficiently sharing appropriate information to the benefit of customers and communities in a low-cost standardized blockchain-enabled information framework that minimizes waste and eliminates high-cost, non-value-added transactional layers of an optimized healthcare ecosystem. The movement of healthcare in this direction requires a new brand of leadership that innovates without fear of legacy industry structures.

## TECHNOLOGY, MARKET, STAKEHOLDER, AND LEADERSHIP CONSIDERATIONS

Table 17.1 summarizes the three MSs in the context of technology, market, stakeholder, and leadership considerations. Technology encompasses any type of software, hardware, or communication platforms, as well as critical infrastructure, such as networks and security protocols. Technology is implemented by health provider organizations to run day-to-day business operations and meet the regulatory pressures related to health data sharing or health information exchange. As discussed by Vest et al. (2022), most health provider organizations participate in the exchange of information outside of their own business purely on a tactical and regulatory basis. Commonplace in other industry sectors but uncommon in the health provider sector, Stage 3 health provider organizations utilize select internal strategic data assets to form partnerships, co-opt with competitors, and generate new businesses.

### TABLE 17.1. HEALTHCARE PROVIDER STAGES OF TECHNOLOGY EVOLUTION

| STAGE | TECHNOLOGY CONSIDERATIONS | MARKET CONSIDERATIONS | STAKEHOLDER CONSIDERATIONS | LEADERSHIP CONSIDERATIONS |
|---|---|---|---|---|
| Stage 1 | Core transactional clinical and administrative platforms in place<br><br>Basic IT infrastructure in place via in-house or sourced relationships | Technology focuses on cost management and maintaining current revenue streams and customer base. | Operational management orientation: Individual and/or community-level consumer strategies meet regulatory requirements and are secondary to traditional models of care delivery. | Optimize resources. Assure adequate productivity and a low threshold for risk; the focus is on transactional success only at the cost of lost innovation |
| Stage 2 | Transform transactional data into management information<br><br>Expand traditional infrastructure and transactional systems to include best practice technologies proven in other economic sectors | The use of organizational systems and information guides responses to environmental shifts and regulatory changes. | Customer orientation: Analysis of organizational information guides the development of early consumer and population health management strategies in response to changes in customer needs and/or regulatory requirements. | Increased stakeholder acknowledgment and engagement; moderate threshold for risk |
| Stage 3 | Core IT platforms and relationships are optimized. Calculated risk in innovative health and/or industry transference technologies facilitates the support of innovative programs, partnerships, or businesses to support the mission. | Technologies and data transformed into information are governed as assets and enable the organization to become a market leader and/or disruptor in select strategic areas. | Generative orientation: Consumers, communities, and stakeholder ecosystems (partners, regulators, co-opted behavior with competitors) guide growth and sustainment strategies. | Innovation focused: High risk necessitates appropriate risk-taking using integrity and ethics; highly visible accountability; demands effective change management skills |

IT, information technology.

Market considerations are also part of staged technology evolution. Traditionally, health provider markets in the United States have been preordained by regulatory requirements and brick-and-mortar strategies involving the growth of hospitals and referring physicians. In the new health economy, virtual health delivery capabilities will likely integrate public and population health modeling, dissolving provider health organizations and market boundaries. External factors, such as rising pharmaceutical costs and global health concerns postpandemic, push organizations toward new and creative partnerships and alignments, such as partners in the retail economic sector. It is forecasted that continued global disruptions and economic globalization will continue to catalyze increasingly creative partnerships across sectors of the digital consumer economy (Dube et al., 2022).

As discussed by Dorrance and Clement (2021), healthcare is an essential service that has yet to fully optimize the levels of digitization ubiquitous in other industries. The reasons for this are complex and historical, dating back to paternalistic models of healthcare delivery. We see outdated software applications, such as secure information and portals written in the language, utilized by healthcare providers, not consumers of health services. As we evolve past systems and technologies that serve only the internal needs of health organizations, we see disruptors entering the health provider economy with an eye on the evolving needs of the 21st-century health community consumers. Stage 3 provider organizations seek calculated risk-based opportunities to experiment in developing these new models of health delivery, leveraging the capabilities of the global digital economy.

Savvy leaders who find the optimal balance across all three stages and integrate the three stages with a strategic consumer-facing focus create the pathway to sustained efficient operations, innovation, and growth. These leaders will propel their organizations to the forefront and create unprecedented service to the patients and communities they serve.

Innovative technology products and services can disrupt an existing market. Technologies that focus on care expansion via an integrated experience and generating data to improve individual patients' and population health will continue to gain momentum. Thriving health organizations will leverage effective technology and facilitate business strategies present in other industries. Those who ignore these changes will eventually be left behind. The rapid testing and deployment of vaccines and the increase in telemedicine service delivery during the COVID-19 pandemic is just one pendulum swing that has disrupted archaic healthcare practices. Figure 17.1 provides example scenarios of the crossover between MSs.

**FIGURE 17.1.** Modular stage model of optimal adoption.

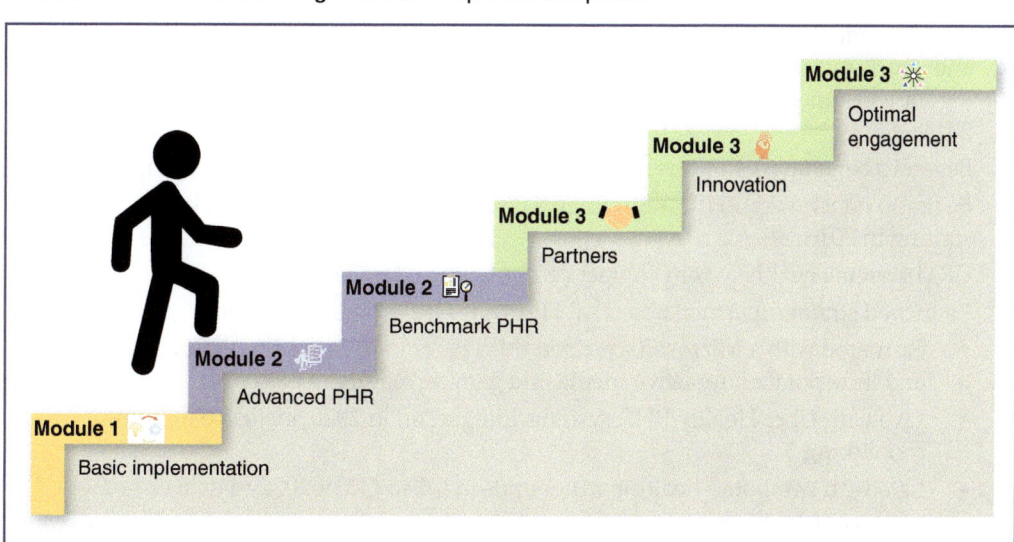

## CASE STUDY 17.1: HEALTH PROVIDER ORGANIZATION SCENARIO A (STAGES 1 AND 2)

Background: Health system with three community hospitals, 200 employed physicians, a long-term care partner, and 10 urgent care centers in their service area
   Technology Topic: Personal Health Record (PHR)

- Implemented patient-provider messaging for 20% of the patient population as required by the federal government in 2013
- Studied health system portal and nonportal health system use and users beginning in 2014; continued to conduct focus groups and consumer surveys regarding PHR use and preferences
- Progressively developed and marketed advanced PHR functions such as direct routine office scheduling and paying bills online, integrated PHR/ambulatory kiosk fast check-in and check-out technologies and online visits, and integrated PHR tele-home monitoring for consumers with chronic illnesses such as coronary heart disease and diabetes
- Began to benchmark PHR use to peer health provider organizations beginning in 2018
- Currently, the use of PHR services by health system consumers has plateaued at approximately 48% of eligible users.

## CASE STUDY 17.2: HEALTH PROVIDER ORGANIZATION SCENARIO B: (STAGES 1 AND 2 AND 3)

Background: Health system with three community hospitals, 200 employed physicians, a long-term care partner, and 10 urgent care centers in their service area
   Technology Topic: PHR

- Implemented patient-provider messaging for 20% of the patient population as required by the federal government in 2010 when CMS Phase III program guidelines were clear
- Implemented bill pay online in 2011 to mitigate operational costs of per person, per year portal software fees
- Progressively developed and marketed advanced PHR functions such as direct routine office scheduling and paying bills online, integrated PHR/ambulatory kiosk fast check-in and check-out technologies and online visits, and integrated PHR tele-home monitoring for consumers with chronic illnesses such as coronary heart disease and diabetes by 2014
- Began to benchmark PHR use to peer health provider organizations beginning in 2015
- Began to benchmark PHR use to financial service portal used by a similar customer base starting in 2016
- CRM systems health system contact center launched in 2017.
- Launched strategic partner-based All Health (PHR) program in 2018
    - Partnered with a Microsoft-certified third party to improve the PHR user interface and incorporate interactive media and gaming features in 2019
    - Live with Uber Health-PHR systems integration in 2020, inclusive of home monitoring
    - Live with two home health partner apps in Q1 to Q3 of 2022 to deliver home services, connected visits, and brick-and-mortar consumer medical ride-sharing

- Live with three retail partner food and consumer health goods home delivery apps in Q4 of 2022
- Live with health system geo mapping and consumer navigation platform in 2023

Currently, the use of All PHR services by health system consumers has an 89% total eligible engagement rate with a steady 2% annual growth.

## CONCLUSION

Provider organizations' ability to execute Stage 3 of the technology maturity evolution depends upon alignment between the information technology (IT) function and the strategic functions of the provider organization. This alignment requires reinforcement from the strategic planning process and **advanced leadership skills**. For a health organization to become a generative contributor to a new health economy, technology functions and investments must align completely with the strategic imperatives of the organization. In this mindset, effective management of technology and data occurs as a partnership in a thriving organization. The short- and long-term strategic technology planning should include engagement from a multidisciplinary team. Unification across IT, strategic, operational, and financial leadership creates a spectrum of alignment that facilitates the achievement of technology and data innovation across all three stages.

## END-OF-CHAPTER RESOURCES

### CRITICAL THINKING QUESTIONS

- What are the most prevalent needs of consumers that health provider organizations should address in the next 5 years?
- Describe three specific challenges that an academic provider health system, comprised of hospitals, physician practices, long-term care, and rehabilitation organizations, as well as home for services, might face when deploying a CRM strategy to maintain their regional market share.
- Discuss the reasons why a small community hospital might be unable to move from Stage 1 of technology advancement 5 years after deploying its EHR platform.
- List five attributes of a perceptive community health system CEO who holds their CIO accountable for Stage 3 technology advancement.
- Why is the field of change management a critical element of moving through technology stages?
- How do innovative healthcare leaders leverage Stage 3 technology advancement to address workforce concerns?
- Discuss the risks and proposed mitigation strategies associated with a high-volume internal medicine practice based in an urban setting deploying online health visits for non-acute illnesses.
- What digital functions do community health consumers expect from organizations that provide healthcare services?
- How can innovative Stage 3 healthcare provider organizations partner with regional employers to leverage technology and improve workforce health?
- Discuss the composition of multidisciplinary teams needed to develop a Stage 3 healthcare provider technology strategy.

### LEARNING ACTIVITIES

**CourseConnect ▸**

To access self-assessment questions and interactive, competency-based learning activities for this chapter, visit www.springerpub.com/courseconnect. See inside front cover and tear-out card for CourseConnect details.

### REFERENCES

Aggarwal, D., Chaturvedi, V., Ramachandran, A., & Singh, T. (2024). Managing talent among healthcare human resource: Strategies for a new normal. *Journal of Health Management*, 26(2), 384–393. https://doi.org/10.1177/09720634231218769

Akbarzadeh Janatabad, A., Sadegheih, A., Lotfi, M. M., & Mostafaeipour, A. (2022). Determining the tariffs of physicians using a combined model of data mining techniques and fuzzy logic in health insurance. *International Journal of Industrial Engineering & Production Research*, 33(1): 1–9. https://doi.org/10.22068/ijiepr.33.1.13

Baashar, Y., Alhussian, H., Patel, A., Alkawsi, G., Alzahrani, A. I., Alfarraj, O., & Hayder G. (2020). Customer relationship management systems (CRMS) in the healthcare environment: A systematic literature review. *Computer Standards & Interfaces*, 71, 103442. https://doi.org/10.1016/j.csi.2020.103442

Boyce, L., Harun, A., Prybutok, G., & Prybutok, V. R. (2024). The role of technology in online health communities: A study of information-seeking behavior. *Healthcare*, 12(3), 2227–9032. https://doi.org/10.3390/healthcare12030336

Breuer, S., Braun, M., Tigard, D., Buyx, A., & Müller, R. (2023). How engineers' imaginaries of healthcare shape design and user engagement: A case study of a robotics initiative for geriatric healthcare AI applications. *ACM Transactions on Computer–Human Interaction, 30*(2), 1–33. https://doi.org/10.1145/3577010

Centers for Medicare & Medicaid Services. (2024). *NHE fact sheet*. https://www.cms.gov/data-research/statistics-trends-and-reports/national-health-expenditure-data/nhe-fact-sheet

Dorrance, K. A., & Clement, B. D. (2021). Transforming the provision of healthcare through emerging technology: A strategic transformation. *Families, Systems, & Health, 39*(1), 158–162. https://doi.org/10.1037/fsh0000597

Dube, O., Simuka, J., & Chitumba, C. (2022). Exploring strategic innovation in the success of private health care business: A conceptual model. *Journal of Research and Innovation for Sustainable Society, 4*(2), 190–199.

Esmaeilzadeh, P. (2020). Use of AI-based tools for healthcare purposes: A survey study from consumers' perspectives. *BMC Medical Informatics and Decision Making, 20*(1), 170. https://doi.org/10.1186/s12911-020-01191-1

Johnson, M., Albizri, A., & Harfouche, A. (2023). Responsible artificial intelligence in healthcare: Predicting and preventing insurance claim denials for economic and social wellbeing. *Information Systems Frontiers, 25*(6), 2179–2195. https://doi.org/10.1007/s10796-021-10137-5

Mauro, T. G., & Borges-Andrade, J. E. (2020). Human resource system as innovation for organisations. *Innovation & Management Review, 17*(2), 197–214. https://doi.org/10.1108/INMR-03-2019-0037

Nguyen, V., Ara, P., Simmons, D., & Osuagwu, U. L. (2024). The role of digital health technology interventions in the prevention of type 2 diabetes mellitus: A systematic review. *Clinical Medicine Insights: Endocrinology and Diabetes, 2024*(17), 1–11. https://doi.org/10.1177/11795514241246419

Pardamean, B., Soeparno, H., Budiarto, A., Mahesworo, B., & Baurley, J. (2020). Quantified self-using consumer wearable device: Predicting physical and mental health. *Healthcare Informatics Research, 26*(2), 83–92. https://doi.org/10.4258/hir.2020.26.2.83

Parsons, A., McCullough, C., Wang, J., & Shih, S. (2012). Validity of electronic health record-derived quality measurement for performance monitoring. *Journal of the American Medical Informatics Association, 19*(4), 604–609. https://doi.org/10.1136/amiajnl-2011-000557

Poquiz, W. A. (2022). Blockchain technology in healthcare: An analysis of strengths, weaknesses, opportunities, and threats. *Journal of Healthcare Management, 67*(4), 244–253. https://doi.org/10.1097/JHM-D-22-00106

Schulman, K. A., Nielsen, P. K., Jr., & Patel, K. (2023). AI alone will not reduce the administrative burden of health care. *JAMA: Journal of the American Medical Association, 330*(22), 2159–2160. https://doi.org/10.1001/jama.2023.23809

Sieja, A., Kim, E., Holmstrom, H., Rotholz, S., Lin, C. T., Gonzalez, C., Arellano, C., Hutchings, S., Henderson, D., & Markley, K. (2021). Multidisciplinary sprint program achieved specialty-specific EHR optimization in 20 clinics. *Applied Clinical Informatics, 12*(2), 329–339. https://doi.org/10.1055/s-0041-1728699

U.S. Department of Health and Human Services. (n.d.). *Guidance portal*. https://www.hhs.gov/guidance

Vest, J. R., Freedman, S., Unruh, M. A., Bako, A. T., & Simon, K. (2022). Strategic use of health information exchange and market share, payer mix, and operating margins. *Health Care Management Review, 47*(1), 28–36. https://doi.org/10.1097/HMR.0000000000000293

CHAPTER

# DATA MANAGEMENT AND ANALYTICS IN HEALTHCARE MANAGEMENT

Elizabeth K. McNutt and Bankole Olatosi

## LEARNING OBJECTIVES

- Articulate the importance of data in healthcare and recognize sources.
- Differentiate between types of data.
- Describe how data is analyzed to determine patterns, develop best practices, and produce predictive models for strategic intelligence.
- Demonstrate how to query, judge, and consume data for decision-making.
- Establish data competency and areas for growth.

## KEY TERMS

- Artificial intelligence
- Data analytics
- Data cleaning and preprocessing
- Data life cycle
- Data visualization
- Machine learning

## INTRODUCTION TO DATA ANALYTICS IN HEALTHCARE

Data collection and use in healthcare is growing at an enormous rate. Years from now, imagine your morning alarm going off. In examining your wearable health dashboard, you see that you have slept 7.14 hours and snored an unusual amount, a note that will be shared with your primary care practitioner if it recurs. Your blood sugar is slightly lower than your physician would like, so a message pops up with suggestions for how to best start your day. During your morning workout, your heart rate and other vitals are tracked. Examining data over the past several months, it was determined that walking, yoga, and lifting light weights provided the most benefits for you personally. In the afternoon, a wearable device captures some arrhythmia and not only suggests a call to your physician but also can predict tests you will likely need and scan registration options against your personal calendar to suggest the date and time that works best. It is Tuesday, so your favorite Mediterranean lunch is ordered and delivered to the office. At the end of the day, you read a summary of your stats to see how your sleep, exercise, stress, and choices that day might have affected your health. When you do go in for your tests, the results are compared against those of other patients, and a possible care plan is suggested to the clinician who interprets your results.

At the healthcare facility where you work, there are ongoing issues with staffing shortages, revenue generation, and quality of care. Similar to every other healthcare organization, your department is challenged with doing more for less, while transforming health outcomes. Your organization's robust systems have data from human resources on your clinicians' and nurses' productivity and the acuity of patient care provided. There is extensive data from electronic health records about all aspects of the patient encounter, billing, and claims. A real-time healthcare revenue cycle analytics management (RCM) system is also available to you. In addition, your organization has invested in various types of "data lakes," ensuring that data is available for driving and guiding decision-making. Your biggest challenge is knowing where to use data to solve your unit and organizational-level issues.

Elsewhere, oncology patient outcomes are correlated to clinical data to help develop best practices, refining clinical pathways that one day may save your own life. Medications are prescribed and dosed based on patients' personal genetics, evaluated for effectiveness and cost efficiency, assessed for risk factors, monitored to avoid adverse drug reactions, and delivered to patients. In your county, social determinants of health data help set community priorities, and technological advancements provide new treatment avenues for all population subgroups.

While some of these options are not widely adopted yet, they are all examples of ways we can use data to improve healthcare decisions and outcomes. Today, understanding data and working with it is becoming a necessary and valuable skill that requires both science and a little bit of art (intuition and experience), much like medicine has always entailed. In this chapter we discuss the types of healthcare data, characteristics, sources, working with data, and assessing your competencies around data.

Early data collection has paved the way for advances in healthcare analytics, epidemiology, clinical outcomes, payor management, and evidence-based management. Later in the chapter, we discuss some of the specific data types captured.

## DATA ANALYTICS

**Data analytics** is the science and art of using tools and processes to extract information, knowledge, and insight to deliver intelligence from collected sources of information to drive operational decisions.

Leveraging data, future trends can be modeled, decisions evaluated, and performance measured to improve patient care, strategic planning, and population health. As a result of ongoing technological, organizational, and methodological advances, combined with the rapid increase in health data, it is now possible to identify more patterns and correlations in data to improve decisions. It has the potential to reduce runaway healthcare costs and improve outcomes. For example, ambulatory care data is helpful in predicting no-show patients whose slots can be filled by other patients, thereby reducing wasted capacity. Similarly, inpatient readmissions, penalties, and costs could be significantly reduced by using data to predict patients most at risk for readmission in real time. Types of health analytics are discussed in detail later in the chapter.

These complexities and the nature of healthcare data require organizations to build effective organizational capabilities in business analytics (BA) to improve performance and create a competitive advantage. Current estimates show that the U.S. healthcare system's effective use of big data could generate more than $300 billion annually through the extraction of intelligence and automated analysis of operational and clinical outcomes (Roski et al., 2014).

*Take away:* Data comes from a variety of sources, and the more integrated it becomes, the more we are able to see patterns, connections, and identify opportunities.

## TYPES OF HEALTHCARE DATA

Before working with data, it is essential to understand its characteristics and how data are collected, stored, and analyzed. It is also essential to be aware of secondary data sources separate from those collected within organizations. Healthcare data can be structured (administrative claims, billing, financing, genotype, phenotype, etc.) or unstructured (memos, clinical notes, prescriptions, medical imaging, lifestyle, etc.). It can be well defined or incomplete and imprecise. Here are some categories of data you will come across in the healthcare industry:

### ADMINISTRATIVE

*Accounting data* can show the financial health of an organization and how they utilize resources. It provides information to investors and governance boards and can be benchmarked against other organizations. *All-payor claims* include billing and claims that allow for tracking patients across providers and facilities regardless of their payor. It is often physician centric and does not represent 100% of claims, so while helpful, it is incomplete. This data is often used to estimate market share, especially on the ambulatory side of care. *Longitudinal claims* data account for all care touchpoints across a provider's patient population but are specific only to a single payor. This data can be used to track patient care across the continuum and identify gaps in care. It can also be used to predict the need for care in a population. Finally, *finance/billing data* shows us billing information, costs, denials, and payments (profit and loss) at a patient level.

### OPERATIONS AND STRATEGY

*Market data* is collected at the state level and focused on the inpatient, ED, and same-day surgery populations. It is useful for calculating market share and identifying trends; however, it has a lot of the data "blinded" or hidden from users. *Electronic health records data* in a decision support system combine patient demographics, payor and finance information, clinical visit information, quality outcomes, and physician/facility information. They are internal to an organization and the most accurate and current data. They are helpful in examining performance across service lines, patient groups, facilities, and physicians over time but only within that organization.

### CLINICAL

*Clinical trials data* produce large amounts of data in an experimental setting. While not unbiased, it can offer insight into the safety and efficacy of healthcare treatments. *Disease management data* is utilized to study disease categories. Examples include pharmaceutical data, personal health habits, and clinical technologies' impact on disease management. The Geisinger Food Farmacy (Feinberg et al., 2018) is an ongoing case example where data analytics is being used to improve the health of diabetics and reduce healthcare utilization by providing them with free, nutritious food and a comprehensive suite of medical, dietetic, social, and environmental services. *Disease registries* contain data about patients with a specific disease. These registries can be hospital specific (e.g., the Smilow Cancer Hospital at Yale-New Haven and Yale Cancer Center Tumor Registry; Boffa et al., 2017), population based (e.g., Surveillance, Epidemiology, and End Results [SEER]; National Cancer Institute, 2018), or patient/community registries (e.g., the Pulmonary Fibrosis Foundation [PFF] registry). Data from these registries can be used to provide insights and support clinical care.

An ever-increasing need exists for quality metrics, built using *data on outcomes and quality*. Understanding how effective a drug may be for a condition and its side effects allows patients and their doctors to plan for treatments. Tracking hospital readmission rates, length of stay (LOS), and infection rates allows administrators to know if they are improving outcomes. *Pharmacy data* is useful when examining what medications are administered and to whom, and tracking outcomes and side effects helps pharmaceutical companies plan for their production and use of medications. Likewise, companies might track who is prescribing their medications, who is taking the medications, what alternative options are available, what competitors offer, and how they compare against these other options. *Omics* includes data generated by biospecimens such as blood and tissue samples. It involves all biological studies ending with -omics, such as genomics (genes), proteomics (proteins), and transcriptomics (RNA molecules like mRNA in enzymes and vaccines), and is powerful for predictive medicine. *Patient self-reported data* are incorporated into large-scale analyses known as patient-reported outcomes (PRO). MedWatch, as an example, is a program used by the Food and Drug Administration (FDA) for reporting reactions or issues with medical products, including products such as drugs and cosmetics (Getz et al., 2014).

The 21st Century Cures Act, partially enforced through the information blocking rule, now mandates all providers to give access to their electronic medical records (EMR) free of charge (Leonard et al., 2023). This has led to interactive *patient portals* through which patients can input and access health data (Magid et al., 2022). The portals serve a variety of roles in healthcare today. *Consumer wearables* and smart devices also track ever-increasing amounts of data, everything from how much you snored last night to your resting heart rate and blood glucose level after eating a bagel. It can help track gait and balance and identify patients at risk for falls or other healthcare use cases.

## CONTEXTUAL

*Social determinants of health data* include factors that impact a patient's overall wellbeing and ability to maintain health, including factors such as access to care, transportation, homelessness, and food insecurity. Public Census data helps track population in terms of size but also provides information on migration patterns, race percentages, education status, and much more. Data from the Centers for Disease Control and Prevention (CDC) and other sources share local, national, and even international data on many factors tracking the health of a population. *Environmental data* includes data on environmental factors including air/water quality, pollution, and the built environment (e.g., bike lanes, safe neighborhoods) that impact patient's health. *Behavioral health data* includes data on factors impacting the mental health and behaviors of patients, including social support systems and lifestyle habits (e.g., substance use, exercise, access to healthy foods). *Public health initiatives data* include policy data that help promote health and prevent diseases, such as vaccination programs/guidelines, tobacco control, opioid misuse, antidiscrimination, and health equity programs. Figure 18.1 displays the data types just discussed into the four categories.

**FIGURE 18.1.** Four types of healthcare data and examples of each.

| Healthcare data types | |
|---|---|
| **Administrative**<br>Claims data<br>Longitudinal claims<br>Finance/billing<br>Accounting | **Operations and Strategy**<br>Market data<br>Patient records<br>Community demographics<br>Disease management<br>Disease registry |
| **Clinical**<br>Pharmacy<br>Patient-reported outcomes<br>Clinical trials<br>Electronic health records<br>Omics<br>Quality and outcomes<br>Smart devices | **Contextual**<br>Census data<br>Demographic projections<br>Utilization projections |

## DATA CHARACTERISTICS

In addition to the sources and descriptions of data mentioned earlier, data has characteristics that refer to what is collected, how often, how quickly, and how accurately. These characteristics include volume, variety, velocity, veracity, and value.

- *Volume* refers to the amount of health data generated. Estimating the ever-changing amount of data is difficult due to the dynamic nature of data creation, collection, and storage. Current projections show healthcare data will exceed 10 zettabytes by 2025 (Rehman et al., 2022). Healthcare is already generating the world's largest volume (approx. 36% by 2025) of data by compound annual growth rates (CAGR; L.E.K. Consulting, 2023).
- *Variety* refers to the different types and heterogeneous nature of healthcare data, particularly structured and unstructured.
- *Velocity* is the speed with which real-time clinical and operational data is being generated and the need for continuous data collection, management, and analytics.
- *Veracity* refers to the accuracy of data obtained from multiple systems, emphasizing data reliability based on missing data, data temporality, fraud, duplication, and latency.
- *Value* represents the cost-benefit to the organization measured through the insight discovery and patterns (business intelligence) obtained and the ability to make impactful clinical and operational data-driven decisions.

## TYPES OF ANALYTICS

There are four types of analytics commonly used in healthcare, namely, descriptive, diagnostic, predictive, and prescriptive. *Descriptive* analytics allows you to understand "what is happening" through historical patterns using traditional statistical measures like counts, means, medians, percentages, variance, and standard deviation. You can use these measures to track changes over time. For example, monitoring no-show rates after introducing an intervention, monitoring room occupancy, or tracking revenue collection rates are all descriptive statistics. *Diagnostic* analytics builds on descriptive analytics and helps you understand "why something is happening" through a deeper dive into the data. For example, descriptive analytics might show fluctuations in daily volume for a particular unit but does not provide any pointers as to why. Diagnostic analytics works best when interpretable data mining techniques (e.g., decision trees, random forests) are combined with domain knowledge (domain experts such as clinicians, business analysts, etc.) and are applied to information extracted from historical data.

Predictive analytics allows you to investigate and anticipate future scenarios based on historical data. It allows you to understand what may happen, identify potential outcomes, and plan for the future. For example, you can predict demand, workforce capacity utilization, occupancy rates, and reasons for visits/diagnoses. With predictive analytics, you can use historical data to train predictive models and predict future events using powerful techniques like machine learning. Some of these machine learning models include advanced forecasting techniques and predictive modeling including least absolute shrinkage and selection operator (LASSO) regression, neural networks, and others. For example, you can use historical data to model future risk scores for the following diseases/conditions: frailty, falls, or sepsis. Such predictive models will allow you to assign patients with the appropriate risk score and allocate the right resources. *Prescriptive* analytics is the highest level of healthcare analytics and allows you to examine what can be changed to further improve the predictive model. It can be used to test specific changes regarding treatment processes and strategic operations and to improve efficiency/efficacy. To illustrate this, prescriptive analytics could help assign the best stent to a patient based on genetic makeup, reduce/stop preventable hospitalizations, or determine optimal drug dosing based on patient physiological characteristics. It does this by optimizing the machine learning processes in the predictive analytics stage.

You may also hear the term *personalized* analytics, which is data aggregated at the individual level using mobile devices and wearables, for example. *Operational* analytics uses aforementioned data to specifically track the performance of health systems and their many departments. Figure 18.2 demonstrates the four characteristics of data described earlier.

**FIGURE 18.2.** Four types of data analytics and what question each answers.

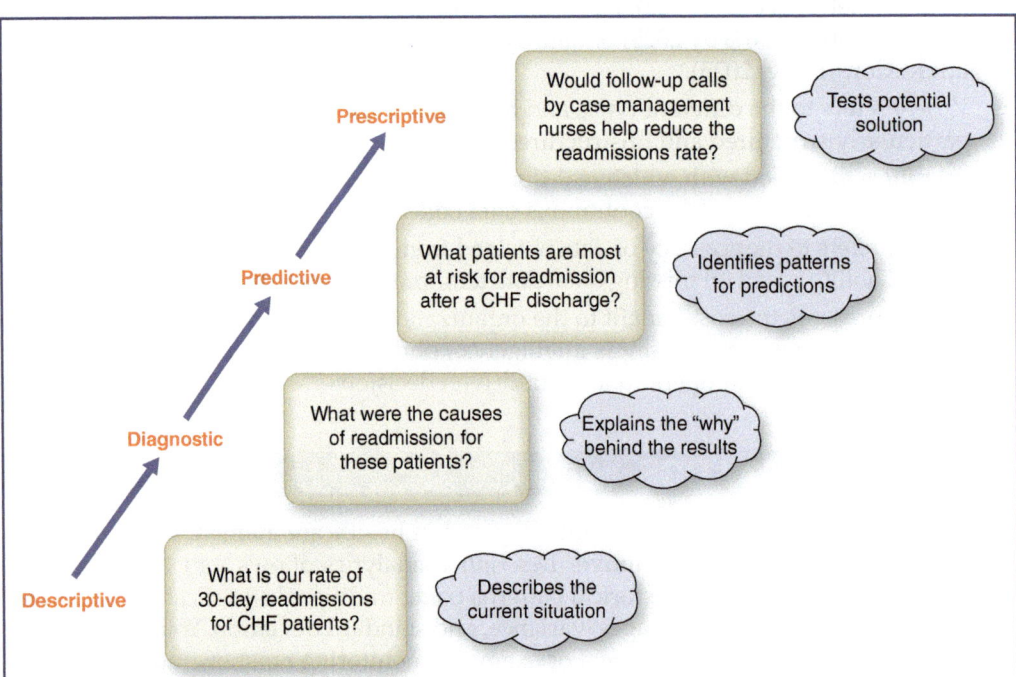

CHF, congestive heart failure.

# WORKING WITH DATA

## DATA COLLECTION

Data must be collected before it can be analyzed. Most often, you will not be collecting the data but may be prepping it, running the analysis, or merely consuming the findings from someone else's analysis. Regardless of how you work with data, you should understand where the underlying data comes from in order to grasp its strengths and weaknesses. If you are not sure, ask questions.

Data can be captured automatically or entered at a point of contact. It can be quantitative (such as a patient's blood pressure or diagnoses codes on a record) or qualitative (such as physician notes or open-ended survey responses), and some data may be more reliable while other requires interpretation to be analyzed. Understanding the data being used is essential for assessing how dependable the results are. For example, grant or licensure applications may request data on patients by race. This is a requirement with the best intentions, as it examines how closely a patient population mirrors the service area population. However, in order to report on it, the data must first be collected, and this can be difficult if patients are not comfortable reporting it at registration. Even worse, it can be incorrect if registrars guess the answer and fill it in on behalf of a patient.

The reporting is much more accurate for data that is close to 100% captured, such as those on EHRs. Even then, there can be errors and omissions or multiple ways of looking at the data. The famous saying "garbage in, garbage out" is very true in healthcare. Your analysis is only as good as the data that you use.

## DATA CLEANING AND PREPROCESSING: PREPARING DATA FOR ANALYSIS AND CONSUMPTION

When data is received, it is often not ready for immediate use. Before diving in, someone will prepare the file to make it easy to work with, a process known as **data cleaning and preprocessing**. The preparation may start with removing titles and footnotes that come with the file. Data may also be in an incorrect format—for example, dates are exported as unrecognizable numbers, or first and last names may appear in the same cell when they need to be separated. Table 18.1 shows data before and after it was prepped for analysis.

Initial checks save a lot of time and frustration down the line. A *data dictionary* can help orient the user to the data by providing definitions of what each data element is. Performing basic analyses on the data can identify missing or incorrect data that cannot be seen by looking at the data in rows and allows for the opportunity to correct the data before a lot of time is lost on the analysis. If the data is dated, examining trends (month to month or year over year) can identify if the totals appear reasonable. Large shifts in the data could mean either missing data or including data that should not be there. Comparing data to prior reports could also identify discrepancies. The more familiar you are with the data being examined, the more comfortable you will be recalling where errors have occurred in the past and testing for those.

On the other hand, if you are the recipient of data in reports or a presentation, take the time to read titles and notes. Give the analysis a gut check—does it make sense? If you are being shown a report that each patient visited the dentist on average 18.2 times a year, you should recognize that to be incorrect. When presenting data, it is very important to check over reports. Do they make sense and tell a story? Are results reasonable? Are there gaps or changes in the data that are not accounted for? Can someone speak to the trends displayed, where the data came from, and how it was analyzed? Do other sources of data

### TABLE 18.1. SAMPLE DATA SET PREPARED FOR ANALYSIS

| EXTRACT FROM SOURCE SYSTEM |
| --- |
| 13-Jul-23 |
| Orthopedic patients |
| Birthday, Last Name, First Name, Admit Date, Patient Type |
| Mar. 11, 2008, Yao, Finley, 44941, Emergency |
| Jan. 22, 2017, Moyer, Phoenix, 44981, Outpatient |
| Mar. 29, 2013, Wainwright, Amari, 45015, Inpatient |
| Sep. 7, 2010, Arden, Dakota, 45028, Same Day Surgery |
| Nov. 5, 2006, Peltier, Remington, 45051, Outpatient |
| Nov. 12, 2009, Blue, Oakley, 45096, Emergency |
| Sep. 17, 2018, Fogarty, Sage, 45111, Inpatient |
| Oct. 2, 2020, Harlow, Rory, 45152, Inpatient |

| BIRTHDAY | LAST NAME | FIRST NAME | ADMIT DATE | PATIENT TYPE |
| --- | --- | --- | --- | --- |
| Mar. 11, 2008 | Yao | Finley | 15-Jan-23 | Emergency |
| Jan. 22, 2017 | Moyer | Phoenix | 24-Feb-23 | Outpatient |
| Mar. 29, 2013 | Wainwright | Amari | 30-Mar-23 | Inpatient |
| Sep. 7, 2010 | Arden | Dakota | 12-Apr-23 | Same-day surgery |
| Nov. 5, 2006 | Peltier | Remington | 5-May-23 | Outpatient |
| Nov. 12, 2009 | Blue | Oakley | 19-Jun-23 | Emergency |
| Sep. 17, 2018 | Fogarty | Sage | 4-Jul-23 | Inpatient |
| Oct. 2, 2020 | Harlow | Rory | 14-Aug-23 | Inpatient |

support the findings? It is also important to summarize the data into tables or graphs that communicate information and highlight takeaways.

While you may think that analyzing data is the biggest part of using information to yield patterns and reports, that is not the case. Understanding a request is essential. Ensuring that the data needed is properly collected and reliable is a large portion of a data project. Working to ensure the data is accurate, cleaning up any errors, and validating the raw data and findings also occur before running reports. Once there is good, clean data to work with in the proper format, the analysis is the fun part. Using the analysis to tell a story is what converts the data into useful intelligence.

*Take away:* Data analysis starts with data collection, validation, and understanding.

## BENCHMARKING DATA

After data has been collected and analyzed, how do we know whether the results are acceptable or should be improved? How do organizations know what to prioritize? That is done by comparing results to baseline data. This can be established internally—for example, sometimes baseline data is simply the starting point at first measurement and continuously tracked over time for improvement (think about measuring the cost of a service and working to improve its efficiencies over time); or the same data can be examined and compared across service lines to rank quality, profitability, volumes, or any number of measures. Still, another way to benchmark data is to compare it to industry standards. Some data may be publicly reported by organizations such as Leapfrog, the Joint Commission, the CDC, and Healthgrades. Or there are opportunities to join collaborations where members share data with each other for the purpose of understanding how they compare, such as for operating room benchmarking data. However benchmarking data is acquired, it can be important to help prioritize initiatives and know where the focus efforts.

*Ask yourself*: Think of a data element that you encounter; how do you know if it is dependable? Improving or getting worse over time? How might you set a realistic goal?

## VISUAL DISPLAYS OF DATA

An effective way to convey meaning through **data visualization** is to present it using colors, graphs, maps, and other visuals alongside data on a dashboard. Many applications today allow for a more seamless production of visual tools that can be updated by clicking through parts of the graphs or data tables. Filters can allow users to select the exact data set they are looking for, and automatic feeds make what previously was a manual update instantaneous and current. While we do not have time to review all the different ways to visually display data, to learn more about best practices and to see examples, please visit classics including Tufte's *The Visual Display of Quantitative Information* (Tufte, 2001), similar texts/material or online resources such as Tableau's "Visual Best Practices" (Tableau, n.d.).

## HEALTHCARE ANALYTICS LIFECYCLE

To meet business needs and strategic objectives, health organizations must assemble their data teams with the analytic life cycle in mind. While departments work with various data sets, each goes through the same process to make it useful. If you look up the term **data life cycle**, you will find many descriptions of this process. Each describes a process that starts with data being generated, then collected, and eventually converted to useful information. Table 18.2 walks through these steps.

### TABLE 18.2. LIFE CYCLE OF DATA

| STAGE | DESCRIPTION |
| --- | --- |
| Generation | Data generation is constantly occurring. Our blood pressure, daily step count, vitamin regimen, time in front of television, lab results, driving habits, and online activity are all data points that are generated. |
| Collection | Only a fraction of the data that is generated is collected. The collection can occur manually or automatically. |
| Processed/Validated | Acquiring the data, cleaning, formatting, and validating—all of these are involved in processing the data. |
| Storage/Management | Afterward, the data needs to be stored and formatted in a way that can be accessed and updated. |
| Analysis/Visualization | Here is the step where data analysts review the data and use methods to turn the data into information that is consumable. The analysis is what turns raw data into intelligence used for making decisions. |
| Operationalized/Tracked | After the data is shared, decisions are made based on the insights. The data will drive better decisions and continue to be tracked for efficacy. As new data is received, it will be incorporated into the decision-making. |

*Take away:* Data analysis is a continuous cycle. Data is collected, analyzed, and interpreted to produce intelligence that guides decisions. It is constantly refined as more data is incorporated over time.

## APPROACHES TO ANALYTICS

Several approaches/processes exist on how you can operationalize analytics. We provide a description of the common options from the industry, but at their core, they are similar. Statistical Analysis System (SAS) Statistical Institute uses the SEMMA process for data analytics, which stands for **S**ample (construct/define a representative data set), **E**xplore (know, describe, and visualize your data), **M**odify (change/transform your data as needed), **M**odel (build statistical models), and **A**ssess (score or rank model performance). Another approach is knowledge discovery in databases (KDD) which includes selection (data definition), preprocessing (data cleaning and management), transformation (dimensionality reduction), data mining (pattern identification), and interpretation/evaluation (model evaluation). Another common data approach is the Cross Industry Standard Process for Data Mining (CRISP-DM). It consists of six phases, namely, business understanding, data understanding, data preparation modeling, evaluation, and deployment. The final relatable model is the commonly used Six Sigma DMAIC approach, which includes define, measure, analyze, improve, and control approaches.

## ESTABLISHING A COMPETITIVE ADVANTAGE USING ARTIFICIAL INTELLIGENCE AND DIGITAL TRANSFORMATION

A recent industry survey of thought leaders showed a growing trust and dependence on using **artificial intelligence** (AI) for strategic management, planning, and value alignment (PricewaterhouseCoopers [PwC], 2024). To gain a competitive advantage in this area, healthcare organizations must leverage advanced analytics to utilize data-driven business processes that yield quicker (agile) solutions while building mature internal and customer-facing technologies. While you may hear them used interchangeably, AI refers to a field aimed at creating machines that can perform tasks typically requiring human intelligence and reasoning/problem-solving. **Machine learning** is a subset of AI, focusing on developing algorithms and statistical models that would enable machines to learn from data and help make projections and predictions.

To maintain a competitive advantage, healthcare organizations must leverage digital transformation and multiply value by rethinking business process analytics and AI. The analytics value add must flow from the backend to the frontlines to improve patient health and organizational operations.

## CHALLENGES WITH ANALYTICS AND ARTIFICIAL INTELLIGENCE

As healthcare proceeds into the new future with analytics, traditional challenges remain of which managers and leaders must be aware to overcome them. A recent industry panel identified some of the concerns outlined in the following paragraphs (Rosen, 2024).

Potential for *bias and ethics* remain prevalent. Algorithmic bias, population bias, and other factors could impact patients and systems significantly through errors. It is essential that trained humans (including multiple domain experts [e.g., clinicians, nurses, and frontline staff]) are involved in interpreting analytics results and providing valuable input and guidance. Managers and leaders must not trivialize or discount organizational concerns about *trust* and the validity of new analytic tools. Clinicians are traditionally wary and suspicious of new tools that are not explainable. Future state leaders and managers must proactively champion, transparently manage, communicate, and address challenges around trust in new algorithms and analytic products for it to succeed.

While *automation* issues persist, COVID-19 changed how we offer and access services, particularly in healthcare. Telehealth, remote human resources workforce analytics, startups, and new providers now thrive in a digital transformation space and provide solutions to known issues with automation specific to healthcare. Successful applications exist within providers, insurers, pharmaceuticals, and technology companies. Healthcare analytics relies on *multidisciplinary* work and includes multiple domain experts (clinicians, administrators, IT, analysts, etc.) working together as a team to optimize solutions. Creating analytic solutions through such multidisciplinary teams increases trust in technology across the team and/or organization. Multidisciplinary teams must be set up early in the analytics life cycle to help with validation and interpretation.

## TOOLS FOR DATA ANALYSIS

New tools and models are continuously developed. However, here are some tools that you should be aware of and familiarize yourself with:

- *Microsoft Excel:* A powerful spreadsheet software a part of the Microsoft Office suite; it is widely used and often the first application data analysts use
- *SAS/Minitab/QI Macros:* Statistical software or add-ons used for data analysis and quality improvement offering a range of analytical capabilities from comprehensive analytics to statistical process control and Excel-based quality improvement tools
- *Tableau:* A leading data visualization tool that allows analysis of larger data sets than Excel and provides increased visual dashboards that can be made interactive for users
- *Power BI:* A business analytics service by Microsoft that provides interactive visualizations with a simple interface for users
- *Python:* A programming language popular due to its readability, libraries, and community support
- *R:* A programming language and environment designed for statistical computing and graphics
- *Structured query language (SQL):* A software suite used for advanced analytics
- *Not only SQL (NoSQL):* A class of database management systems designed to handle a variety of data models known for their flexibility and scalability when dealing with large volumes of unstructured or semistructured data
- *Large language models (LLMs):* Systems capable of understanding and generating human language, which can be leveraged for data analysis. LLMs can identify patterns, extract insights, and generate comprehensive reports. They can automate tasks like data classification, coding, sentiment analysis, and predictive analytics, offering a powerful tool for businesses.

## COMPETENCY MODELS

The World Health Organization's Data Management Competency Framework publication describes data competencies in data generation, processing, analysis, and usage in detail. By examining proficiency levels across dimensions, you can examine where you currently fall and how to increase competencies and comfort (World Health Organization,

### TABLE 18.3. DATA MANAGEMENT COMPETENCY FRAMEWORK

| LEVEL | COMPETENCIES |
| --- | --- |
| 5. Strategic project leader | **Competencies of data driver and:**<br>Able to lead team of data analysts<br>Can prioritize operational questions and make requests that yield intelligence, leading to strategy implementation |
| 4. Data driver | **Competencies of data analyst and:**<br>Able to determine series of data needs for a project<br>Strong communicator and refine requests and scope<br>Work with leadership to refine presentations<br>Comfortable presenting findings to audience |
| 3. Data analyst | **Competencies of data novice and:**<br>Strong understanding of data sets<br>Able to ask appropriate questions to refine requests<br>Knowledge of where to collect data from<br>Competent in performing data analysis in any number of applications |
| 2. Data novice | **Competencies of introductory student and:**<br>Exposure to data collection methods<br>Data analysis through coursework or entry-level job |
| 1. Introductory student | Display curiosity for data and information<br>Strong math and analytical foundation<br>Initial exposure to data sets |

Regional Office for the Western Pacific, 2023). Table 18.3 shows a simplified description the authors of this chapter have outlined to more quickly establish competency levels.

To improve your competencies in data analytics, you can enroll in classes that target these skills in your program or at a local or online university. You can purchase textbooks and self-study, as well as watch videos such as those on YouTube, LinkedIn Learning, Coursera, or other online learning service. Finally, many schools offer online asynchronous learning or tracks, and some sources, such as edX and Khan Academy, offer many options for free lessons. The more you expose yourself to data analytics, and approach it with a learning and curious mindset, the more comfortable you will become with it.

### CASE STUDY 18.1: UTILIZING DATA TO IMPROVE OUTCOMES AND EQUITY

Healthcare outcomes are a key component in evaluating the quality of care and services that are provided by a healthcare system. Pressure ulcers are an indicator of nursing care and patient safety, reflecting on effectiveness of preventative measures implemented by facilities and units to maintain skin integrity, keep patients safe, and promote their overall well-being.

According to the Agency for Healthcare Research and Quality (AHRQ, 2017), the additional hospital inpatient cost for a patient with a pressure ulcer is estimated to be $14,506. Pressure ulcers are also estimated to contribute to 41 excess deaths per 1,000 pressure ulcer cases. In addition to the costs and negative health outcomes, studies have shown race/ethnic disparities in primary pressure ulcer (PPU) hospitalization mortality, length of stay (LOS), and inflation-adjusted charges (IAC; Bazargan-Hejazi et al., 2023).

RWJBarnabas Health (RWJBH) system in New Jersey recognized an opportunity to improve equitable patient care and set out to run a rigorous data analysis methodology to identify incidence by stage of pressure ulcer wounds over 3 years across race, ethnicity, payor types, and RWJBH facilities. They looked at data for all adult inpatients and identified those who were coded with one or more pressure wounds that were not present on admission (POA).

Several statistical analyses were run on the data:

- Logistic regression was used to estimate the probability of an event occurring.
- Odds ratios (ORs) were calculated to compare groups of patients.
- $p$-Values were used to determine any statistically significant associations between the outcome and demographic categories.
- Chi-square tests were conducted to determine if there was a significant association between two categorical variables (e.g., race versus occurrence of pressure wounds).
- Cramer's $V$ was used to indicate the strength of the association (effect size) between two categorical variables as part of the Chi-square tests.

The results showed a statistically significant difference in outcomes across patient groups within race, facility, and payor, especially when compared against Black people, several of their hospitals, and Medicare or Blue Cross patients specifically. The strength of association between occurrence of pressure wounds and these demographic categories was not strong, however. Since the literature suggests that most pressure ulcers are the result of deep tissue injuries (DTI), it led the team to conclude that some DTIs may not have been detected, diagnosed, or coded appropriately among patients with darker pigmented skin as compared to those with lighter skin.

The data team shared these findings with system leaders and clinicians. As a result, job aid materials were updated in the electronic medical records (EMR) system to provide more information on DTIs and pressure injuries. The updated guide highlights who may be more at risk for ulcers, requires providers to document any concerns within 24 hours of admission, and includes pictures of pressure wounds at all stages for both light and dark skin tones. The team continues to track the data and identify additional patient safety indicators to analyze.

## END-OF-CHAPTER RESOURCES

### CRITICAL THINKING QUESTIONS

- What is an example of a career a data analyst can enter in the field of healthcare?
- Name three examples of healthcare data that are currently available today.
- What are some of the various ways that data is collected?
- Identify one source of public data and one that would be available internally to an organization.
- What are some questions that you should be able to answer when consuming data?
- Describe an example of data use through the phases of descriptive, diagnostic, predictive, and prescriptive analytics.
- Where do you fall on the data competency model? What can you do to grow your skills?
- What are the five Vs of data? Provide definitions for each and discuss how they work together.

### LEARNING ACTIVITIES

**CourseConnect >**

To access self-assessment questions and interactive, competency-based learning activities for this chapter, visit www.springerpub.com/courseconnect. See inside front cover and tear-out card for CourseConnect details.

### REFERENCES

Agency for Healthcare Research and Quality. (2017, November). *Estimating the additional hospital inpatient cost and mortality associated with selected hospital-acquired conditions*. Agency for Healthcare Research and Quality. https://www.ahrq.gov/hai/pfp/haccost2017-results.html

Bazargan-Hejazi, S., Ambriz, M., Ullah, S., Khan, S., Bangash, M., Dehghan, K., & Ani, C. (2023). Trends and racial disparity in primary pressure ulcer hospitalizations outcomes in the US from 2005 to 2014. *Medicine, 102*(40), e35307. https://doi.org/10.1097/MD.0000000000035307

Boffa, D. J., Rosen, J. E., Mallin, K., Loomis, A., Gay, G., Palis, B., Thoburn, K., Gress, D., McKellar, D. P., Shulman, L. N., Facktor, M. A., & Winchester, D. P. (2017). Using the National Cancer Database for outcomes research: A review. *JAMA Oncology, 3*(12), 1722–1728. https://doi.org/10.1001/jamaoncol.2016.6905

Feinberg, A. T., Hess, A., Passaretti, M., Coolbaugh, S., & Lee, T. H. (2018). Prescribing food as a specialty drug. *NEJM Catalyst, 4*(2). https://catalyst.nejm.org/doi/full/10.1056/CAT.18.0212

Getz, K. A., Stergiopoulos, S., & Kaitin, K. I. (2014). Evaluating the completeness and accuracy of MedWatch data. *American Journal of Therapeutics, 21*(6), 442–446. https://doi.org/10.1097/mjt.0b013e318262316f

L.E.K. Consulting. (2023, December 4). *Tapping into new potential: Realising the value of data in the healthcare sector*. https://www.lek.com/insights/hea/eu/ei/tapping-new-potential-realising-value-data-healthcare-sector

Leonard, S. M., Zackula, R., & Wilcher, J. (2023). Attitudes and experiences of clinicians after mandated implementation of open notes by the 21st Century Cures Act: Survey study. *Journal of Medical Internet Research, 25*, e42021. https://doi.org/10.2196/42021

Magid, S. K., Cohen, K., & Katzovitz, L. S. (2022). 21st Century Cures Act, an information technology-led organizational initiative. *HSS Journal®, 18*(1), 42–47. https://doi.org/10.1177/15563316211041613

National Cancer Institute. (2018). *Surveillance, epidemiology, and end results program. SEER*. https://seer.cancer.gov/

PricewaterhouseCoopers. (2024). *PWC's 27th annual global CEO survey*. PwC. https://www.pwc.com/gx/en/ceo-survey/2024/download/27th-ceo-survey.pdf

Rehman, A., Naz, S., & Razzak, I. (2022). Leveraging big data analytics in healthcare enhancement: Trends, challenges and opportunities. *Multimedia Systems, 28*, 1339–1371. https://doi.org/10.1007/s00530-020-00736-8

Rosen, H. (2024, August 12). Council post: Top five opportunities and challenges of AI in healthcare. *Forbes*. https://www.forbes.com/councils/forbesbusinesscouncil/2023/02/07/top-five-opportunities-and-challenges-of-ai-in-healthcare/

Roski, J., Bo-Linn, G. W., & Andrews, T. A. (2014). Creating value in health care through big data: Opportunities and policy implications. *Health Affairs, 33*(7), 1115–1122. https://doi.org/10.1377/hlthaff.2014.0147

Tableau. (n.d.). *Visual best practices*. Help.tableau.com. https://help.tableau.com/current/blueprint/en-us/bp_visual_best_practices.htm

Tucker, T. C., Durbin, E. B., McDowell, J. K., & Huang, B. (2019). Unlocking the potential of population-based cancer registries. *Cancer, 125*(21), 3729–3737.

Tufte, E. R. (2001). *The visual display of quantitative information* (2nd ed.). Graphics Press.

World Health Organization, Regional Office for the Western Pacific. (2023). *Data management competency framework*. WHO Regional Office for the Western Pacific. https://iris.who.int/handle/10665/367502

# CHAPTER 19

# INTRODUCTION TO HEALTHCARE COMPLIANCE

Tina Batra Hershey and Natalie C. Bulger

## LEARNING OBJECTIVES

- Identify the seven essential elements of an effective compliance program.
- Explain the difference between fraud, waste, and abuse (FWA).
- Describe the history of compliance programs.
- Understand the major federal fraud and abuse laws and enforcement agencies.
- Understand and apply solutions associated with a real-life compliance incident.

## KEY TERMS

- Compliance
- Corrective action
- Ethics
- Fraud, waste, and abuse
- Just culture
- Mitigation
- Oversight
- Regulation
- Reporting
- Risk management

## HEALTHCARE COMPLIANCE OVERVIEW

### WHAT IS COMPLIANCE?

In the healthcare industry, **compliance** means providing healthcare services within applicable laws, regulations, and policies set by federal and state governments, as well as those instituted by private insurers and government contractors. Compliance also encompasses following the organization's internal policies, procedures, and code of conduct, all of which should be rooted in the higher level rules and **regulations**, but which may apply additional requirements to employees, stakeholders, and third-party contractors.

## WHY IS COMPLIANCE IMPORTANT?

As one of the most highly regulated industries in the United States, healthcare entities are required to comply with numerous statutes, regulations, and policies. Healthcare compliance professionals and programs are tasked with preventing, detecting, and correcting violations of these regulations in order to ensure effective and efficient use of resources and the provision of high-quality care. Healthcare spending in the United States reached $4.3 trillion in 2021, accounting for 18.3% of the gross domestic product (Centers for Medicare and Medicaid Services.[CMS], 2021). Government officials have estimated that up to 10% of this spending can be attributed to **fraud, waste, and abuse** (FWA; U.S. Department of Justice [DOJ], 2020). Moreover, in FY 2022, the government obtained more than $2 billion of settlements and judgments involving fraud and false claims (DOJ, 2022). Thus, a major component of compliance is associated with FWA laws, discussed in more detail in the following section.

*Fraud* is generally defined as knowingly and willfully executing, or attempting to execute, a scheme or artifice to defraud any healthcare benefit program or to obtain (by means of false or fraudulent pretenses, representations, or promises) any of the money or property owned by, or under the custody or control of, any healthcare benefit program (18 U.S.C. § 1347). Waste means direct or indirect overutilization of services or practices that result in unnecessary costs to the healthcare system, including Medicare and Medicaid programs. Abuse involves payment for items or services when there is no legal entitlement to that payment and the individual or entity has not knowingly and/or intentionally misrepresented facts to obtain payment.

## WHAT IS A COMPLIANCE PROGRAM?

A compliance program is an infrastructure of rules, procedures, trainings, penalties, and protocols designed to prevent, detect, respond to, reduce, and report instances of noncompliance with laws and **ethics** rules. A compliance program must include certain elements, discussed later in this chapter, in order to be effective.

## BENEFITS OF COMPLIANCE PROGRAMS

Compliance programs offer a variety of benefits to healthcare organizations, including the stakeholders and the patients they serve. First, they demonstrate good corporate citizenship, which enhances public image and reputation. They also serve as a clearinghouse and one-stop shop for legal and payor requirements. Compliance programs encourage employees to report misconduct, which can help staff feel empowered to ask questions, thereby allowing entities to react quickly and effectively to reports by providing methods to address misconduct and protocols for investigations. In many cases, misconduct or potential compliance violations are first detected by those intimately involved in the associated processes or by individuals immediately impacted. Ensuring safe and reliable **reporting** from those with firsthand knowledge can strengthen a compliance program immensely. Finally, an effective compliance program reduces exposure to a wide range of civil and criminal legal penalties.

## HISTORY OF COMPLIANCE PROGRAMS

Today, healthcare entities are expected to operate effective compliance programs. However, this expectation has evolved over time and can be traced back to other industries. In the 1980s, defense contractors became the subject of investigations and prosecutions regarding procurement schemes against the federal government, leading to voluntary initiatives throughout the industry to combat this rampant fraud. In 1991, the U.S. Sentencing Commission (USSC) created the Federal Sentencing Guidelines for Organizations (the Guidelines) to establish consistent criminal sentencing for noncompliance (USSC, n.d.). The Guidelines, revised in 2021, lay out the key elements for an effective compliance program, discussed in more detail later in this chapter (USSC, 2021).

In 1998, the Department of Health and Human Services Office of the Inspector General (HHS-OIG) issued the Compliance Program Guidance for Hospitals, leaning heavily on the Guidelines and indicating that providers who lacked effective compliance programs would risk receiving harsher sanctions (Office of Inspector General [OIG], 1998). HHS-OIG continued to release compliance program guidance and supplemental guidance documents for various types of healthcare entities (e.g., nursing homes, ambulance suppliers, pharmaceutical manufacturers) until 2008 (OIG, n.d.). As new healthcare services and care settings develop, this additional guidance is challenged to keep up with an ever-evolving industry in an effort to close the gap between new potential compliance loopholes and the ability to detect them. In April 2023, HHS-OIG announced plans to improve and update the existing Compliance Program Guidances (CPGs) and introduce new CPGs for newly emerged segments of the healthcare industry (Federal Register, 2023).

## SEVEN KEY ELEMENTS OF AN EFFECTIVE COMPLIANCE PROGRAM

As mentioned earlier, HHS-OIG established the seven elements of an effective compliance program, built upon the Guidelines; they remain the foundation upon which compliance programs are built (Murtha & Brandt, n.d.). The seven essential elements are listed in Figure 19.1. *Note*: There are a few variations of the seven elements as modified by professional organizations that are also available to review. These include versions that combine education and communications while splitting apart investigation, enforcement, and response into three separate elements. For the purposes of this text, the HHS-OIG seven elements will be reviewed.

**FIGURE 19.1.** The seven essential elements of an effective compliance program in association with risk management and culture.

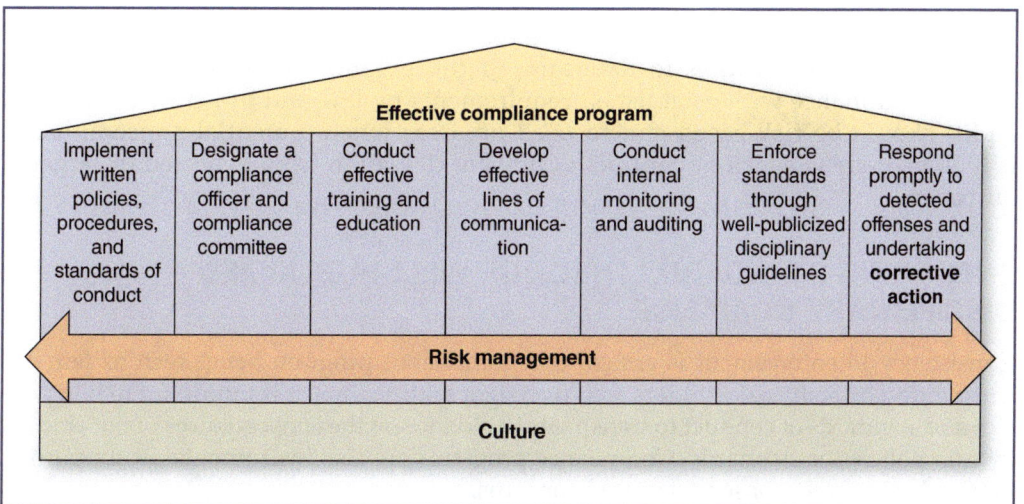

## IMPLEMENTING WRITTEN POLICIES, PROCEDURES, AND STANDARDS OF CONDUCT

Most healthcare organizations have a code of conduct or a similar fundamental document that outlines compliant and ethically acceptable behavior for all staff, contractors, and volunteers of the organization. In addition, to this document, it is imperative to include written policies and standard operating procedures into the operations of the organization.

## DESIGNATING A COMPLIANCE OFFICER AND COMPLIANCE COMMITTEE

Each healthcare organization should have a designated individual tasked with facilitating organizational **oversight** and ownership of the compliance program operations. In smaller organizations, this individual may wear multiple hats but conflicts of interest must be avoided with respect to management roles. The organization must also establish a compliance committee that is responsible for reviewing compliance trends, reports of noncompliance, and alignment of any strategic changes with known regulations or laws.

## CONDUCTING EFFECTIVE TRAINING AND EDUCATION

The compliance officer and the compliance program are responsible for educating employees, leadership, contractors, and others (e.g., vendors) on the rules and regulations associated with operations and any specifically impacting unique job roles as appropriate. The education and training must be effective, responsive to deficiencies, and accessible to all required to participate.

## DEVELOPING EFFECTIVE LINES OF COMMUNICATION

Organizations are required to maintain systems that track reports of potential noncompliance; these systems must allow for anonymous reporting. This is often met through the establishment of a compliance hotline where compliance, privacy, and other concerns can be reported.

## CONDUCTING INTERNAL MONITORING AND AUDITING

The compliance program is responsible for establishing auditing and monitoring plans for the organization to determine if the organization's operations are, in fact, in compliance with established requirements by law and policy. Monitors and audits should be risk based and focused on areas where potential noncompliance is high or there is a lack of controls to prevent deviation from expected or targeted outcomes.

## ENFORCING STANDARDS THROUGH WELL-PUBLICIZED DISCIPLINARY GUIDANCE

Consistency in enforcement is critical to a compliance program being seen as fair and trustworthy by staff, stakeholders, and oversight bodies; thus, it is important to link policies and standards of conduct to transparent guidance on the consequences of not abiding by said policies or standards. Compliance programs are also instrumental in supporting nonretaliation in response to reported concerns.

## RESPONDING PROMPTLY TO DETECTED OFFENSES AND UNDERTAKING CORRECTIVE ACTION

In tandem with enforcement and auditing is the ability to detect offenses and to establish actions to remediate those offenses in a timely and effective fashion. Reports of potential noncompliance made through the communications channel established by the organization must be reviewed and investigated, if warranted, and either substantiated or unsubstantiated, with proper documentation and retention of records.

## POSSIBLE AREAS OF REGULATORY OVERSIGHT TO INCLUDE IN COMPLIANCE PROGRAMS

There are many oversight areas that can be covered by a compliance program. Exactly what topics are covered will depend upon the type of entity involved and the services they provide. Common areas include the following:

- Billing and coding
- FWA
- Antitrust
- Privacy and security
- Tax
- Emergency Medical Treatment and Active Labor Act (EMTALA)
- Research and grants
- Employment and labor issues
- Quality and safety

Since many compliance risks in the healthcare arena focus on the FWA laws, they are often emphasized in compliance programs and trainings and are discussed in greater detail in this chapter. Other laws, however, are also important to healthcare compliance, and entities should carefully consider what to include in their compliance programs.

## FRAUD, WASTE, AND ABUSE LAWS

A significant area of concern for healthcare entities and, therefore, their compliance programs is FWA. Business practices that may be acceptable in other industries are prohibited in the healthcare sphere by laws at the federal and state level. The major *federal* FWA laws are described in the following section. It is important to recognize that such laws also exist at the state level and private payors may also have rules related to FWA that may be relevant.

The False Claims Act (FCA), described in more detail in Chapter 23, "Healthcare Law and Ethics," is the federal government's main tool to combat FWA. The FCA imposes liability upon any person who knowingly submits, or causes to submit, false claims or makes a false record or statement in order to secure payment of a false or fraudulent claim by the federal government.

The Anti-Kickback Statute (AKS), also described in more detail in Chapter 23, prohibits giving or receiving payment for patient referrals in federal healthcare programs. The AKS is an intent-based statute, requiring a person to act *knowingly and willfully* regarding their intent to induce or reward referrals.

Due to the complexity of the AKS and questions related to the application of its safe harbors, the HHS-OIG offers the opportunity to request a formal advisory opinion regarding proposed or current arrangements regarding the application of the AKS. While the HHS-OIG's opinion is applicable only to the requesting party, such opinions offer insight into how the HHS-OIG would view similar arrangements. See https://oig.hhs.gov/compliance/advisory-opinions/process/ for more information regarding the advisory opinion process. Advisory opinions are published in a searchable database: https://oig.hhs.gov/compliance/advisory-opinions/browse/.

The HHS-OIG occasionally publishes other guidance documents in the form of Special Fraud Alerts and Special Advisory Bulletins to address relationships or conduct the HHS-OIG has identified as potential sources of FWA.

The Civil Monetary Penalties Law, 42 U.S.C. § 1320a-7a, is an administrative fraud remedy that is often used to enforce potential AKS violations through civil fines and program exclusions. The HHS-OIG has the authority to impose a variety of CMPs; the list of authorities, including implementing regulations, can be found at https://oig.hhs.gov/Fraud/enforcement/cmp/cmpa.asp.

The Physician Self-Referral Law, 42 U.S.C. § 1395nn, commonly referred to as the Stark Law after the law's champion, prohibits a physician from referring Medicare patients to an entity for designated health services if the physician (or an immediate family member) has a financial relationship with the entity unless an exception applies. There are no criminal penalties associated with Stark Law violations; however, penalties are still harsh and include denial of payment for the services, repayment of any payment made, civil penalties up to $25,000 per claim, and program exclusion. When Stark Law violations are enforced under the FCA, the penalties become even more severe.

## THE ENFORCEMENT ENVIRONMENT

### MAJOR ENFORCEMENT AGENCIES

At the federal level, there are a number of agencies that regulate compliance in the healthcare arena. The DOJ is the federal agency tasked with U.S. law. It is led by the Attorney General who is appointed by the President and confirmed by the Senate. The DOJ has more than 40 separate component organizations, including 93 federal districts with a U.S. Attorney's Office led by a United States Attorney, the Federal Bureau of Investigations, and the Drug Enforcement Administration (DEA). If criminal charges are possible, the DOJ will take over an investigation from other federal agencies.

The U.S. Department of Health and Human Services (HHS) has 12 operating divisions, several of which are relevant to healthcare compliance, including CMS, the Food and Drug Administration (FDA), the Centers for Disease Control and Prevention (CDC), the Office for Civil Rights (OCR), and HHS-OIG. Other federal agencies also have an impact on compliance matters, including the Departments of Labor, Defense, and Veterans Affairs, as well as the Federal Trade Commission (FTC).

In addition to the federal agencies listed earlier, states also have agencies that regulate matters pertaining to healthcare compliance. With respect to the Medicaid program, Medicaid Fraud Control Units (MFCUs) investigate and prosecute Medicaid provider fraud as well as abuse or neglect of residents in healthcare facilities and nursing homes and of Medicaid beneficiaries in other settings. MFCUs, which are typically part of the State Attorney General's office, operate in each of the 50 states, the District of Columbia, Puerto Rico, and the U.S. Virgin Islands. HHS-OIG has oversight over the MFCUs. Finally, private payors and private citizens also play a role in combating FWA.

### ENFORCEMENT INITIATIVES

The Health Insurance Portability and Accountability Act of 1996 (HIPAA) required the establishment of a national Health Care Fraud and Abuse Control Program (HCFAC), under the joint direction of the Attorney General and the Secretary of the HHS, acting

**FIGURE 19.2.** Medicare strike force locations.

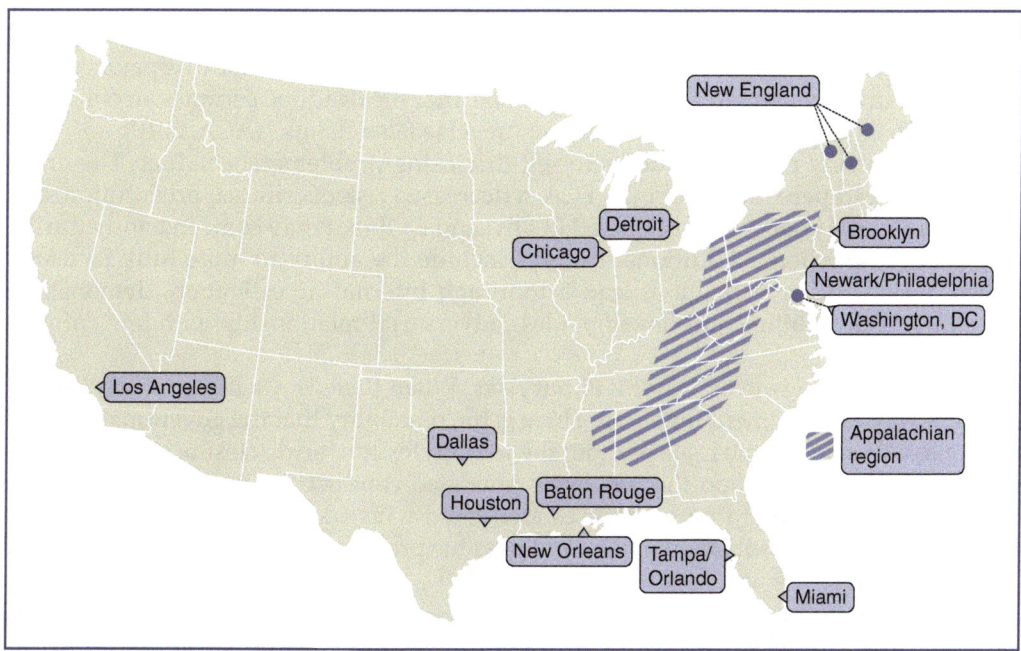

*Source:* U.S. Department of Health and Human Services. (2022). *Medicare fraud strike force.* https://oig.hhs.gov/fraud/strike-force/.

through HHS-OIG. The HCFAC program is designed to coordinate federal, state, and local law healthcare fraud enforcement activities. An annual report is required each year outlining the program's activities and accomplishments, including major enforcement activities and amounts recovered via judgments and settlements. HCFAC reports can be found at https://oig.hhs.gov/reports-and-publications/hcfac/index.asp.

The Medicare Fraud Strike Force is a multiagency team of federal, state, and local investigators first established in 2007 that uses data analysis, community surveillance, and traditional investigation techniques (e.g., wiretaps) to prevent and combat FWA. Current Strike Force locations are illustrated in Figure 19.2.

The Healthcare Fraud Prevention and Action Team (HEAT) was established by the DOJ and HHS-OIG in 2009 to build and strengthen existing programs combatting Medicare fraud, such as the Medicare Strike Force, while investing new resources and technology to prevent and detect FWA. HEAT targets healthcare fraud *hot spots* around the country.

Following major upheavals in the healthcare industry, enforcement actions will often focus on those extreme circumstances, such as the honing in on COVID-19 fraud schemes following the COVID-19 pandemic. Such enforcement action were announced in April 2023 (https://www.justice.gov/opa/pr/justice-department-announces-nationwide-coordinated-law-enforcement-action-combat-covid-19), April 2022 (https://www.justice.gov/opa/pr/justice-department-announces-nationwide-coordinated-law-enforcement-action-combat-health-care), and May 2021 (https://www.justice.gov/opa/pr/doj-announces-coordinated-law-enforcement-action-combat-health-care-fraud-related-covid-19).

## REPAYMENTS AND SELF-DISCLOSURES

Determining whether a billing error is a simple mistake that merely requires repayment or is more indicative of a larger issue that might lead to liability exposure under the fraud laws is a complex question faced by healthcare providers. The decision to make a repayment or disclosure is based on a variety of legal authorities that either create a repayment obligation or directly link the underlying violation to financial penalties. For example, the Patient Protection and Affordable Care Act (ACA) requires that a person who has received an overpayment must report and return it within 60 days of the date the overpayment was identified. An overpayment retained by a person after the deadline becomes an obligation that could trigger potential FCA liability for "reverse false claims" (ACA, 2010).

There are many possible benefits to self-disclosing problematic conduct. They may include reduced penalties under the FCA, a decreased risk of criminal prosecution, and the generation of good will with the HHS-OIG and DOJ that may come in handy during settlement discussions. Additional benefits include the ability to more fully focus the issues during the investigation, lead a thorough internal investigation, demonstrate corporate responsibility, and develop a less adversarial relationship with law enforcement officials.

Self-disclosure, however, is not without risks. When there is a self-disclosure, there is almost always a repayment involved. There is the possibility that the government would never have discovered the issue without the self-disclosure; the disclosure itself may trigger additional investigation that uncovers unrelated conduct that may be problematic. Further, there are little to no guarantees associated with a self-disclosure; the provider may still be subject to substantial fines and possible prosecution.

## CORPORATE INTEGRITY AGREEMENTS

Corporate Integrity Agreements (CIAs) and Integrity Agreements (IAs) are tools used by the HHS-OIG to enforce fraud and abuse laws. Such documents outline the obligations the entity has agreed to as part of a civil settlement with the HHS-OIG in exchange for the HHS-OIG's agreement that it will not seek to exclude the entity from participation in Medicare, Medicaid, or other federal healthcare programs.

CIAs have been common since the mid-1990s when the government began strengthening its efforts to enforce federal healthcare statutes and recoup funds lost as a result of FWA. Since that time, HHS-OIG has entered into more than 1,000 CIAs and IAs. Noncompliance with the terms of a CIA can lead to monetary penalties, referred to in CIAs as stipulated penalties. A material breach of the CIA constitutes an independent basis for the provider's exclusion from participation in federal healthcare programs. Current CIAs and IAs are publicly available at https://oig.hhs.gov/compliance/corporate-integrity-agreements/cia-documents.asp.

## CULTURE AND RISK MANAGEMENT

With so much to digest when it comes to **risk management**, it may seem impossible to pinpoint where to start when engaging with a compliance program. As discussed so far in this chapter, there are many rules and regulations that inform a compliance professional's goal posts for things such as auditing and monitoring, education, and investigation. However, depending on what segment of healthcare an individual is in, the focus of those efforts may look a little bit different. Underlying everything that a compliance professional does are two things, culture and risk. A compliance program will only be as strong as the culture that supports it. This means leadership at all levels of the organization speaking with a consistent tone at the top on what it means to act with integrity and how important compliance is in the everyday actions of all employees and stakeholders.

One of the key factors associated with many qui tam cases is an inconsistent tone at the top, a lack of trust in leadership, and potential retaliatory practices. These factors have an adverse impact on having a culture that fosters appropriate reporting and response when compliance violations or concerns are detected and reported. This then leads to the need to involve external entities in order to pursue response and resolution. A supportive compliance culture may be established as a part of other culture-driven initiatives such as **just culture** or creating a *high-reliability organization* and can even be nested in the way that strategic planning is approached or in the setup of communication plans. What a strong compliance culture is not comprised of is a *gotcha game*. While it is in incredibly important for a compliance program to be able to detect and correct the wrongdoing of an individual or a group of individuals, it is even more important to address the prevention aspect of the wrongdoing by getting to the heart of systemic gaps and errant processes and addressing behavioral changes (OIG—HEAT, n.d.)

This is where risk management must be recognized as a critical variable to the success of a compliance program. In order to know where the highest risk for noncompliance lies, a program must partake in a risk assessment and subsequently absorb that information into their approach to the seven elements. Compliance risk management can be very narrow in scope in that it looks at the operations of the compliance program itself and then implements necessary **mitigation** plans to address processes or objectives that are at high likelihood for failure and would result in significant harm or impact to the organization. However, risk practices become much more powerful when the compliance program is seen as a part of the organization's operations and risks are not viewed in silos but as an interwoven and integrated set of processes and outcomes. This allows for compliance to reflect where, in broader operations, the highest risks for noncompliance exist. It also brings more value to the compliance program as it becomes seen as a critical and integrated part of the organization's operations.

Organizations can also utilize risk assessments to determine when it is appropriate to pursue potential risks as the return on investment and associated positive outcomes outweigh the risk of not taking action or remaining stagnant. This is often where innovation comes into play. For example, when the pandemic began escalating in severity, many organizations decided to rapidly pursue the expansion of telehealth services because meeting the needs of patients while protecting the safety of all involved became more important than it had in the past. The ability to pursue these formerly *riskier* endeavors was supported by the rollback of some of the stricter rules and regulations associated with telehealth and ultimately led to new delivery pathways for many services. Compliance officers were often highly involved in those discussions and became powerful partners in determining how billing and coding associated with the rapid change in delivery would be implemented and monitored, how privacy concerns would be addressed, and how to ensure that licensure rules for clinicians would still be followed when necessary. Postpandemic, some of the waived rules and regulations were reestablished, which required compliance professionals to support their organizations with change management in bringing processes back into compliance with regulations and assisting with change management communications (McGowan et al., 2023).

It is critical for compliance programs to be involved in organizational risk assessments, reviewing gaps and opportunities in the ability of the organization to meet its strategic goals and objectives. The risks that are deemed to be of highest priority are then integrated into the organization's approach to the seven elements of compliance. This integration may be seen through new standing committee reports, the development of new audits and monitors, the establishment of new or modified educational programs, and potentially even result in marking potential wrongdoing reports with an additional flag if they happen to be associated with a high-risk area to indicate a higher priority investigation. This allows compliance to be integrated but still act as an objective and independent service in the organization. Ensuring the connection from the tone at the top, through the completion of risk assessments and consideration of the seven elements along with other clinical and regulatory requirements, is one of the most critical yet overlooked components of a successful compliance program.

## CASE STUDY 19.1: HEALTHCARE COMPLIANCE OFFICER

A new and relatively young compliance officer was orienting to their new duties overseeing privacy at a small organization with approximately 10 in-house physicians. The physicians were faced with highly complex pediatric cases that sometimes were complicated by custody matters, the foster care system, or the caregivers' attempts to navigate additional social services needed to fully support the wellness of the child. Requests for release of information were prevalent and many times came from a multitude of different directions, including from the legal system. The compliance officer determined that not only was the organization at high risk for breaching HIPAA simply due to the volume of requests and sensitive nature of the types of records maintained but also that there had not been recent training for the physicians on what to do when a request was made directly to them during a visit, particularly if it was made by someone other than the child's legal guardian. The organization determined that records printed and released at the point of care may have lacked appropriate documentation pertaining to the release; sometimes, the incorrect records were being released to families, creating an immediate breach of privacy as well as fostering a lack of trust in the organization's processes. The compliance officer met individually with each physician after gaining the support of the Chief Medical Officer (CMO) to understand each physician's knowledge of HIPAA and explore where in the process the breakdown in required procedures and documentation was occurring. They took the opportunity to coach the physicians and educate each based on their individual circumstances and, when necessary, formally documented their part in any breach of protected information.

To create a collaborative environment around a difficult topic, it was important to acknowledge the situation at hand and the importance of resolving the deficiencies. This meant partnering with those involved to develop the solution. Doing so created buy-in, and brought a feeling of personal responsibility to all of those involved to ensure the same outcome did not happen again. They actively contributed to the **corrective action**, complied with receiving additional training, and ultimately understood that when release of information requests were made, they had an entire records management team to rely on to support the processing of those requests. Ultimately, breaches decreased over time, but physicians also noted that this allowed them to redirect their energies toward actual patient care. Further, they trusted that if they self-reported a compliance violation, they would not immediately be punished as the first response to the report.

Over the next 6 years, the compliance officer was able to build trust with all of the physicians, and when new physicians were brought on board, the compliance officer was one of the first people to orient them so that they knew who they were, what they could support them with, and that the organization would take their compliance with laws and regulations seriously. All this was made possible because the organization's leadership, including the CMO, empowered the compliance officer to act in an objective and independent fashion, spoke with a consistent voice and tone, and became a partner in resourcing and supporting actions necessary to resolve the deficiency once identified. Compliance professionals can often be stereotyped as part of the *gotcha* program, simply out to catch people doing the wrong things. In reality, a good compliance professional spends the majority of their time and energy on relationship building, education, and prevention while maintaining consistency when enforcement and action is required. Without trust, compliance programs will fail.

## END-OF-CHAPTER RESOURCES

### CRITICAL THINKING QUESTIONS

- Are there any downsides to developing a robust corporate compliance program?
- Which of the seven elements of compliance do you think is the hardest to achieve?
- What are some ways you can translate complicated legal and regulatory statutes so that all healthcare employees and patients can understand them?
- How can you help a compliance program become more proactive and less reactionary?
- What value add does a compliance program provide to a healthcare organization beyond "keeping leadership out of jail?"

### LEARNING ACTIVITIES

**CourseConnect**

To access self-assessment questions and interactive, competency-based learning activities for this chapter, visit www.springerpub.com/courseconnect. See inside front cover and tear-out card for CourseConnect details.

### REFERENCES

18 U.S.C. § 1347 (2021). *Health care fraud*. https://www.law.cornell.edu/uscode/text/18/1347

42 U.S.C. § 1320a-7a (2021). *Civil money penalties*. https://www.law.cornell.edu/uscode/text/42/1320a-7a

42 U.S.C. § 1320a-7b(a). Centers for Medicare and Medicaid Services. (2013). *Medicare managed care manual chapter 21—Compliance program guidelines*. https://www.cms.gov/Regulations-and-Guidance/Guidance/Manuals/Downloads/mc86c21.pdf

McGowan, J., Wojahn, A., & Nicolini, J. R. (2023, January). Risk management event evaluation and responsibilities. Updated February 6, 2023. In *StatPearls* [Internet]. StatPearls Publishing. https://www.ncbi.nlm.nih.gov/books/NBK559326/

Federal Register. (2023, April 25). *Modernization of compliance program guidance documents, 88 FR 25000*. https://www.federalregister.gov/documents/2023/04/25/2023-08326/modernization-of-compliance-program-guidance-documents

Murtha, F. L., & Brandt, K. (n.d.). *Compliance program effectiveness*. Health Care Compliance Association Resources Library. https://assets.hcca-info.org/Portals/0/PDFs/Resources/library/ComplianceEffectivenessPresentation.pdf

Office of Inspector General. (n.d.). *Compliance guidance*. https://oig.hhs.gov/compliance/compliance-guidance/

Office of Inspector General. (1998). *Compliance program guidance for hospitals*. https://oig.hhs.gov/documents/compliance-guidance/798/cpghosp.pdf

Office of Inspector General. (2013). *Special advisory bulletin on the effect of exclusion from participation in federal health care programs*. https://oig.hhs.gov/exclusions/files/sab-05092013.pdf

Patient Protection and Affordable Care Act. (2010). https://www.congress.gov/bill/111th-congress/house-bill/3590

U.S. Department of Justice. (2020). *Criminal resource manual § 976*. https://www.justice.gov/archives/jm/criminal-resource-manual-976-health-care-fraud-generally

U.S. Department of Justice. (2022). *Press release, february 7, 2022: False Claims Act settlements and judgments exceed $2 billion in fiscal year 2022*. https://www.justice.gov/opa/pr/false-claims-act-settlements-and-judgments-exceed-2-billion-fiscal-year-2022

U.S. Sentencing Commission. (n.d.). *An overview of the organizational guidelines*. https://www.ussc.gov/sites/default/files/pdf/training/organizational-guidelines/ORGOVERVIEW.pdf

U.S. Sentencing Commission. (2021). *Guidelines manual*. https://www.ussc.gov/sites/default/files/pdf/guidelines-manual/2021/GLMFull.pdf

# CHAPTER 20

# CASE: HEALTHCARE FINANCE, SERVICE LINE DEVELOPMENT, HEALTH OUTCOME, AND QUALITY INITIATIVE

Laura Griffin, MariaRita Genovese, and Shashank Rao

## LEARNING OBJECTIVES

- Summarize the different types of access challenges for patients seeking timely, convenient, and affordable healthcare.
- Examine the relationship between a patient's overall health and the ability to access timely, convenient, and affordable healthcare.
- Evaluate and rank the initiatives that the health system has proposed to address barriers to patients accessing care.
- Formulate alternative strategies for consideration to address the health system's challenges.

## KEY TERMS

- Access to healthcare
- Clinical trials
- Patient experience
- Telemedicine

## INTRODUCTION

This case focuses on the challenges of providing access to timely and affordable healthcare. The aim is to enhance care for cancer patients in the Denver metropolitan area.

## MAJOR CHALLENGES AND DILEMMA

Access to timely and affordable healthcare has been a challenge for many patients across the nation. Even though many appointments are underutilized, patients are waiting longer than ever to see providers, especially those seeking specialty care. As it relates to the cancer patient population, **access to healthcare** can be a significant issue for several reasons.

### FINANCIAL CONSTRAINTS

Cancer treatment can be extremely expensive, including surgeries, chemotherapy, radiation therapy, medications, and follow-up care. Many cancer patients struggle with medical bills, especially if they do not have adequate health insurance coverage. Even with insurance, co-payments, deductibles, and out-of-pocket expenses can be substantial.

### INSURANCE COVERAGE

Not all health insurance plans cover all aspects of cancer treatment, or they may have limitations on certain treatments or medications. This can result in patients not being able to afford necessary treatments or having to choose between treatments based on what they can afford rather than what is most effective.

### GEOGRAPHIC BARRIERS

In some areas, especially rural areas, access to specialized cancer care facilities may be limited. Patients may have to travel long distances to reach a cancer center or specialist, which can be burdensome in terms of time, money, and logistics.

### TIMELY DIAGNOSIS AND TREATMENT

Delays in diagnosis and treatment can have a significant impact on cancer outcomes. Some patients may face barriers to timely diagnosis due to lack of access to screening services or delays in receiving referrals from primary care providers.

### PSYCHOSOCIAL FACTORS

Cancer diagnosis and treatment can take a toll on patients emotionally and psychologically. Access to mental health support services, such as counseling or support groups, may be limited or not readily available to all patients.

### IMPACT AND EXPECTATIONS

An inability to access timely healthcare diminishes the patient's experience and can have a negative impact on a patient's health and well-being. In addition to patient experience, access challenges impact an organization financially as well. Access is the initial entry into the revenue process at many healthcare facilities; it is also the gateway to providing quality care.

The expectation from patients is to receive care when they want it and where they want it. For many healthcare organizations, access to care has become a strategic priority to address to drive improved patient and financial outcomes. This has led many healthcare organizations to look inwardly at their processes with intent to develop innovative initiatives to give patients the ability to access care more quickly.

## ORGANIZATIONAL OVERVIEW

Greater Medical Center (GMC) provides a range of specialty cancer care services to patients throughout the greater Denver, Colorado area. GMC is one of the most respected centers focused on cancer patient care, education, and prevention. One of the most important decisions a patient will need to make is where to go for their cancer treatment.

Founded in 1910, the GMC began focusing on cancer treatments and cellular research in the late 1950s. GMC received its National Cancer Institute (NCI) designation in 1995 and its designation as a comprehensive cancer center in 2004. As a comprehensive academic medical center, it offers a full range of cancer care—from screening and early detection to treatment and recovery—at several locations, as well as treatment for other conditions that may develop due to cancer or a preexisting condition. GMC employs over 300 physicians and clinical researchers who are dedicated to eliminating cancer by having a multidisciplinary approach to treatment. A multidisciplinary team can consist of specialists from different disciplines such as surgery, radiation oncology, medical oncology, nursing, nurse navigation, social work, pathology, radiology, and nuclear medicine. All are working together to discuss the best options for the treatment of their patients. This is the gold standard in cancer care. The GMC team of cancer care providers is recognized for its leadership in cancer research, treatment, and complex diagnoses and is committed to providing compassionate, high-quality care.

In addition, as part of treatment, patients can participate in a clinical trial if they meet certain criteria within offered studies. Clinical trials are studies of new treatments and diagnostic approaches. Almost every advance that has been achieved in cancer treatments and has improved patients' lives has occurred as a result of clinical trials. If a provider feels a patient is a candidate for a clinical trial, they will speak with the patient and review the opportunities that are available to them.

The areas of research at GMC consist of the cancer biology program, which performs laboratory research, fortifying the comprehension of molecular and genetic research and therapies. GMC's translational research consists of innovative research in oncology therapeutics, cancer, immunotherapeutics, and hematologic malignancies. Translational research focuses on developing strategies for cell and gene therapies. These programs translate clinical research and laboratory monitoring into patient care.

The GMC is a comprehensive cancer center designated by the NCI. This is the gold standard for cancer center programs and is awarded to the nation's top cancer centers. This recognition states that the GMC cancer center has renowned physicians, clinical teams, and researchers who administer team-based, patient-centered research to create the latest groundbreaking technologies and treatments to address patient needs. As a result, people who come to GMC for cancer care have access to hundreds of clinical trials in all phases.

As an NCI-designated comprehensive cancer center, GMC is recognized for its expertise and commitment to patient care; cancer research, including clinical trials; and education. The rapid discovery and early accessibility of many new cancer treatments at NCI-designated comprehensive cancer centers give GMC an edge in offering cancer patients access to the latest therapies and treatment options.

The GMC team believes that there are four components to the healing process: physical, mental, emotional, and financial health. That is why they offer a full range of supportive services, including social work, behavioral health, financial counseling, genetics, and patient education programs.

*Mission:* To provide the best cancer care in the region by offering the newest technology and cutting-edge treatments with excellent outcomes

*Vision:* To be a leader in cancer treatment and prevention while promoting innovation in care delivery, leading to improved patient health outcomes

*Core values:* Caring, safety, integrity, innovation, service excellence, and stewardship

Annually, GMC encounters approximately 150,000 patients seeking cancer treatment. In addition to inpatient care, GMC performs approximately 1 million outpatient visits; 15,000 surgeries; 6 million pathology/lab procedures; and 320,000 diagnostic imaging procedures.

## ACCESS TO CARE

Accessibility to care is defined by four main categories: location, timeliness of care, facility navigability, and affordability.

- *Service location:* Services are in areas where patients seeking care can conveniently access and obtain care without traveling unmanageable distances.
- *Timeliness of care:* Services are available in a timely manner that meets a patient's scheduling needs and preferences.
- *Facility navigation:* Facilities are designed so that patients and family members can move throughout them efficiently and comfortably.
- *Affordability:* Services are not so expensive that patients cannot afford to seek treatment or opt out of some or all treatments and support services.

By the year 2024, the American Cancer Society estimated that the national number of cancer incidences will rise to 2 million (Collins, 2024). Advancements in cancer treatment and continued research in the industry have positively impacted survivorship; the American Cancer Society also estimated a rise in cancer survivors to 19 million by 2024. The rising number of both incidences and survivors increases the need for access to cancer care and follow-up treatment.

In addition to the rising number of patients, the complexity of cancer care treatment and the growing number of treatment options play a role in impacting access to care. Patients are also often required to coordinate appointments with other providers to ensure treatment of multiple comorbidities. For this vulnerable population, timely, convenient, and affordable care is critical to health outcomes and overall patient satisfaction.

## CLOSING THE GAP ON ACCESS TO CARE

GMC serves some of the most vulnerable patients, and improving access to care is a critical strategic priority for the organization. The organization is preparing its 3-year strategic plan and has received a $10 million grant dedicated to improving access to cancer care for patients across the state of Colorado. The grant parameters are that all interventions must demonstrate an impact on quality and patient experience outcomes, as well as be financially sustainable beyond the grant.

GMC has outlined a few different opportunities for improvement to close the gap for their patients to access care. However, they need to prioritize initiatives and begin to develop plans to operationalize those that obtain final approval from the board of directors. Some of the initiatives are outlined in the following.

## EXPANDED CALL CENTER HOURS

Expanding call center hours provides additional access for scheduling appointments to patients. Patients who are unable to call during traditional business hours will now have enhanced opportunities to schedule important appointments at their convenience rather than trying to make special arrangements to call throughout the busy workday. Expanding hours helps to reduce delays in care by addressing barriers for patients whose schedules do not align with that of the GMC call center for scheduling critical appointments.

## TEMPLATES FOR PHYSICIAN SCHEDULES

The creation of standard scheduling templates for physicians reduces the variability in the number of open appointments that may be available. Standard templates eliminate the ability for offices to block certain spots or create their own appointment times. This also allows the call center to see all open appointment slots for providers in the same format.

## UTILIZATION OF TELEMEDICINE

Telemedicine provides the opportunity for patients to see their provider without needing to travel to a specific hospital or office. While telemedicine is not appropriate for all types of appointments, it can be used for follow-up care and day-to-day care management of patients. Telemedicine appointments are typically shorter in length and offer the flexibility for providers to open up additional appointments.

## RN-STAFFED CLINICAL TRIAGE UNIT—7 DAYS A WEEK

Patients who have been diagnosed with cancer, especially those newly diagnosed, often decide without consulting their provider to visit hospital emergency departments for symptoms that do not warrant that type of care (Hong et al., 2023). Opening a 7-day-a-week RN-staffed clinical triage unit can help to manage patients with non-life-threatening health concerns while simultaneously eliminating unnecessary emergency department visits.

# END-OF-CHAPTER RESOURCES

## CASE OBJECTIVES

1. Assess and discuss the challenges to accessing timely, convenient, and affordable cancer care in the greater Denver, Colorado area.
2. Prioritize current initiatives and outline others that will help GMC improve access to care.

## LEARNING ACTIVITIES

### CourseConnect >

To access self-assessment questions and interactive, competency-based learning activities for this chapter, visit www.springerpub.com/courseconnect. See inside front cover and tear-out card for CourseConnect details.

## REFERENCES

Collins, S. (2024, January 17). *2024 Cancer Facts & Figures—First year the US expects more than 2M new cases of cancer*. https://www.cancer.org/research/acs-research-news/facts-and-figures-2024.html

Hong, A., Hughes, A., Courtney, D. M., Fullington, H., Craddock Lee, S. J., Sweetenham, J. W., Sadeghi, N., Zhang, S., Bazzell, A., & Halm, E. A. (2023, September 14). Characteristics of self-triaged emergency department visits by adults with cancer. *The American Journal of Managed Care, 29*(9). www.ajmc.com/view/characteristics-of-self-triaged-emergency-department-visits-by-adults-with-cancer

# SECTION III: LEADERSHIP THEORIES, APPLICATION, AND ACTIONS IN HEALTHCARE MANAGEMENT

# CHAPTER 21

# JOURNEY OF A HEALTHCARE LEADER

William Tuttle and Patrick Grusenmeyer

## LEARNING OBJECTIVES

- Assess the current healthcare career environment.
- Develop a personal mission, vision, and values and assess against the mission, vision, and values of a prospective healthcare employer. Assess congruity (fit) between employee and organization.
- Identify stages in a healthcare administration leaders' career.
- Discuss competencies required at each career stage and how the execution of those competencies changes with the stage.
- Devise a career plan.

## KEY TERMS

- Career framework
- Career stages
- Competencies
- Early career
- Encore career
- Mentor
- Mid-career
- Senior career

## INTRODUCTION

When talking with current students of healthcare administration, the topic of what they want to do in their careers often comes up. This is often a challenging question for someone who has spent their entire life as a student whose limited exposure to careers in healthcare administration may be part-time jobs and a summer internship.

There is no *typical* healthcare career progression. Each career progresses and sometimes regresses at its own pace due to circumstances unique to the individual, the organizations in which they work, changes in national healthcare policy, the macro-U.S. economic environment, and oftentimes, sheer luck—good or bad.

The individual's knowledge, skills, abilities, and competencies will have a significant impact on their career progression, as will their emotional intelligence and people skills. Changes in national healthcare policy can potentially make certain skills less valuable in the marketplace and thus less promotable. For example, if someone developed a broad breadth of knowledge and experience in a service line or segment, such as value-based care, changes in policy away from value-based care can make that knowledge and skill less viable. Downturns in the U. S. economy (and healthcare reimbursement policies) can substantially affect organizations' revenue and bottom line, requiring personnel cutbacks that impact careers. Clearly, luck has played a positive role in our careers; some of it is being in the right place at the right time. However, preparation improves performance.

This chapter provides a brief review of how healthcare and healthcare careers have changed. It discusses the rapidly changing healthcare environment and how "continuous white-water rapids" are the new normal. Navigating that future will not be easy for the healthcare leader.

The chapter presents four career stages: early career, mid-level career, senior career, and encore career. It reviews key positions and roles of each stage and competencies required or highly utilized during that period.

## HEALTHCARE IN LIMINAL TIMES: BETWEEN OUR PAST AND FUTURE

### WHAT IS PAST IS PROLOGUE

What does the profound Shakespearean adage "what is past is prologue" mean? It is a reflection on the idea that one must draw to some extent on the past when considering the current environment and to be in league with the future. In the context of healthcare, the notion of understanding past trends, policies, and practices reveals a pattern of advances in scientific knowledge that has changed at an astounding rate during the last several decades.

These changes have resulted in a profound impact on the practice of medicine and the delivery of healthcare services. Although the achievements have been spectacular, so too have been the strains. The U.S. healthcare system is at the threshold of transformation with the old and new coexisting; a time of betwixt and between, neither fully within the old state nor entirely within the new one. Such points in history can be referred to as a liminal space and time whereby individuals and organizations are caught between the past and facing a future of uncertainty, change, and opportunity.

### CHAOS THE NEW NORMAL

Seismic shifts in social, economic, and political systems have, and are, taking place within the United States. Additionally, advances in scientific knowledge have grown exponentially, almost beyond belief. The dynamics of these changes are unavoidably enmeshed with the provision of healthcare services. The culmination of these factors is that healthcare leaders must contend with an ever-evolving and increasingly turbulent environment where chaos has been ingrained in its fabric.

The current chaotic environment and other new complexities faced in the future will unquestionably require leaders to embrace change, as well as demonstrate the expertise

| **TABLE 21.1. REFLECTIVE INSIGHTS** | |
|---|---|
| **Become A Chaos Virtuoso** | Whether it is shifting regulations, emerging technologies, or changes in patient expectations, healthcare executives must embrace chaos and be agile as well as adaptable in their decision-making. |
| **Insure Financial Resilience** | Infuse the heritage of healthcare delivery with renewed vitality and broaden the vision to maximizing health and providing equitable care to everyone while minimizing resource consumption. |
| **Establish Goal Clarity** | Have plans that define short-term and long-term career goals and the steps needed to achieve them. Without clear goals, it is easy to get lost in the daily grind. |
| **Embrace Data Innovation** | Understand and utilize data analytics to make informed decisions that can improve patient outcomes, reduce cost, and enhance the quality of care. |

required to navigate the complex healthcare ecosystem. This will require leaders to understand how to make a difference in whatever setting they are involved in and to have the right mindset and approach to adjust quickly to accommodate unanticipated events.

## NAVIGATING THE FUTURE TERRAIN

Stakeholders leading through this in-between space and time should recognize this is a natural part of the evolving landscape of healthcare services. This state of perpetual transition requires leaders to navigate the myriad of settings where healthcare is delivered with the blurring of traditional boundaries, constant flux, and uncertainty. It is not enough to know just what is going on today; tomorrow counts even more.

The importance of formulating well-structured plans is critical to avoid efforts to just prop up existing systems and programs or put Band-Aids on issues. Such planning will require the mutual interchange of ideas and a breadth of perspective to address the tremendously significant challenges with which healthcare is confronted. The challenges are substantial and must be addressed with vision, a broad perspective, ingenuity, creativity, and the realization that no healthcare organization can be an island unto itself (Table 21.1).

# CHARTING A COURSE: ENHANCING EFFECTIVENESS OF HEALTHCARE LEADERS

## IDENTIFYING YOUR CORE WHY

Why do you get up in the morning? What are you passionate about? Who do you want to be? Such questions are not just about some vague platitude about building character. Aristotle once said, "Knowing yourself is the beginning of all wisdom." Such words underscore the importance of understanding the core *why* of what leads individuals to enter and remain in the challenging profession of healthcare administration.

Knowing why you do what you do in healthcare is not just about a career; it is about understanding one's true self. It takes courage to be honest with yourself and embarking on the journey to discover your core *why* may not be an easy task. Some tend to believe it finds you. Others have deeply personal reasons that may reflect the impact of profound or pivotal life events that have shaped their past and present situation. What is important is understanding why you chose a path and let that understanding guide your actions and decisions so that you can reach your highest potential.

## CULTIVATING MENTORS

Who are you surrounding yourself with? Who do you admire and aspire to be like? A **mentor** can serve as a beacon of experience, knowledge, and motivation to help dream dreams that might otherwise be overlooked. Such individuals will help you navigate the complexities of the healthcare industry by challenging you, affirming your strengths, and nurturing your abilities.

The path to success in healthcare administration is not a journey to be walked alone and involves skills in building relationships with key individuals who can serve as a mentor. Along the way, developing the art of discernment is critical in engaging and finding such select individuals. Nurture such relationships with care and gratitude, and never stop learning from the wisdom and guidance mentors can provide. The importance of building a team of trusted mentors and cultivating such relationships throughout a career cannot be overstated.

## CREATING A ROADMAP

It takes more than desire to achieve a destination that moves you forward. A conviction to take action to develop and regularly update a career plan and strategy is crucial to help navigate your journey. Such a plan aligns itself with your special circumstances and provides a structured approach to match the critical elements of goal setting and skill development.

Establishing a roadmap for career success requires a combination of factors and a prioritized approach. Focus on where you want to go and do not set a low bar of achievement that you can always jump over. Develop high-bar goals and action plans that you may occasionally fall short of achieving and potentially experience bumpy parts of the journey. One of the marks of success is being prepared to pivot; reset, readjust, restart, and refocus as many times as you need.

## DEVELOPING THE KNOW-HOW

The complexity associated with leading today's healthcare organizations necessitates individuals to have appropriate education and experience to address the confluence of issues facing the complex and evolving landscape. Some of the knowledge and experience factors for a successful career have changed little over the course of time. Others are in flux and require greater prominence in today's healthcare leader's skill profile.

Practitioners of healthcare leadership must commit to developing the required talents and having a keen awareness of the ever-evolving nature of the industry. This will be an ongoing process and will require a combination of education, expertise, and adaptability. Individuals will be in a perpetual state of learning throughout their careers. The real test of developing the know-how is not who you are when you graduate from college but who you will become 10 or 20 years out (Table 21.2).

### TABLE 21.2. REFLECTIVE INSIGHTS

| | |
|---|---|
| Prioritize Ethical Leadership | Insist that decision-making nurtures a culture of integrity and a commitment to aligning goals with ethical principles and actions. |
| Excel in Knowledge Learning | Stay informed about the latest developments, regulations, and technology in and outside of healthcare. |
| Commit to Networking | Build a strong professional network to collaborate, seek mentors, and establish connections within and outside of healthcare. |
| Practice Disengagement | Consider your personal life in how it aligns with your career goals and ambitions. Take time to rest, read, reflect, and recover from work-related stress. |

# A FRAMEWORK FOR THE JOURNEY: CAREER STAGES AND COMPETENCIES

We can think of the typical healthcare management or leadership career in four distinct stages: early career, mid-career, senior career, and encore career. As stated earlier, no career is typical; each follows its own course. However, this **career framework** provides a way to think about career progression. One may spend longer or shorter periods at any given stage, possibly even skipping a stage, or staying in one stage for the remainder of their career. In part, this depends on the individual with their capabilities, competencies, and preferences. In part, it also depends on the context of their career.

While these **career stages** occur in most careers, we believe that a career in healthcare leadership, caring for people who are at one of the most vulnerable points in their lives, is a special calling. When people find themselves in unfamiliar situations, lacking the knowledge and vocabulary needed to understand and make important decisions, they rely on healthcare professionals for their physical health and safety. This relationship is built on trust and requires reverence and respectful caring from the healthcare leader. A healthcare leader's compassionate understanding sets this field apart from others.

The four stages encompass differing roles, responsibilities, and competencies (Table 21.3). Often a higher level of competency attainment leads to advancement in the later stages of a career. This section discusses the four stages and essential competencies for each stage. These competencies have been identified by major healthcare management organizations including the American College of Healthcare Executives, the Commission on Accreditation of Healthcare Management Organizations, the Association of University Programs in Healthcare Administration, and the National Center for Healthcare Leadership.

**TABLE 21.3. COMPETENCIES BY CAREER STAGE**

| CAREER STAGE | COMPETENCIES |
|---|---|
| **Early Career**<br>Often works as manager, director, assistant administrator; responsible for a program, service line, or department | • Project management<br>• Human resources<br>• Information management and analysis<br>• Quality and safety<br>• Performance improvement<br>• Financial management<br>• Communication<br>• Relationship development and management, especially with clinical staff |
| **Mid-Career**<br>Often holds a title such as vice president or administrator; leads major components of an organization such as a service line, institute, or center | • Leadership<br>• Human resources and people development<br>• Strategic planning and management organizational direction setting<br>• Financial management<br>• Legal/ethics/compliance |
| **Senior Career**<br>Leads an organization, major portions of an organization, or subsidiary of an organization; Often acts as a chief officer, such as executive (CEO), operations (COO), finance (CFO), clinical care (CMO, CNO), quality and safety (CQ&SO), information (CIO), strategy (CSO), president, executive vice president, senior vice president | • Leadership; development of organizational culture, especially patient safety, and clinical quality<br>• People development<br>• Strategic planning, implementation, and management; organizational direction setting<br>• Financial management; making the big decisions<br>• Legal/ethics/compliance<br>• Mergers and acquisitions<br>• Board development and relations<br>• Community relations |

*(continued)*

| TABLE 21.3. COMPETENCIES BY CAREER STAGE (*CONTINUED*) ||
|---|---|
| **CAREER STAGE** | **COMPETENCIES** |
| **Encore Career**<br>Consultant, executive in residence at an academic program, lecturer, faculty member, community volunteer | • Leadership<br>• Organizational development<br>• People development; mentoring<br>• Varies depending on role |

*Note:* Titles vary significantly between organizations and roles. The roles, responsibilities, and breadth of responsibility in terms of the numbers of employees, budgets, and decision-making responsibilities vary substantially across organizations.
CEO, chief executive officer; CFO, chief financial officer; CMO, chief medical officer; CNO, chief nursing officer; COO, chief operating officer; CQO, chief quality officer; CSO, chief safety/strategic officer.

## EARLY CAREER

What does an **early career** look like? People entering healthcare on a leadership path often enter at levels with titles such as manager, assistant director, director, assistant administrator, or similar. They are often responsible for managing a specific program or department within a service line or institute.

New leaders are often responsible for the performance of the program or department, including patient care, relationships with staff and physicians, quality and safety, and financial performance. The new manager is also learning specific details of the program or department (e.g., clinical treatments and patient flow), even as they begin to lead it.

This can be challenging. Often with limited "real-world" work experience, new leaders need to make an adjustment from academia to the work world. One of the challenges is to understand and perform within this new environment with differing expectations and rules. Unlike academia, which may have provided a structured environment with specific assignments and timelines, rubrics for assignment grading, and periodic grades, in the work environment, new employees are often asked to complete a task or project with limited information, strict timelines, and the expectation to successfully "make it happen." This requires the new leader to quickly develop new skills, develop new relationships, start to understand their own competencies, and determine when to seek assistance from peers or supervisors and when to proceed on their own.

A common challenge for new leaders is human resource management. Most new managers have never hired, disciplined, or terminated an employee. Acquiring human resource skills is vital. Hiring the best can be a challenge and poor hiring choices can be an obstacle to overall unit performance. Learning how to have difficult conversations regarding performance improvement, which can include discipline, is even more critical and it is almost impossible to learn these skills in academia. While healthcare administration education programs include courses on human resources and organizational behavior, actually sitting in front of another human being leading a disciplinary action is nearly impossible to simulate adequately. At the end of the simulation, no one lost their job. A new leader must develop this skill to succeed. Hiring and personal action is an area where an organization's mission, vision, and values can guide the manager. The manager can use these to begin any performance improvement review.

Early career can also be a time to explore different roles and opportunities and work to determine the "best fit" for their talents and competencies within a particular organization. It can also be a time to embrace patient-centered care.

## MID-CAREER

What does a **mid-career** look like for a healthcare leader? With titles such as vice president or administrator, and with responsibilities leading major components of an organization such as a service line, institute, or center, their scope of responsibility is larger and broader than for those in the early career stage. Because they manage larger programs with broader clinical scope, more staff, and bigger budgets, it is critical that they start to develop a broader sense of the organization, how their units fit into it, and how their responsibilities for the larger organization are developing.

In addition, mid-career often sees a shift from data management and analysis to decision-making. The mid-careerist must assure that the right data and the right amount of data are analyzed before a decision is made. They also must make decisions with incomplete information. Judgment and decision-making play a much greater role as one moves into mid-career.

It is also important for mid-careerists to not only manage direct reports but also the organization's senior executives, a concept known as managing up. While this may have occurred earlier in their career, it becomes an important competency in mid-career. Often, senior leaders do not have an in-depth understanding of the areas managed by the mid-careerist. Perhaps they developed their own career in a different service line or functional area, such as finance or strategy, leading to knowledge gaps that need to be filled, delicately, by the person in their mid-career.

## SENIOR CAREER

What does a **senior career** look like? Senior leaders are responsible for the performance of the entire organization, or significant parts of an organization, everything it does or fails to do. They are responsible for clinical care, quality and safety, human resources, legal, compliance, strategy, vision, culture, board development, community relations, and fiscal performance, amid a myriad of other responsibilities. Because of the complexity of their roles, effective senior leaders recognize their own strengths and acknowledge when to bring in others with different skills and perspectives in order to manage a large and complex organization.

A critical role and one of the most difficult for senior leaders is to create and maintain an organizational culture supportive of putting patients first and maintaining quality and safety. Senior leadership has a primary role regarding patient safety and the quality of patient care. Unless senior leaders take responsibility and lead the organization's efforts, it will likely fall short in this critical area. Consequently, senior leaders play an important role in performance improvement.

Senior leaders are responsible for the organization's strategic planning and direction; its mission, vision, and values; and determining what activities the organization should undertake, stop doing, or perform differently. Senior leaders also have the role of developing community relations and developing the board of directors.

A challenge for senior leaders can be to manage with incomplete information, relying on the expertise of others. Whereas in earlier stages in their career, the leader was often the subject expert, at this point in the career, their responsibilities are so broad it is impossible to have expertise across all areas.

## ENCORE CAREER: SUCCESS TO SIGNIFICANCE

What does an **encore career** look like? The options for the encore career are almost limitless, constrained only by the individual's imagination and capabilities. Having attained a significant degree of career success, many executives look for a way to give back to the profession. Encore careers can also provide significant satisfaction and purpose for the healthcare leader and support the organization served.

Many executives seek out a role as a consultant or start their own consulting business to take advantage of the significant knowledge and skills they have acquired in their careers. Initiative, project management, organizational development, financial management, and analytics are often critical to the consultant.

Some executives will seek to pass on their knowledge of healthcare leadership through academic training programs, serving as faculty or executives in residence at academic healthcare administration programs. Many Bachelor of Health Administration, Master of Health Administration, and executive doctoral programs make use of executives in residence who provide academic and career advice, counseling, mentoring, and guest lectures for students. They may also serve on advisory boards. Healthcare leaders can also serve as faculty members, teaching courses and conducting research. Faculty positions at accredited university programs often, although not always, require a doctoral degree.

In addition, some healthcare executives may serve on boards of directors/trustees for healthcare organizations or not-for-profit organizations serving the community. The skills they have honed as healthcare leaders can be extremely helpful to often resource-constrained community-based organizations.

## OPPORTUNITIES, ROADBLOCKS, AND POTENTIAL PITFALLS IN A CAREER JOURNEY

### NOT A GOOD MATCH BETWEEN THE ORGANIZATION AND THE LEADER

In some cases, individuals may find that there is not a good match between the leader and the organization. Often, this occurs when there are differences or even conflicts in mission, vision, and values between the individual and the organization. The organizational culture may not be a good fit for the individual. In cases of this nature, it is often necessary to find a different organization for which to work, as organizational cultures are not easily changed, and then only by significant, sustained work from senior leadership.

### LACKING SPECIFIC COMPETENCIES

In some cases, an individual may lack specific **competencies** or levels of achievement in required competencies to perform well in their current role or desired next role. Sometimes, leaders may be thrust into an environment or role in which they lack a needed competency. It is critical that individuals accurately self-assess throughout their career and make use of supervisors and mentors to guide them and offer advice in difficult situations. Any career in healthcare requires a commitment to life-long learning. Leaders must affirmatively plan learning activities in self-assessed areas of need.

### CAREER STANDSTILL

It is possible for individuals who have achieved satisfaction with their current role to eventually find that the role is no longer challenging, that going to work is no longer invigorating and exciting, and lack a sense of achieving personal and/or professional accomplishment. When these points are reached, it may be necessary to seek new opportunities within one's current organization or look outside of their current organization to find their next career role.

## THE GOAL: SATISFACTION AND CONTRIBUTION

Neither a roadblock nor a pitfall, this is an ideal time in one's career, when one has found both satisfaction and competency in their current role in an organization and stage of career. They enjoy the colleagues with whom they work and find the work deeply satisfying on both a personal and professional level. Individuals may be content to spend a significant portion of their career in such a role.

As one progresses through their healthcare leadership journey, lifelong learning plays a critical role in preparing the professional. Healthcare is rapidly and constantly changing. Failure to keep up with those changes can drastically limit one's career. Lifelong learning opportunities are available in a myriad of ways including through professional associations, professional and popular press, and formal and continuing education, to name a few.

An important part of any healthcare career includes the role of mentorship throughout the career, including availing oneself to a mentor and becoming a mentor for others. Never stop learning and never stop helping others to learn and progress.

## CONCLUSION

The career journey of a healthcare leader typically starts in early career as the individual graduates from college and starts their first job and progresses through multiple stages of mid-career, senior career, and in some cases, encore career. Healthcare leaders manage different responsibilities and spans of control throughout their career, typically starting smaller and growing, as responsibilities, areas under direction, number of employees, and budgets grow. Consequently, a leader's knowledge and competencies must grow and expand, becoming adept at new competencies and refining and becoming more effective at other competencies.

Healthcare leaders must learn to deal with rapid change and ambiguity as the world around them changes and the specifics of healthcare change. Leaders can be guided by their own personal ethics; their core *why* for choosing a career in healthcare; and by the organization's mission, vision, and values. In the best of circumstances, a leader's personal ethics are reflected in the organization's mission, vision, and values.

Emerging healthcare leaders will find that mentors who are more senior can assist them in their career journey, providing advice, guidance, and in some cases, career opportunities. Leaders should strive to be mentors to others as they advance in their career, paying it forward to the next generation of leaders.

A career in healthcare will likely be both incredibly challenging and incredibly fulfilling. It will require hard work and continuous learning. In the end, our experience has been that a career as a healthcare leader is also incredibly rewarding.

## END-OF-CHAPTER RESOURCES

### CRITICAL THINKING QUESTIONS

1. How do responsibilities change throughout a healthcare career and how do competencies change?
2. How might the fit between an organization and a leader affect the leader and the organization?
3. Why are ethics important to a healthcare leader?
4. How might changes in the general, reimbursement, and healthcare environment affect one's career?
5. Why is adapting, facilitating, and encouraging change important in a healthcare career?
6. How can mentors affect a career?
7. Who are current or desired mentors?
8. How can networking affect a career?
9. What steps can be taken to develop or clarify your core *why*?

### LEARNING ACTIVITIES

**CourseConnect ▸**

To access self-assessment questions and interactive, competency-based learning activities for this chapter, visit www.springerpub.com/courseconnect. See inside front cover and tear-out card for CourseConnect details.

### BIBLIOGRAPHY

Gamble, M. (2020, August 29). Career impatience: The No. 1 worry hospital CEO's have about the next generation of healthcare leaders. *Becker's Hospital Review.* https://www.beckershospitalreview.com/hospital-management-administration/career-impatience-the-no-1-worry-hospital-ceos-have-about-the-next-generation-of-healthcare-leaders.html

Gupta, A., Howell, S. T., Yannelis, C., & Gupta, A. (2021). Does private equity investment in healthcare benefit patients? Evidence from nursing homes. [NBER Working Paper No. 28474]. *National Bureau of Economic Research.* http://www.nber.org/papers/w28474

Hartman, M., Martin A. B., Whittle, L., Catlin, A., & National Health Expenditure Accounts Team. (2024). National health care spending in 2022: Growth similar to prepandemic rates. *Health Affairs, 43*(1). Pharmaceuticals, Opioid Use, Health Spending & More. https://www.healthaffairs.org/doi/epdf/10.1377/hlthaff.2023.01360

The Health Management Academy. (2022) *[Research Brief] Trends and profiles of new leading health system CEOs.* https://hmacademy.com/resource/2023-new-leading-health-system-ceo-report/

Sullivan Cotter. (2023) *Executive Workforce Trends— [Infographic] from 2023 health care management and executive compensation survey report.* https://sullivancotter.com/wp-content/uploads/2023/10/SullivanCotter_2023-Executive-Workforce-Trends-Infographic.pdf

Witt/Kieffer (2017). *Emerging millennial healthcare leadership: Views and reflections from the new generation.* [White paper].

# CHAPTER 22

# LEADERSHIP THEORIES AND APPLICATIONS IN HEALTHCARE MANAGEMENT

Lee Bewley and Matthew P. Ayers

## LEARNING OBJECTIVES

- Understand how leaders achieve results through the path-goal theory application.
- Identify considerations leaders apply following contingency theory principles.
- Describe prime leadership approaches of the situational leadership theory.
- Explain how followers are grouped by applying leader-member exchange theory.
- Identify decision-making pathways should leaders consider applying the normative decision-making model of leadership.
- Understand the prime constructs of the transformational leadership theory.
- Explain the application of leadership theory to modern problems and opportunities.
- Explain the three domains of leadership development.

## KEY TERMS

- Contingency
- Leader-member exchange
- Leadership development
- Normative decision-making
- Path-goal
- Situational
- Transformational

## INTRODUCTION

The 21st century began with the world wondering what unknown, unseen effects of simple computer coding errors may have on practically every element of our existence tied to technology. Ultimately, the "Y2K" or Year 2000 phenomenon proved to be but a brief blip in our national and world reality, but the extreme pervasiveness of potential impact did serve as a foreboding prelude to a series of events that challenged and continues to vex leaders in all fields, including healthcare. Y2K also served as a precursor for the tsunami-like impact of the internet, computing power, and worldwide information effects on leaders' time to act, amount of information to process, and complexity of socioeconomic considerations.

The events of September 11, 2001, and the associated series of terrorist actions following the main attacks shocked the country and world and strained the capacity of healthcare systems to respond, particularly when elements of the healthcare delivery team were victims, and the supporting resources were impacted by attacks. Similarly, a whole series of national disasters—including hurricanes in the Atlantic and Gulf of Mexico; tornadoes in Kansas, Missouri, and Kentucky; flooding, heat waves, and severely cold weather—generated sudden and substantial mass casualty events while damaging or incapacitating elements of the healthcare delivery system. Clearly, the global pandemic comprehensively stressed America's health system along with the rest of the world and caused casualties of health providers and teams in the provision of healthcare while communities and the nation debated the efficacy or sometimes the legitimacy of practical points of preventive medicine strategies. Finally, the underlying foundational elements of socioeconomic inequities and injustices matched with profound schisms of perspectives and experiences within communities exploded on the streets of cities and across our national and international news outlets, leading in many cases to violent demonstrations, riots, assaults, shootings, and mass murders. On many occasions, metropolitan-based health facilities were at the center of conflict, treating patients and trying to serve the community, sometimes with temporary security measures including blockades, armed security, and armored vehicles, shockingly like facility protection measures in active war zones.

The continuing aggregate effects of these events coupled with generational transition impacts result in an aging population and retiring providers, and health professionals are stressing healthcare organizations and the communities served. Burnout, "quiet quitting," and resignations from healthcare teams have become pressing concerns for health systems and organizations across the country. Community members seeking healthcare question healthcare practices, access, and whether financing for healthcare will be available given the varying policy effects of healthcare reform, state activities, and the short-term pandemic measures expiring. Looking forward, the 21st-century healthcare leader must be prepared to serve as a leader for both their own organization and the community served to achieve higher levels of both organizational outcomes and population health.

The study of leadership theory provides healthcare leaders and the organizations and communities served a basis for explanation, prediction, development, and evaluation of leadership application in healthcare management toward better outcomes, higher levels of performance, and enhanced health. Having an enhanced level of knowledge of leadership theory and associated leadership development techniques drives competency development of individual healthcare leaders as well as healthcare teams. The following chapter provides an overview of foundational leadership theories, contemporary leadership theories for current healthcare management practice, and a framework for leadership development to translate theory into practice.

## ANCIENT, EARLY, AND NICHE LEADERSHIP THEORIES AND MODELS

The study and practice of leadership are inextricably rooted and intertwined with the existence of mankind. Ancient discussions of leadership are included in the works of Plato, Caesar, and Plutarch as they sought to provide leadership development guidance for future generations by studying and describing the actions of successful leaders, developing a line of the great man theory of leadership. In the *Iliad*, Homer identifies four sets of successful leadership traits exemplified by various characters: justice/judgment, Agamemnon; wisdom/council, Nestor; shrewdness/cunning, Odysseus; and valor/action, Achilles (Homer, 1961). Machiavelli's *The Prince* prescribed leadership lessons for rulers at the end of the Middle Ages through modern times. The introduction of the word *leader* in English language was recorded circa 1,300, while the term *leadership* only became prevalent in the early 19th century among writings about political power associated with members of the British Parliament.

Research in the United States has been the primary source of knowledge on leadership and leadership development for American enterprises in the modern age. Identifying and applying common leadership traits dominated the first half of the 20th century as academics and practitioners sought to discover specific leadership traits associated with successful outcomes. The second half of the century was marked by a dramatic increase in academic studies and the development of leadership theory. Notable examples of these theories include Theory X, Theory Y, and charismatic leadership. Theory X and Theory Y posited a line of thinking that leaders employed leadership styles based on their assessment of follower motivation. Charismatic leader theory suggests that elements of a leader's personality or other personal characteristics predict the likelihood of follower commitment and support to direction and guidance ordered by the leader. Finally, throughout its history, the U.S. Armed Forces have developed and evolved leadership models to meet the requirements of national defense and security (Bass, 1981; Ledlow & Coppola, 2014; United States Army, 1999).

## MODERN LEADERSHIP THEORIES

### PATH-GOAL THEORY

**Path-goal** theory establishes a set of foundation principles and enabling techniques for leaders to achieve organizational goals. The primary foundational principles include matching rewards to achievements; providing clear, focused paths to goal achievement; and removing and moderating obstacles, barriers, and points of friction that followers may encounter in the process of taking action to achieve organizational goals. The specific actions or approaches that a leader may take to apply path-goal theory include directive, supportive, achievement, and participation.

In many ways, modern healthcare management practices in human resources (bonuses, promotions, awards-team, awards-individual, etc.) and quality improvement (total quality management, path diagrams, root cause analysis, transaction cost analysis) reflect the prime elements of path-goal foundations. Clearly, leaders should seek to understand appropriate incentives, rewards, and consequences that match appropriately, in level and magnitude, to desired outcomes and goals and take actions to develop and provide accordingly. Similarly, leaders should seek to establish clear plans that offer a path with instructions, guidelines, and match resources to facilitate follower achievement. Finally, leaders who can observe; predict obstacles, challenges, and shortfalls; and develop contingency plans or moderate and eliminate disruptions to follow progress toward goal achievement are more likely to succeed.

The way leaders apply the fundamental elements of path-goal theory (Figure 22.1) varies depending on the ability and capacity of the leader and followers, as well as circumstances associated with achieving the targeted goal. In occasions that require timely action and a leader who is both competent and confident, a directive approach would likely provide the most effective way toward goal achievement. Circumstances that allow

**FIGURE 22.1.** A goal-focused model of the path-goal theory.

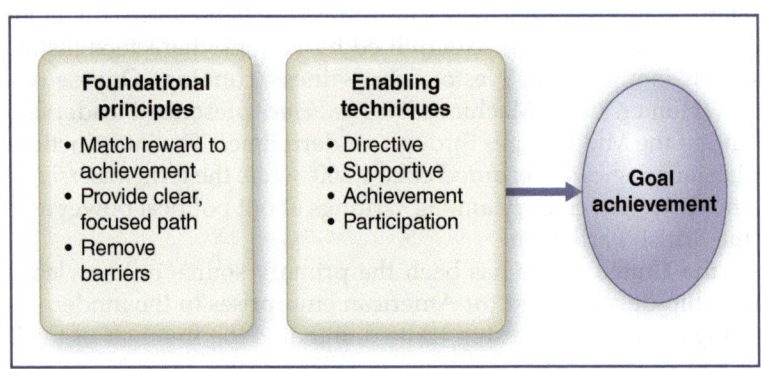

more time and the need for coaching followers and developing plans would call for a supportive approach. An achievement-based approach matches effectively with a clear goal that the team of followers is readily developed, prepared, and motivated to succeed. Finally, if conditions require the active joint participation of the leader with followers to achieve targeted goals, then a participative approach is warranted.

One clear example of the path-goal theory applied is manifest in the many ways that hospitals and health systems conduct quality assurance and total quality management. Leaders throughout healthcare delivery organizations set clear goals, levels of achievement, and performance and enable team members with tools, training, information, rewards, and consequences on both individual and group bases. An organization that evaluates the process and outcomes of every patient encounter, contract negotiation, or medical logistic transaction employs elements of the theory. Consider the four path-goal-enabling techniques: directive, supportive, achievement, and supportive. Each technique is appropriately matched to stages and levels of development in a total quality management process, spanning initial indoctrination and implementation through fully implemented and established processes of excellence (Fabac et al., 2022; House, 1971).

## CONTINGENCY THEORY

The author's graduate health administration didactic phase was filled with volumes of literature reviews, outstanding guest lectures, excellent instruction, great colleagues sharing the pursuit of healthcare management knowledge to lead effectively, and a common mantra for the most difficult set of strategic choices in analysis: "It depends." Our class carried the principles of contingency theory through our courses, residency, and into our careers, applying the theoretical framework to serve our country, patients, and healthcare community, being ever mindful that we must understand ourselves, our team, and the circumstances tied to our tasks to make the most effective decisions and take definitive actions most likely to succeed.

The contingency theory of leadership consists of one factor associated with leader considerations, including their preferred leadership style, conditions of followers, organizational behaviors, the nature of the task, and environmental conditions. The second factor of the contingency theory is the leader's choice framework which includes the nature of relationship with followers, circumstances of the task, and the amount or level of power and available resources for the leader to employ toward goal achievement.

Effective application of the contingency theory of leadership (Figure 22.2) requires that leaders have a clear and unbiased assessment of their own strengths, weaknesses, limitations, and capacity, as well as those of their team and the organization tasked with

**FIGURE 22.2.** A goal-focused model of the contingency theory.

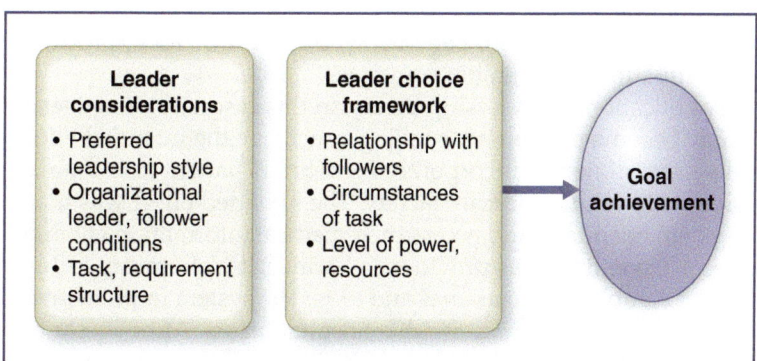

achieving a targeted goal. In a way, a leader should always have a working value chain analysis of their own operational element of the organization then find ways to leverage value-producing strengths and moderate the effects of weaknesses by developing and implementing plans that align with task requirements and available resources.

A health system that aims to "meet employees where they are" in the process of employee engagement incentives, recognition, and workforce development applies elements of contingency theory on a regular basis. Employees, individually and collectively, may evolve concerns, goals, and ambitions in concert with operating conditions, the market environment, and the circumstances of similar employees across the industry; consequently, leaders who understand the needs and requirements of their teams, as well as the limits and bounds of their own leadership styles and available resources, may develop initiative and transactions to drive employee productivity, retention, and commitment toward organizational goals by applying a contingency approach. The contingency theory approach is more likely to be successful when applied by leaders with experience who possess a richer and more profound sense of potential actions matched with consequences or outcomes, as well as intervening considerations within the organization and market environment, weighing likelihoods, benefits, and costs of action alternatives (Fiedler, 1971; Monehin & Diers-Lawson, 2022).

## SITUATIONAL LEADERSHIP THEORY

**Situational leadership theory** aims to achieve organizational goals and objectives by applying fundamental assessments of followers' ability to conduct necessary tasks and actions, as well as followers' willingness or commitment to achieving organizational goals and objectives. By assessing these two prime factors of follower success generation, willing and able, leaders may choose appropriate approaches matched with the status of followers. Leader approaches include telling, selling, delegating, and participating.

Consider a situation where follower status ranks "high" on both willing and able dimensions, indicating a high competence level and extraordinary motivation to achieve. In this situation, a leader simply needs to communicate or tell the team what is expected. Somewhat alternatively, in a similar situation, a highly competent team of followers rating high on the able dimension but low on the willing dimension would require a leader to sell the team on the benefits and value of action toward achieving organizational goals.

Another set of situations could be based on a state where the able levels are lower with follower teams not fully or appropriately trained or developed to take action to achieve organizational goals. If the follower group possesses a relatively high level of willing, then a competent, able leader could directly participate with this team providing coaching and examples to enable the team to succeed. On the other hand, if a team low on the able factor is also low on the willing factor, then delegation, bringing in additional resources to both train and extol achievement benefits, would serve as an appropriate action for a leader following situational leadership principles.

Appropriate application of leadership theory, in this case, situational leadership theory (Figure 22.3), may become evident after failing to achieve the intended effects. Recently, a major hospital system aimed to incorporate "real-time" patient care data access at every patient's bedside within the healthcare facility. The intended effect was that every patient admitted to a system hospital could access their medical information entered into their patient medical record in real time as providers, pharmacists, laboratory technicians, and diagnostic specialists completed procedures and tests. The system implemented the initiative with one of its most recognized and capable hospital teams. After 1 year of implementation, the health system leadership team temporarily halted the initiative and reconsidered their implementation approach as providers, support staff, and patients expressed consistent dissatisfaction and ambivalence toward the project. In retrospect, the clinical and administrative capabilities of the healthcare team were clearly in the middle to high range of the "able" scale aligned with the situational leadership framework, but the "willing" dimension of the team was more likely low to middle range because the healthcare team not clearly see the compelling need or could readily answer the "why?" of the initiative; consequently, system leaders incorrectly assessed the situation as a simply "telling" dimension application where capable, motivated leaders and teams would readily implement to significant effect. At the same time, the more appropriate situational leadership approach of "selling" would inform and clarify the benefits and value for teams of competent, engaged professionals to pursue (Hall et al., 2023; Hersey & Blanchard, 1988; Vecchio et al., 2006).

## LEADER-MEMBER EXCHANGE THEORY

Leader-member exchange theory establishes principles for leaders to follow to achieve desired organizational outcomes and objectives by perpetually evaluating and grouping followers based on the state of relationship with the leader and then matching leadership

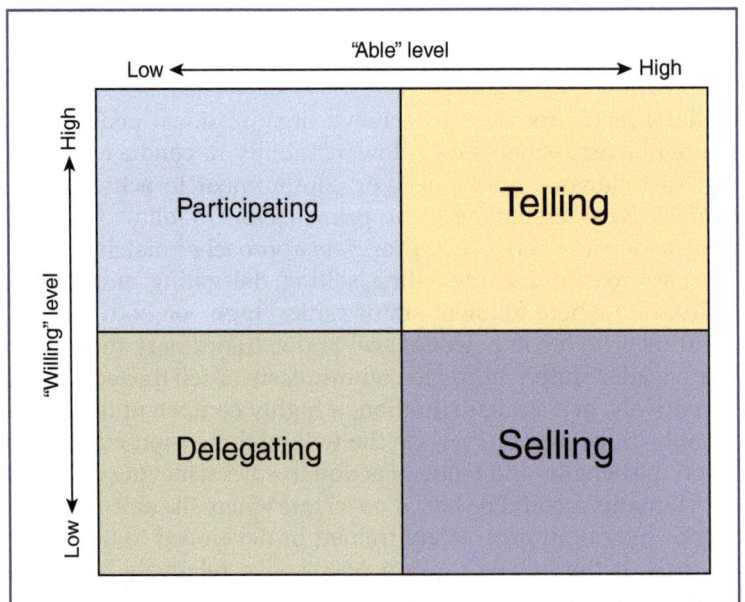

**FIGURE 22.3.** A decision matrix model of the situational leadership theory.

actions based on group standing. Leaders evaluate whether followers, individually and/or collectively, are in a group that is committed, dedicated, or loyal to the actions, directions, and ways of the leader or whether they are comparatively uncommitted, not dedicated, or not loyal to the leader.

The actions or style of leadership that a leader will employ with a group of dedicated followers would be materially different from those not dedicated to the leader. If each action, order, or request that a leader posits would be considered a transactional exchange between leader and follower(s), then the resources necessary to consummate a successful exchange would generally be expected to be in varying rates across the groups requiring constant evaluation and bargaining.

Leader-member exchange theory (Figure 22.4) predicts that individuals and groups may change over time and some individuals or groups may straddle or hedge their allegiances to leaders based on their own assessments of organizational conditions or the value of leader exchanges within the organizational setting. Additionally, a leader's application of leader-member exchange principles requires the expenditure of resources to maintain a loyal group and to stimulate action in followers grouped among those that require extraordinary consideration to achieve organizational goals.

Leader-member exchange theory is frequently and effectively applied across the healthcare industry in merger integrations and similar group onboarding, partnering, and alliance developments. Each leader's tenure in a managerial role exists as an aggregation of experiences, challenges, setbacks, successes, and outcomes shared with individuals and groups that create a shared basis of knowledge, appreciation, and understanding of actions necessary to create conditions for organizational achievement. Individuals, groups, and leaders with shared experience naturally develop the "in group" basis of the leader-member exchange approach, and the actions that a leader may take to achieve organizational goals will likely be different for an individual or group (e.g., "out group") that becomes a part of the greater organizational collective through merger, alliance, new hire, or some other organizational activity; however, in time and with accumulated shared experiences, all members of the organization may evolve from an "out group" to "in group" standing. For instance, an organizational leader aiming to implement a new strategic initiative may consider applying different informational and incentive approaches for a newly acquired hospital rather than a long-standing hospital within the system, as varying levels of trust and past experiences will likely impact the initiative implementation success (Erdogan & Bauer, 2014; Kim et al., 2023).

**FIGURE 22.4.** A goal-focused model of the leader-member exchange theory.

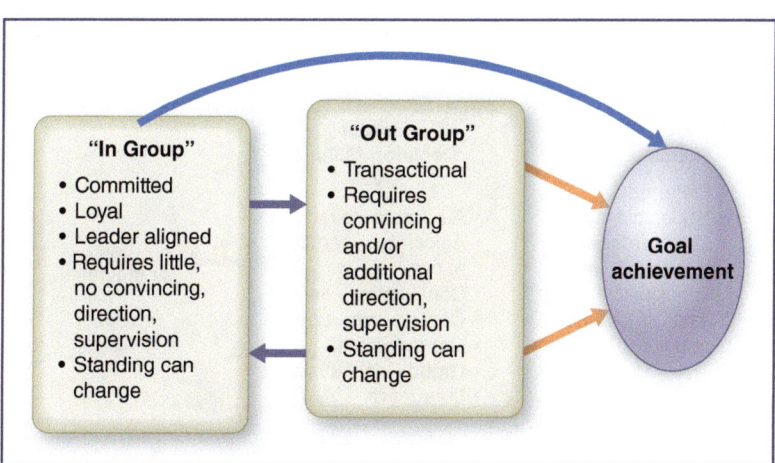

## NORMATIVE DECISION-MAKING MODEL

The **normative decision-making model of leadership** is predicated on fundamental leader considerations of organizational state and the appropriate application of the decision-making style most likely to generate organizational goal achievement. The primary leader considerations include their own preferred leadership style, conditions of leader-follower relationships, the nature of task, and the associated operational environment. The choices that leaders may follow regarding decision-making generating action to achieve organizational goals include variations of autocratic, consultative, group, and delegative.

Application of normative decision-making model principles begins with leaders understanding their preferred leadership style as well as potential areas of risk or friction following their own style or choosing a style not normally suited toward their development. Leaders must consider whether they are comfortable or will accept sharing decision-making. An associated and sequential consideration for leaders is assessing the nature of relationships with followers regarding level of trust, capabilities, experience of followers, and past experiences of the team. Finally, leaders should evaluate the nature of the task and environment in terms of complexity, time considerations, and available resources.

The leader following the normative decision-making model (Figure 22.5) principles will extend their assessment of fundamental considerations to how decision-making will be conducted in the process of working toward achieving organizational goals. In some circumstances requiring expedient execution of tasks, leaders may follow an autocratic decision-making style with all decisions made directly by the leader or a modified form that may include asking close followers for input prior to making decisions. A consultative approach to decision-making in a limited or open format would be matched with conditions of ample time and capable and experienced followers. Finally, on occasions with ample time, resources, and competency levels of followers, leaders may follow group and delegated decision-making processes.

Healthcare leaders manage organizations with highly educated, trained professionals on a perpetual basis, requiring understanding and ability to apply elements of the normative decision-making leadership approach on a regular basis. The normative decision-making approach is predicated on an effective assessment of current organizational dynamics and requirements, then matching appropriate decision-making styles in operational execution. Leaders who inappropriately assess organizational circumstances as

**FIGURE 22.5.** A goal-focused model of the normative decision-making theory.

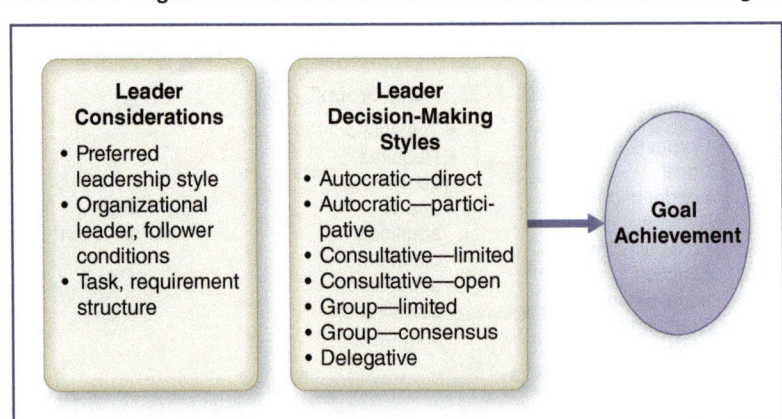

emergent, risk laden, and resource poor, for instance, may apply an autocratic-direct style of leadership decision-making that drives capable professionals to become resistant to directives and create conditions for organizational failure. Often, healthcare leaders find that highly capable and dedicated teams may operate most efficiently and effectively with opportunities for input and decision-making on both individual and collective bases. For instance, one healthcare system developed an information system response that sends a "thumbs-up" symbol and "We heard you!" message each time employees send suggestions or recommendations for improvements through the online message board (Islam et al., 2022; Vroom & Yetton, 1973).

## TRANSFORMATIONAL LEADERSHIP THEORY

The final contemporary model of leadership theory of this chapter, **transformational** leadership, is perhaps the most complex and often the most appealing for application in healthcare. Transformational leadership theory's foundations are drawn from other leadership theories, industrial-organizational psychology principles, and organizational politics. The primary constructs of transformational leadership include charisma (leader), intellectual stimulation, individual consideration, and inspirational motivation. Leader implementation considerations include contingencies, situational analysis, and leader-member exchange perspectives to achieve intended organizational goals. Transformational leadership is very strongly aligned with the core principles of the servant-based leadership approach (Burns, 1978).

The appealing nature of transformational leadership theory (Figure 22.6) in healthcare is likely to manifest in constant change and evolutions in the field, requiring elements of transformation to survive and have aspirations of thriving in ever-changing operational environments. Healthcare organizations are principally staffed by highly educated and trained professionals through the full range of team members, including physicians, allied health professionals, nurses, administrators, technicians, and associates, who appreciate, and may even seek, intellectual stimulation of applied leadership direction communicated effectively by a leader who intentionally seeks to make individual and group connections and builds commitments toward organizational goals. Furthermore, particularly given the frequent incongruences between societal community demands for health services and available resources and healthcare supply, health professionals, individually and collectively, require motivational and inspirational initiatives to bolster morale and positively orient team activities.

**FIGURE 22.6.** A goal-focused model of the transformational leadership theory.

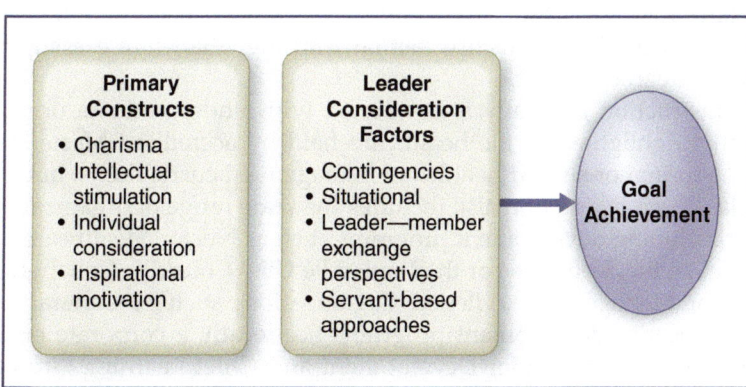

Implementation of leadership initiatives through applied healthcare management following a transformation leadership framework combines multidimensional considerations of contingencies, situational analyses, and elements of organizational political net benefit calculus. These are aligned with leader-member exchange principles to choose appropriate actions and manners of application most likely to achieve intended effects, resulting in anticipated and expected transformation and achievement of organizational goals.

Effective application of the transformational leadership approach enables substantial potential organizational benefits and facilitates the expansion of organizational capabilities for achievement requires investments and leaders with exceptional competency strengths in communication and interpersonal understanding and dynamics. A board of directors seeking to infuse higher levels of organizational performance of a health system staffed by capable providers, administrators, and associations but lags operational performance and community impact of peer systems in the marketplace may seek to hire a chief executive officer (CEO) and top management team to enable higher levels of performance by moving the capable and compliant team of teams toward higher levels of achievement through bolstered and collective commitment. The new CEO and top management team applying transformational leadership approaches would simultaneously evaluate the personalities, organizational citizenship behaviors, and achievement orientation while developing clear, productive lines of communication and professional relationships within the organization. Evaluation of organizational dynamics could include both formal and informal assessments. Still, the nature of communications would most effectively be applied directly and frequently, albeit on varying levels of individual and group bases, given time and opportunity to communicate. The perpetual combinations of constant evaluations and communications will shape both leadership and followership actions and reactions as understanding, and shared appreciation of essential elements of motivation drive healthcare team performance. The transformational leadership approach, effectively applied, will ultimately evolve the organization toward a new shared identity aligned with the goals and expectations of the leadership team (Baluti et al., 2024; Clarke et al., 2014; Greenleaf, 1977).

## TRANSLATION OF LEADERSHIP THEORY TO PRACTICE THROUGH LEADERSHIP DEVELOPMENT

Leadership theories provide a basis for individuals and organizations to consider approaches for application as well as to guide processes of development to achieve intended outcomes and to facilitate efficient and effective healthcare management practices. Leadership development approaches may include formal and informal methods. The scope of development may be individual-based development to complex, interactive group and team processes. Leader development processes include higher education instruction, developmental relationships, action learning, challenging assignments, team training, and 360-degree feedback.

Classroom instruction generally is associated with undergraduate or graduate programs, typically highlighted in the healthcare field by accredited Master of Science in Health Administration or similar healthcare management curriculums, but leader development via classroom instruction also includes the wide range of organizational internal and external continuing development programs such as Norton Healthcare's Leadership Academy in Louisville, Kentucky, or the Louisville CEO Council's Collaborative Healthcare Institute for Managerial Excellence. Organizations such as General Electric have long-established leader development programs headed by a corporate executive identified as Vice President for Leader Development and Chief Learning Officer. The goals of these programs are generally designed to improve the level of leadership within the organization and to develop a group of leaders to vie for the corporate leadership posts in the future.

Developmental relationships in the form of mentoring and coaching are employed both formally and informally to develop leaders. Informal developmental relationships are generally initiated voluntarily between staff members on a dyadic mentor-protégé basis where the mentor guides or assists the protégé in achieving proficiency or success within a professional career context. Some organizations opt to formalize developmental relationships by assigning mentors and coaches to individual staff members rather than relying upon social\professional chance or circumstance, generating developmental relationships.

Action learning enables organizations to conduct enterprise operations while simultaneously employing intensive leader development activities. Activities such as new market penetration, off-site brainstorming sessions, or focused strategic initiatives are conducted with the intent of yielding immediate organizational return, identifying specific leader development shortcomings, and enhancing existing leadership competencies. Organizational adaptive responses to pandemic challenges yielded an abundance of action-learning opportunities, as leaders responded to necessary immediate requirements related to operating capacity management, environment of care maintenance, and logistics challenges.

Leader development through challenging job assignments exists as the most enduring approach for building leader competencies. The process for assigning developmentally challenging assignments is typically characterized by assignments involving diverse tasks and an incrementally progressive level of responsibility and rigor as the individual demonstrates increased leadership proficiency. A CEO of a hospital who entered the healthcare administration profession as an administrative resident or fellowship then systematically progressed through the hierarchy of health administration, including clinic administrator, department administrator, and chief operating officer, prior to being selected as CEO serves as an example of leader development via challenging job assignments.

The increased importance of teams within organizational processes has resulted in team training serving as a valuable mechanism for leader development, particularly in an environment requiring multifunctional skill sets operating in complex environments. Leader development is facilitated as team members interact with members from across the organization, bringing different experiences, competencies, and organizational knowledge to team processes. The team develops leader competencies as members alternatively or by selection manage the team. Often, services or departments will generate ad hoc teams to focus on specific tasks, including implementation of a strategic initiative, facility transfer, or accreditation preparation, which provide team members opportunities to lead based on their background, development, or assigned role. Additionally, the nature of team interactions provides a dual basis for practicing alternating roles of leadership and followership among colleagues focused on a common task. The opportunity to practice followership among colleagues may enable enhanced leadership competencies by providing ample opportunities for observing, experiencing, and communicating the effects of various leadership techniques and practices derived from leadership theories and approaches.

The final major leader development technique involves multidimensional feedback regarding an individual's developmental successes, failures, and opportunities through 360-degree feedback. The feedback process involves obtaining critical and thorough developmental evaluation of job performance and leadership competencies from supervisors, peers, and subordinates. This approach may also employ both formal and informal approaches. Formal approaches include periodic reviews and evaluations, while informal means may be as simple as direct oral communication of performance in process and/or following application of leadership.

Application of elements or whole factors of leadership development has generating, maintaining, and expanding effects. In some cases, particularly for early careerists or professionals with little or no experience in a particular area of applied leadership development, individuals will generate new competencies and capabilities in leadership while another professional experiencing the same developmental activity may be maintaining, reinforcing, or even substantially expanding capacity for effective leadership building upon prior development.

## A MODEL OF LEADERSHIP DEVELOPMENT

The practice of leadership development exists within three interconnected domains: training and education, interpersonal interaction, and job performance. Training and education include all formal educational and training activities ranging from undergraduate and graduate education to continuing education and training seminars. Interpersonal interaction encompasses mentoring and 360-degree feedback, where the primary basis for leader development is predicated on developmental communication between people. Finally, the job performance cluster of leader development includes those approaches (action learning, challenging job assignments, and team training) that are actively conducted within the normal job performance process (Bewley, 2005; Bewley & Yarbrough, 2009).

Figure 22.7 illustrates a model of leader development arrayed in three domains of development approaches. Additionally, the model demonstrates interconnected associations between clusters. For instance, although mentoring and challenging job assignments fall under separate development clusters, there is clearly an intuitive and theoretically supportable association between the approaches. An example of this interconnected

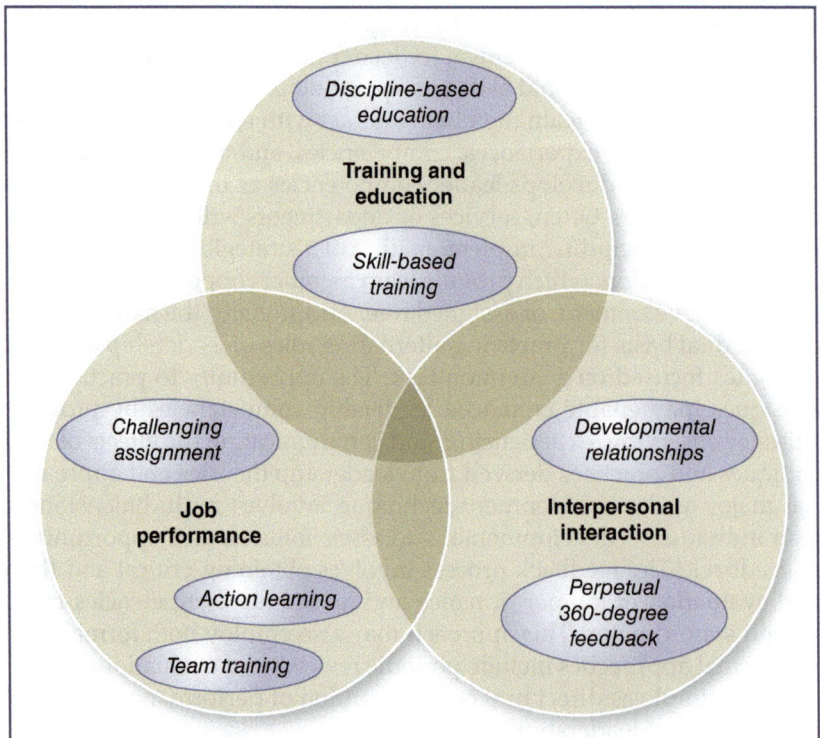

**FIGURE 22.7.** A multidimensional model of leadership development.

association is when a challenging job assignment is directed by a mentor to facilitate protégé leader development.

An extended applied point of this leadership development model is that an individual could consider the model to be a form of map or graphical depiction of their leadership development and associated capacity for application. For many years and currently, mobile phone carriers have often advertised their capacity and mobile phone network with maps of the United States showing comparative strength of coverage through shaded or pixelated graphs. Similarly, the strength of an individual's leadership development could be illustrated or depicted by evaluating the quality and magnitude of development of each indicator and each factor of leadership development showing areas of substantial strength or areas needing further development. Furthermore, individuals and organizations may use leadership development evaluations to consider risk levels assuming and/or assigning tasks and initiatives based on assessed capabilities while also considering forward-looking plans for supplemental and continuing leadership development.

## CASE STUDY 22.1: CONTEMPORARY APPLICATIONS OF LEADERSHIP THEORY IN HEALTHCARE MANAGEMENT: A REAL-WORLD APPLICATION

Consider the following scenario: A modern healthcare system operates in the heart of the largest metropolitan area within the state. The system's flagship hospital is a wonder of modern medical marvels and employs thousands of healthcare professionals within the county and from outlying communities within a 1-hour drive. The downtown hospital is known for top-tier clinical quality, receiving national and regional accolades while consistently meeting accreditation and service line certifications. The health system enjoys a well-earned favored position within the community as an employer of choice with high morale and low turnover while being viewed as a good neighbor sponsoring youth sports, local universities and colleges, and community outreach programs. Financially, the nonprofit health system generates operating surpluses consistently, even during periods of federally managed reductions in reimbursement rates and the pandemic, and maintains an excellent credit rating and low to scarce financial leverage. Despite this rosy, aspirant market standing, the board of directors has recently considered strategic and operational risks to meeting the mission, achieving vision, and adhering to every element and the spirit of the health system's revered values. Practically within the shadows of the downtown medical center's towers and not more than 5-minute drive to the emergency department, several historically marginalized, economically and socially, communities numbering about 75,000 citizens have life expectancies of nearly 1 decade less than the rest of the city. This health desperate downtown enclave reflects substantially different demographic content than the rest of the city: 80% people of color (versus 75% White rest of the city), higher unemployment rates, and majority eligible or enrolled in Medicaid. Recent needs assessments and community outreach surveys indicate that the members of this subset of the community are highly more likely to utilize the health system's services on an emergent or critical care basis than routine or preventative, and most troubling, as a group, these citizens report having low to moderate levels of trust or recognition of the health system's quality rankings. Finally, in a brief review of the health system team demographics, less than 10% of employees overall and only 5% of providers reflect people of color.

Given this scenario, how might leaders within this health system employ leadership theory and leadership development elements to address current and contingent challenges within the community?

## SUMMARY

Our present century brings fundamentally profound challenges and opportunities for healthcare leaders due to expedited time expectations, prodigious generation of information, and an enormous groundswell of socioeconomic equity, access, and inclusion. The United States of America dedicates nearly one fifth of our economic activity toward healthcare, while nearly 10% of our citizens have no consistent health financing and a substantial portion of our country has medical financing but inadequate access to healthcare. Competent and effective healthcare leadership from an organizational and community-based perspective is essential. By understanding and applying leadership theory in singular or combination manners and utilizing leadership development frameworks to generate and extend leadership and healthcare management competencies, we may aspire to achieve higher levels of population health and pursuits of happiness across our communities and society.

# END-OF-CHAPTER RESOURCES

## CRITICAL THINKING QUESTIONS

- What are the differentiating elements of leadership theories?
- What aspects of leadership theories demonstrate consistency in approaches?
- How might leadership theory application vary based on socioeconomic factors?
- How does consideration of legal and ethical standards affect leadership theory application?
- What combinations of leadership theories do you judge most appropriate in 21st-century markets and environments?
- What contemporary factors or conditions should leaders consider when choosing single or combination leadership theory approaches?
- What considerations should organizations incorporate in leadership development in hiring actions, promotions, and assignments?

## LEARNING ACTIVITIES

**CourseConnect ▸**

To access self-assessment questions and interactive, competency-based learning activities for this chapter, visit www.springerpub.com/courseconnect. See inside front cover and tear-out card for CourseConnect details.

## REFERENCES

Baluti, M., Santos, S. B., Tubastuvi, N., & Astuti, H. J. (2024). Assessing the impact of occupational health and safety, work environment, organizational culture, transformational leadership, and motivation on employee performance in the post-COVID-19 Malawi. *International Journal of Research in Business and Social Science*, 13(1), 157–170. https://doi.org/10.20525/ijrbs.v13i1.3064

Bass, B. (1981). *Stogdill's handbook of leadership: A survey of theory and research*. The Free Press.

Bewley, L. (2005). *Seasons of leadership development: An analysis of a multi-dimensional model of mentoring among career Groups of United States Army Officers*. [Doctoral dissertation]. University of Alabama at Birmingham.

Bewley, L., Yarbrough, A. (2009). *Leadership development, succession planning, and mentoring. strategic human resource management in health services organizations*. Delmar-Thomson.

Burns, J. M. (1978). *Leadership*. Harper & Row.

Clarke, P., Cody, W., & Cowling, R. (2014). Transformative leadership based on nursing science. *Nursing Science Quarterly*, 27(2), 126–131. https://doi.org/10.1177/0894318414522662

Erdogan, B., & Bauer, T. N. (2014). Leader-member exchange (LMX) theory: The relational approach to leadership. In D. V. Day (Ed.), *The Oxford handbook of leadership and organizations* (pp. 407–433). Oxford University Press.

Fabac, R., Kokot, K., & Bubalo, I. (2022). Path-goal theory—Leadership styles and their changes during the COVID-19 pandemic. *Interdisciplinary Description of Complex Systems*, 20(4), 349–374. https://doi.org/10.7906/indecs.20.4.4

Fiedler, F. E. (1971). Validation and extension of the contingency model of leadership effectiveness: A review of empirical findings. *Psychological Bulletin*, 76(2), 128–148. https://doi.org/10.1037/h0031454

Greenleaf, R. K. (1977). *Servant leadership: A journey into the nature of legitimate power and greatness*. Paulist Press.

Hall, M. L., Meyer, C. K., & Clapham, M. M. (2023). Leadership theories and styles understood and synthesized. *Journal of Business and Behavioral Sciences*, 35(3), 93–102. http://asbbs.org/files/2023-24/JBBS_35.3_Fall_2023.pdf

Hersey, P., & Blanchard, K. H. (1988). *Management and organizational behavior*. Prentice-Hall.

Homer. (1961). *The Odyssey*. Translated by R. Fitzgerald. Doubleday.

House, R. J. (1971). A path goal theory of leader effectiveness. *Administrative Science Quarterly, 16*, 321–339. https://doi.org/10.2307/2391905

Islam, R., Abdul Ghani, A. B., Mahyudin, E., & Osman, N. (2022). Impact on strategic leadership of strategic models and development. *Academy of Strategic Management Journal, 21*(3), 1–12. http://echo.louisville.edu/login?url=https://www.proquest.com/abicomplete/scholarly-journals/leadership-theories-styles-understood-synthesized/docview/2900390044/sem-2?accountid=14665

Kim, S., Lee, S., & Son, S. (2023). Why does leader-member exchange ambivalence reduce taking charge? The moderating role of cognitive reappraisal. *Journal of Business and Psychology, 38*, 1355–1369. https://doi.org/10.1007/s10869-023-09899-3

Ledlow, G., & Coppola, M. (2014). *Leadership for health professionals: Theory, skills, and applications*. Jones and Bartlett.

Monehin, D., & Diers-Lawson, A. (2022). Pragmatic optimism, crisis leadership, and contingency theory: A view from the C-suite. *Public Relations Review, 48*(4), 102224. https://doi.org/10.1016/j.pubrev.2022.102224

United States Army. (1999). *FM 22-100: Army leadership*. McGraw-Hill.

Vecchio, R. P., Bullis, R. C., & Brazil, D. M. (2006). The utility of situational leadership theory: A replication in a military setting. *Small Group Research, 37*(5), 407–424. https://doi.org/10.1177/1046496406291560

Vroom, V., & Yetton, P. (1973). *Leadership and decision-making*. University of Pittsburgh Press. https://doi.org/10.2307/j.ctt6wrc8r

CHAPTER 23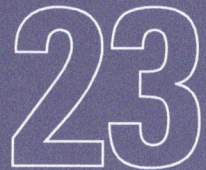

# HEALTHCARE LAW AND ETHICS

Elizabeth Van Nostrand and Nicholas J. Barcellona

## LEARNING OBJECTIVES

- Identify the sources of law.
- Describe the difference between civil and criminal law.
- Define the elements of a negligence action.
- Explain the four pillars of ethics and the role of an ethics committee.
- Recognize legal and ethical principles implicit in the role of healthcare managers.

## KEY TERMS

- Autonomy
- Beneficence
- Civil law
- Criminal law
- Ethics
- Executive branch
- Federalism
- Judicial branch
- Justice
- Legislative branch
- Malpractice
- Nonmaleficence
- Preemption
- Vicarious liability

## INTRODUCTION

This chapter provides an overview of how laws and **ethics** can impact healthcare managers. Law and ethics can *improve the quality of patient care*. For example, the Emergency Medical Treatment and Labor Act or EMTALA (pronounced "em-talla") is a federal law that prohibits "patient dumping" by requiring most hospitals to provide treatment to anyone who presents in the emergency department regardless of their ability to pay (EMTALA, 1986). Trust is an essential component of optimal patient care, but 62% of Americans do not trust their health plans (Ribbon Health, 2022). Incorporating ethical principles of autonomy and justice into healthcare manager practice can improve patient trust and lower healthcare costs (Greene et al., 2019).

Laws and ethics can *shape behaviors* and result in better health outcomes. In the 1950s, about 45% of Americans consumed tobacco, as opposed to about 11% in 2022 (Gallup, 2023). Laws that raised the age for tobacco purchases; created smoking bans; taxed tobacco products; limited cigarette advertising; and prevented a cartoon mascot, Joe Camel, from targeting underage tobacco use shifted societal norms and are credited with the decline in tobacco use. By incorporating ethical principles into their behaviors, healthcare managers can improve workplace cultures and mitigate employee dissatisfaction (American College of Healthcare Executives, 2020).

Laws also *provide protections* for healthcare managers, such as legal protections from retaliation when reporting unsafe work conditions or medical errors (42 USC. § 299 *et seq.*). Workplace ethics can shape a healthcare organization's culture, resulting not only in personal benefits for healthcare managers but also in protecting organizational assets by deterring illegal business practices (Hauser, 2020).

## STATUTES, REGULATIONS, EXECUTIVE ORDERS, AND CASE LAW

> *"Stroke of the pen. Law of the land. Kinda cool."* Paul Begala (a former advisor to President Bill Clinton) commenting on the power of presidential executive orders

A law is an external rule created and enforced by a governmental entity. Unlike a *policy*, which is a practice of an organization or government, laws go through very specific, formalized rulemaking processes. Statutes, regulations, executive orders, and case law all have the force and effect of law, but they differ with respect to which entity can create them, what processes are undertaken before they become "law," and how they can be modified or rescinded after they are established.

U.S. federal and state governments are divided into three coequal branches: the legislative, executive, and judicial branches. Our system of government is based on **federalism**, which means that some powers are reserved for the federal government, some are reserved for state governments, and some fall to local governments. Although this type of governmental structure protects citizens from the threat of one level of government becoming too powerful, having multiple levels of government enacting laws can also create confusion. If two levels of government enact similar laws that can be read together, both laws govern. If they conflict, **preemption** goes into effect. Under the U.S. Constitution's Supremacy Clause, a higher level of government can limit or eliminate a lower level of government's authority to enact a law (i.e., federal law trumps state law, and state law trumps a local ordinance; U.S. Const. art. VI, para. 2). For example, the federal government used preemption to prohibit state governments from enacting their own cigarette warning labels. During the COVID-19 pandemic, some governors preempted local jurisdictions from issuing local mask mandates and disallowed shuttering of schools.

# THE LEGISLATIVE BRANCH ENACTS STATUTES

At the federal level, the *U.S. Congress leads the* **legislative branch**. Congress is divided into two bodies: the House of Representatives (435 elected members, divided among the 50 states in proportion to their population, and six nonvoting members representing the District of Columbia, Puerto Rico, and four U.S. territories) and the Senate (100 members, two from each of the 50 states). The names of state legislative bodies vary—in Pennsylvania, it is the General Assembly; in Massachusetts, it is the General Court; and in North Dakota, it is the Legislative Assembly.

The legislative branch enacts and rescinds *statutes*. The authority to enact statutes is found in the U.S. Constitution. There is no explicit authority for the federal government to enact healthcare laws; however, *implicit authority* is found in two constitutional provisions. Under the Commerce Clause, Congress can enact statutes that regulate commerce between states, foreign governments, and tribal nations (U.S. Const. art. 1, § 8, cl. 3). Congress has used this authority to enact drug labeling statutes (Federal Food, Drug, and Cosmetic Act, 1934) and statutes that regulate controlled substances (Controlled Substance Act, 1970). The Tax and Spend Clause allows the federal legislature to enact laws that penalize certain behaviors it considers to be harmful, such as "sin taxes" on tobacco and alcohol, and provide funds for initiatives that positively impact health, such as Medicare and Medicaid (U.S. Const. art. I, § 8, cl. 1). Powers not explicitly reserved to the federal government fall to the states (U.S. Const. amend. X). States have used this authority to enact laws impacting medical record requirements, prohibiting physicians from being corporate employees and mandating licensure requirements for healthcare facilities.

# THE EXECUTIVE BRANCH PROMULGATES REGULATIONS AND ISSUES EXECUTIVE ORDERS

The **executive branch** is led by the president at the federal level (U.S. Const. art. II) and by governors at the state level. Several federal executive branch agencies that regulate the healthcare industry are part of the Department of Health and Human Services (DHHS): the Centers for Medicare & Medicaid Services, which provides public health insurance to more than 100 million people; the Food and Drug Administration, which regulates drugs, biological products, and medical devices; and the Centers for Disease Control and Prevention, which issues requirements to protect health and safety.

Executive branch agencies promulgate *regulations*, which are rules that implement a statute. For example, the Patient Protection and Affordable Care Act allows a child to remain on their parent's health insurance until age 26 (The Patient Protection and Affordable Care Act, 2010). Congress instructed the DHHS to determine who was considered within the definition of "child." In regulation, DHHS includes married individuals, people with their own insurance, and those who turn down an offer of job-based insurance coverage as "children" who can remain on their parent's insurance coverage until the age of 26 (Code of Federal Regulations, 2015).

An *executive order*, issued by the president or governor, directs an executive branch agency to do something. It can be revoked by the president or governor at any time. Federal executive orders issued during the COVID-19 pandemic included ordering the Secretary of DHHS to identify risks associated with pharmaceutical supply chains (Exec. Order No. 14001, 2021) and mandating masks on commercial aircraft (Exec. Order No. 13998, 2021). States also issued pandemic-related executive orders such as those activating the National Guard (Idaho Exec. Order No. 2002-02, 2022), mandating masks in public places (Rhode Island Exec. Order No. 21-116, 2021), and closing ski slopes (Colorado Exec. Order No. D 2020-004, 2020).

## THE JUDICIAL BRANCH CREATES CASE LAW

The **judicial branch** interprets what laws mean. The Supreme Court is the United States' highest court (U.S. Const. art. III). Supreme Court Justices are appointed by the President, confirmed by the Senate, and are on the bench for life (or until they choose to retire). States each have their own judicial systems composed of trial, appellate, and supreme courts. *Case law* (or "common law") is based on judicial decisions rendered in previous lawsuits. In theory, courts can only deviate from previous court opinions issued within their jurisdictions if there is a compelling reason to do so. If the legislature does not agree with a judicial interpretation of a statute or regulation, it can rescind or modify the law, thereby negating the judiciary's decision.

## HEALTHCARE ETHICS

*"Every human being of adult years and sound mind has a right to determine what shall be done with his own body.* Schloendorff v. Society of New York Hospital (1914).

The World Health Organization defines *health ethics* as "the consideration of values in the prioritization and justification of actions by health professionals, researchers, and policymakers that may impact the health and well-being of patients, families, and communities" (World Health Organization, n.d.). Ethics helps healthcare managers make decisions based on values within legal parameters (Haddad & Geiger, 2024).

Healthcare organizations often have ethics committees to help address challenging questions. An ethics committee should do the following (American Medical Association, n.d.):

- Serve as advisors rather than decision-makers.
- Respect the rights and privacy of all participants.
- Be available for emergent and nonemergent situations.
- Have diverse representatives.
- Adopt policies that govern the committee.
- Draw upon the guidance of professional organizations.

There are four fundamental ethical pillars in healthcare: beneficence, nonmaleficence, autonomy, and justice (Beauchamp & Childress, 1989). The principle of **beneficence** is traced to Hippocrates and comes from the Latin term *beneficenti*a, meaning kindness or generosity. Beneficence is the obligation of healthcare managers to act for the benefit of their organization and its patients by preventing, removing, or mitigating harm.

**Nonmaleficence** is also attributable to Hippocrates. It is the principle that healthcare managers should "do no harm" and weigh the benefits of an action against its burdens. This includes balancing the costs and effectiveness of treatment options with the quality of care. For example, glucagon-like peptide-1 is a pharmaceutical intervention that is being explored to treat and prevent obesity. The debate within a health system around a medication authorization plan design can quickly shift to an ethical debate that balances the effectiveness of a medication with its corresponding cost.

**Autonomy** is the right of individuals to make their own decisions, but sometimes it can be diminished. For example, infants and children lack the legal capacity to act autonomously. People with mental impairments are sometimes considered incapable of making medical decisions for themselves. In Cruzan v. *Director* (1990), the Supreme Court addressed whether there was a constitutional right for a person to refuse medical treatment. Nancy Cruzan was involved in an automobile accident, which left her in a "persistent vegetative state." Her parents wanted to have her feeding tube removed, which would result in her death, but her physicians refused to comply. The Supreme Court held that, based in part on autonomy, patients have a fundamental right to refuse life-sustaining treatment; however, states can decide the circumstances under which such treatment may be withdrawn when a patient is unable to speak on their behalf.

The fourth ethical principle, justice, demands fair treatment and applies to patients and the work environment. *Distributive justice* requires the fair and equitable allocation of healthcare resources. Medicaid and Medicare, two governmental insurance programs, are based on distributive justice. During the COVID-19 pandemic, there was insufficient personal protection equipment to protect all healthcare professionals. The number of people requiring ICU beds, ventilators, and vaccines outpaced their availability. Healthcare managers were faced with the difficult ethical decision of deciding who was entitled to lifesaving equipment.

## CIVIL LAW

*"A lean compromise is better than a fat lawsuit." George Herbert, English poet and orator (1593–1633)*

**Civil laws** address private disputes between individuals, organizations, and business entities to make an injured party "whole" again. It starts when a *plaintiff* (the individual, organization, or business entity who claims they were wronged) files a lawsuit against a *defendant* (the individual, organization, or business entity the plaintiff claims committed the wrong). The plaintiff has the burden of proving their lawsuit by a *preponderance of the evidence*, meaning it is more likely than not that the defendant should be held accountable.

## TORTS

A *tort* is a civil action resulting in an injury to a person or property. A tort can result from committing a wrongful act, such as a nurse improperly inserting a catheter, or failing to act, such as not adhering to reporting requirements. A medical error is one of the most common bases for a tort action (Miziara & Miziara, 2022). High rates of medical errors occur in intensive care units, operating rooms, and emergency departments (Carver et al., 2023).

*Negligence* is the failure to use reasonable care that results in harm. To be successful in a claim for negligence, a plaintiff must prove by a *preponderance of evidence* (i.e., that it was more likely than not) that all four of the following occurred:

- *The wrongdoer owed a duty to the injured person.* A duty is a legal obligation to protect the rights of others.
- *The wrongdoer breached their duty.* This occurs when a person does not act with the same care that a reasonable person would exhibit in the same situation.
- *An injury occurred.* Injuries can include physical harm, emotional distress, or damages to a business or a person's reputation.
- *The breach of duty caused the injury.* There must be a clear connection between what a wrongdoer did or did not do and an injury.

An injured party can be awarded compensatory damages, including money for lost wages, medical bills, and pain and suffering.

An *intentional tort* occurs when a person knowingly causes harm, such as when a physician deliberately fails to obtain a patient's consent before surgery (Valles v. Albert Einstein Medical Center et al., 2000). In addition to the elements that must be proven in a negligence lawsuit, a plaintiff with an intentional tort claim must show by a preponderance of evidence that the defendant acted willfully to engage in a harmful action. If a healthcare provider acts with extreme recklessness or intentionally hurts someone, the injured person can be awarded *punitive damages* in addition to compensatory damages. Punitive damages punish the wrongdoer for their actions and are usually multiples of the compensatory award.

**Malpractice** is a type of negligence that occurs when a professional fails to act in accordance with acceptable standards, which directly causes injuries. In *Downs et al. v. Trias et al. (2009)*, Allison Downs had a family history of breast cancer. As a precaution, she had a bilateral mastectomy, and later, she was diagnosed with uterine fibroids. Her physician, Dr. Trias, told Ms. Downs that despite her family history, she did not have an increased risk of uterine cancer. Unfortunately, about 1 year later, Ms. Downs was diagnosed with late-stage, terminal ovarian cancer. The jury determined that Dr. Trias committed malpractice because he did not inform Ms. Downs of the heightened risk of ovarian cancer and awarded Ms. Downs $4 million in damages.

Under **vicarious liability**, a hospital can be legally responsible for the actions of its employees. For example, if the nurse is a hospital employee and accidentally gives their patient the wrong medication, both the nurse and the hospital could be liable for a negligence claim. However, if a nurse is an independent contractor of a hospital, vicarious liability would not apply.

## THE STARK LAW

Although related to the antitrust laws discussed in the following, the Stark Law is a civil law that prohibits physicians from referring Medicaid and Medicare patients to entities in which they or their immediate family members have a financial interest (unless an exception applies). There is no requirement that the plaintiff must prove that the physician intentionally or knowingly violated the law. Violators of the Stark Law can face fines and exclusion from federal programs (The Stark Law, 2010).

## TORT REFORM

Medical malpractice awards vary tremendously. In 2022, Wyoming had the lowest average medical malpractice award in the United States ($144,300), while Vermont had the highest ($2.18 million). Vermont had two medical malpractice awards, whereas Florida had 845 (U.S. Department of Health and Human Services, 2023). Costs associated with malpractice are frequently cited as contributing to consolidation—a shift of individual practitioners and hospitals into larger health systems. From 2012 to 2023, the percentage of physicians working in private practices fell from 60.1% to 46.7% (American Medical Association, 2023).

*Tort reform* is an attempt to reduce the volume and costs associated with civil claims. Alaska limits most claims against healthcare providers to $400,000 (Alaska Statutes, 2024). In Nebraska, an award cannot exceed $2.25 million (Nebraska Revised Statutes, 2023). Delaware limits fees attorneys can receive in medical malpractice cases (Del. Code Ann., tit. 18, § 6865). In other states like Wyoming, state constitutions prohibit caps on damage awards (WY. Const. art. 10, § 4[a]). In Washington, courts have held that malpractice caps are unconstitutional (Sofie v. Fibreboard Corp., 1989).

As providers increase their focus on value-based care, it is important to understand the implications of medical malpractice law on the practice of defensive medicine. Balancing the competing pressure of reducing overutilization while not exposing a provider to increased malpractice risk is a key focus for administrators and one that grows in importance as tort reform conversations continue.

## CONTRACTS

A contract is a written or oral agreement that creates obligations for two or more parties. To establish a contract, the following elements must be present:

- One of the parties must make an offer (a promise to do or refrain from doing something).
- The person who is offered a contract must accept its terms.
- Something of value, called *consideration*, must be given, like money or the performance of a service.

A *breach of contract* occurs when one of the parties violates one of the contract's terms.

Some healthcare *employment contracts* include a noncompete clause, prohibiting an individual from competing with their employer after they leave their job. A *patient transfer contract* is needed when a patient is moved from one healthcare practice to another. A *healthcare vendor contract* can cover both supplies and equipment and is used when a lease is preferable to a purchase. *Patient contracts* establish the terms of the healthcare provider-patient relationship, including the kind of care a healthcare provider will deliver, risks and benefits of medical procedures, payment for services, and insurance information.

## CRIMINAL LAW

*"If he who breaks the law is not punished, he who obeys it is cheated." Thomas Szasz (Hungarian–American academic and psychologist [1920–2012])*

**Criminal law** sanctions individuals, organizations, and business entities for violating rules that society has determined are necessary to protect the public. A civil and a criminal proceeding can occur at the same time. For example, a physician who leaves an instrument in a patient's body during surgery can be criminally prosecuted for battery (unlawful physical contact) and sued civilly for malpractice by the patient to compensate for pain and suffering, medical bills, and lost wages (and, possibly, an intentional tort). A criminal action is always brought by the government. The standard of proof is much higher than in civil cases and is usually *beyond a reasonable doubt*.

Antitrust laws regulate business practices to ensure competition, protect consumers from high prices and inferior products, and encourage innovative production methods. At the federal level, these laws are enforced by the Federal Trade Commission, and actions for violations are brought by the U.S. Department of Justice, the Federal Trade Commission, or private parties.

Antitrust laws prohibit the following (U.S. Department of Justice, n.d.)

- *Price fixing*: When two or more businesses agree to charge a certain price for their goods and services or agree to not sell something below a given price
- *Bid rigging*: Bidding in a way that ensures that a designated company will be awarded a contract
- *Market allocation*: Collusion between businesses to divide customers, such as by designated geographic areas

## THE FALSE CLAIMS ACT

In 2021, the U.S. Department of Justice recovered more than $5.6 billion in settlements and judgments for fraudulent claims against the federal government (U.S. Department of Justice, 2022). The False Claims Act protects the federal government from being overcharged or fraudulently invoiced for inferior goods or services (The False Claims Act, 1863).

Examples of actions that could give rise to a False Claims Act violation include a physician billing Medicaid for patient services they did not provide, a hospital billing Medicare for supplies it never received, or a psychologist failing to submit overcharges they received in Medicaid reimbursements. Violators can be charged with penalties up to three times the program's loss, penalties between $13,508 and $27,018 per violation, and prison sentences of up to 5 years (Federal Register, 2023).

An individual with knowledge of a violation, like a billing associate who witnesses the submission of false Medicaid reimbursement claims aid, can bring their own False Claims Act action. These witnesses are referred to as "whistleblowers" or "relators," and the action they bring is called a *qui tam action* (Latin for one that sues "for the king as well as for himself"). If the government decides that the relator's claim has merit, the U.S. Department of Justice will prosecute the case. If the prosecution is successful, the relator can be awarded attorney's fees and a percentage of the recovered funds. If the government decides not to pursue the relator's claim, the relator can pursue a lawsuit themselves.

## THE ANTI-KICKBACK STATUTE

In general, it is a crime to give or receive payment for patient referrals in federal healthcare programs (Anti-Kickback Statute, 1935). However, there are certain exceptions, known as "safe harbors," which include certain leasing arrangements of property and office equipment, employee compensation arrangements, and sales of physician practices (Code of Federal Regulations, 2023). Criminal sanctions for violations include fines, jail time, and exclusion from participation in federal healthcare programs. Civil penalties of up to $50,000 per kickback can also be imposed (Anti-Kickback Statute, 1935). As with False Claims Act violations, relators can report a kickback. Violations of both the Anti-Kickback Statute and the Stark Law can be used as bases for False Claims Act actions.

**CASE STUDY 23.1:** NAVIGATING HEALTHCARE LAW IN HEALTHCARE LEADERSHIP—HEALTHCARE LEADERSHIP'S ROLE IN UNDERSTANDING THE STARK LAW IN AN EVOLVING HEALTHCARE DELIVERY SETTING

In a large integrated delivery network (IDN) serving a blend of rural and urban markets with a proud history of being a leading academic medical center, the leadership team is committed to transitioning from value-based care to a capitation model. The engagement and partnership of clinicians are the key success factors, but developing commitment from private practices is a significant barrier, with fee-for-service contracts still driving the financial sustainability of many of these practices.

Jane Smith is a private practice administrator who is excited about the opportunity to expand her practice, her leadership skills, and her career horizons by actively partnering with the large IDN in her market. Jane is a highly skilled and long-tenured administrator who has led her practice successfully through many changes in healthcare. She prides herself on being well respected by the physician partners in the practice while motivating the group to provide high-quality care in an efficient and profitable manner.

Over the past decade, the last remaining independent local hospital and some of the other local private practice groups in town were acquired by a large IDN. Many of the physicians in the group are concerned about the practice's future and question rumors of lavish perks and rich administrative stipends for agreeing to send patients to a competing health system of the IDN. One of the IDN executives recently approached Jane about potentially being acquired by their system and shared their desire to focus on population health and move toward a capitated model.

Around this same time, one of the group's busiest physicians shared the article "Competition or Conflict of Interest—Stark Choices" (Miller et al., 2021) with her. (The article can be found here: https://jamanetwork.com/journals/jama-health-forum/fullarticle/2776935.) The article resonates with Jane because of the challenges of sustainable private practice medicine and the exploration of the potential benefits of self-referrals in a capitated model. It also raised questions about the consolidation of care delivery and how that juxtaposes against the application of the Stark Law.

## CASE STUDY DISCUSSION QUESTIONS

- How does the increasing pace of consolidation in healthcare impact the application and effectiveness of Stark Law?
- What are some of the challenges private practice leaders face in a healthcare environment increasingly focused on moving toward value-based care and, ultimately, capitation?
- What implications do those challenges have on Stark Law, and are there ways the law could be modernized to address them?
- In what ways can the recommendations presented in the article be applied to the challenges Jane is facing to help the practice navigate a path to future sustainability?
- What skills will leaders need to better navigate Stark Law in this changing healthcare environment?

## CASE STUDY CONCLUSION

Jane Smith's experience represents that of many private practice clinical and administrative leaders who aspire to continue to provide excellent care to their patient communities while finding their way to a sustainable future for their organization. By exploring the challenges highlighted in the article, healthcare leaders will have a better understanding of balancing compliance while determining a path forward to a sustainable healthcare model.

## CONCLUSION

Laws are dynamic, and new statutes, regulations, and executive orders are issued daily. Because the beliefs of groups and individuals shift over time, ethics transform, too. But what will not change is the importance of law and ethics in the practice of healthcare management. As technologies emerge and new pharmaceuticals are introduced, healthcare leaders will have to be aware of the role laws and ethics play in addressing new trends. The ongoing implementation of the Patient Protection and Affordable Care Act will also present new legal and ethical challenges for the healthcare community. An awareness of legal principles and ethical considerations can assist healthcare managers in making informed decisions, creating a positive workplace environment, improving healthcare delivery, and mitigating unnecessary costs.

# END-OF-CHAPTER RESOURCES

## CRITICAL THINKING QUESTIONS

- During a federally declared emergency, such as the COVID-19 pandemic, the Secretary of the Department of Health and Human Services can waive certain healthcare restrictions, including those under the Emergency Medical Treatment and Labor Act (EMTALA) and the Stark Law. How would waiving the restrictions in these two laws benefit patients during an emergency?
- Although ethics influences laws, not all laws are ethical. Can you think of some instances throughout history when a law has not been ethical (or has been unethical)?
- Under the VIII Amendment to the U.S. Constitution, the incarcerated population is the only population in the United States who is guaranteed healthcare. About 9% of incarcerated individuals have diabetes. Some correctional facilities require co-pays, but others do not. Is this fair to the rest of the population that does not have a constitutionally protected right to healthcare?
- In addition to the examples in this chapter, what are some other laws you can think of that have improved health outcomes?
- If you were a healthcare manager at a hospital and saw a coworker submit a Medicaid reimbursement claim for a fictional patient, what steps (legal and ethical) would you take to address this issue?

## LEARNING ACTIVITIES

### CourseConnect >

To access self-assessment questions and interactive, competency-based learning activities for this chapter, visit www.springerpub.com/courseconnect. See inside front cover and tear-out card for CourseConnect details.

## REFERENCES

Alaska Statutes, AS 09.55.549 (2024).
American College of Healthcare Executives. (2020, November 16). *Creating an ethical culture within the healthcare organization*. https://www.ache.org/about-ache/our-story/our-commitments/ethics/ache-code-of-ethics/creating-an-ethical-culture-within-the-healthcare-organization
American Medical Association. (2023, July 12). *AMA examines decade of change in physician practice ownership and organization*. https://www.ama-assn.org/press-center/press-releases/ama-examines-decade-change-physician-practice-ownership-and#:~:text=Between%202012%20and%202022%20the,9.6%25%20between%202012%20and%202022
American Medical Association. (n.d.). *AMA Code of Ethics: Opinion 10.7*. https://code-medical-ethics.ama-assn.org/ethics-opinions/ethics-committees-health-care-institutions#:~:text=Be%20structured%2C%20staffed%2C%20and%20supported,one%20or%20more%20community%20representatives
Anti-Kickback Statute, 42 USC. § 1320a-7b (1935).
Beauchamp, T. L., & Childress, J. F. (1989). *Principles of biomedical ethics*. Oxford University Press.
Carver, N., Gupta, V., & Hipskind, J. E. (2023). Medical errors. In StatPearls [Internet]. StatPearls Publishing.
Code of Federal Regulations, 42 C.F.R. § 1001.952 (2023). https://www.ecfr.gov/current/title-42/chapter-V/subchapter-B/part-1001/subpart-C/section-1001.952
Code of Federal Regulations, 45 C.F.R. § 147.120 (2015). https://www.ecfr.gov/current/title-45/subtitle-A/subchapter-B/part-147/section-147.120
Colorado Exec. Order No. D 2020-004 (2020).
Controlled Substance Act, 21 U.S.C. ch. 13 § 801 et seq. (1970).

Cruzan v. Director, Missouri Department of Health, 497 U.S. 261 (1990).
Del. Code Ann., tit. 18, § 6865.
Downs et al., v. Trias et al., Ct. Sup. 13654 (Conn. Super. Ct. 2009) (2009).
Emergency Medical Treatment and Labor Act, 42 U.S.C. § 1395dd (1986).
Exec. Order No. 13998, 86 C.F.R. 7201 (2021).
Exec. Order No. 14001, 86 C.F.R. 7219 (2021).
Federal Food, Drug, and Cosmetic Act, 21 U.S.C. §§ 301-392 (Suppl. 5 1934).
Federal Register, (2023, January 31). 88 Fed. Reg. 5776-01 https://www.govinfo.gov/app/details/FR-2023-01-30/2023-01704
Federal Trade Commission. *Guide to anti-trust laws*. https://www.ftc.gov/advice-guidance/competition-guidance/guide-antitrUSt-laws
Gallup. (2023, August 18). *US cigarette smoking rate steady near historic low*. https://news.gallup.com/poll/509720/cigarette-smoking-rate-steady-near-historical-low.aspx#:~:text=Cigarette%20smoking%20has%20become%20less,high%20of%2045%25%20was%20reached
Greene, J. C., Haun, J. N., French, D. D., Chambers, S. L., & Roswell, R. H. (2019). Reduced Hospitalizations, emergency room visits, and costs associated with a web-based health literacy, aligned-incentive intervention: Mixed methods study. *Journal of Medical Internet Research, 21*(10), e14772. https://doi.org/10.2196/14772
Haddad, L. M., & Geiger, R. A. (2024, January). Nursing ethical considerations. In *StatPearls* [Internet]. StatPearls Publishing. https://www.ncbi.nlm.nih.gov/books/NBK526054/
Hauser, C. (2020). From preaching to behavioral change: Fostering ethics and compliance learning in the workplace. *Journal of Business Ethics, 162*, 835–855. https://doi.org/10.1007/s10551-019-04364-9
Idaho Exec. Order No. 2002-02 (2022).
Miller, B. J., Ehrenfeld, J. M., & Wu, A.W. (2021). Competition or conflict of interest—Stark choices. *JAMA Health Forum, 2*(2), e210150. https://doi.org/10.1001/jamahealthforum.2021.0150
Miziara, I. D., & Miziara, C. S. M. G. (2022). Medical errors, medical negligence and defensive medicine: A narrative review. *Clinics (Sao Paulo, Brazil), 77*, 100053. https://doi.org/10.1016/j.clinsp.2022.100053
Nebraska Revised Statutes, § 44-2825 (2023).
Rhode Island Exec. Order No. 21-116 (2021).
Ribbon Health. (2022). https://go.ribbonhealth.com/research-report-health-plans-can-use-data-to-unlock-better-care
Schoenorff v. Society of New York Hospital, 211 N.Y. 125 (N.Y. 1914).
Sofie v. Fibreboard Corp., 112 Wn.2d 636 (1989).
The False Claims Act, U.S.C. §§ 3729-3933 (1863).
The Patient Protection and Affordable Care Act, 42 USC. § 18001 et seq. (2010).
The Stark Law, 42 U.S.C. § 1395nn (2010).
42 U.S.C. § 299 *et seq*. (1999).
U.S. Const. amend. X.
U.S. Const. art. I, § 8, cl. 1.
U.S. Const. art. I, § 8, cl. 3.
U.S. Const. art. II.
U.S. Const. art. III.
U.S. Const. art. VI, para. 2.
U.S. Department of Health and Human Services. (2023). *National practitioner Data Bank*. https://www.npdb.hrsa.gov/
U.S. Department of Justice. (2022, February 1). *Justice news*. https://www.jUStice.gov/opa/pr/jUStice-department-s-false-claims-act-settlements-and-judgments-exceed-56-billion-fiscal-year
U.S. Department of Justice. (n.d.). *Preventing and detecting bid rigging, price fixing, and market allocation in post-disaster relief projects*. https://www.jUStice.gov/atr/preventing-and-detecting-bid-rigging-price-fixing-and-market-allocation-post-disaster-rebuilding
Valles v. Albert Einstein Medical Center et al., 758 A.2d 1238 (Pa. Super. 2000).
World Health Organization. (n.d.). *Ethics*. https://www.who.int/westernpacific/health-topics/ethics-and-health
WY. Const. art. 10, § 4(a).

# CHAPTER 24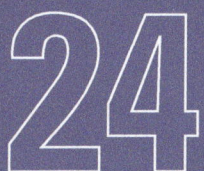

# CRISIS MANAGEMENT IN HEALTHCARE

Aram Dobalian and Pete Brewster

## LEARNING OBJECTIVES

- Identify factors associated with effective crisis management.
- Describe how crises differ and the four phases of emergency management.
- Explain how approaches such as after-action reviews (AARs) and root cause analysis help to identify strategic failures during crises.
- Discuss factors to consider in developing an effective crisis communication plan.
- Identify challenges associated with the COVID-19 pandemic and their implications for future crisis responses.

## KEY TERMS

- After-action reviews
- Crisis communications
- Crisis leadership
- Crisis management
- Disaster
- Emergency
- Pandemic
- Preparedness

## INTRODUCTION

Crises take many forms and may result from natural or human-caused events such as industrial accidents, terrorism, adverse events that cause patient harm or death, or political events. They encompass occurrences as diverse as hostile takeovers, financial catastrophes such as the loss of grants, or employee sabotage or violence. Crises may be classified into natural **disasters**, technological crises, confrontations by social action groups (e.g., boycotts) or malevolence (e.g., cybercrime, product tampering), and management failures like mismanagement and misconduct (Lerbinger 2012). They may occur anytime and to any organization; not all will be predictable. They commonly involve a high degree of instability and uncertainty, have the potential for extremely negative results, and may bring about dramatic change.

Numerous definitions of crises exist. James and Wooten (2005) provide a helpful definition that encompasses many of these components; they define *organizational crisis* as "Any emotionally charged situation that, once it becomes public, invites negative stakeholder reaction and thereby has the potential to threaten the financial wellbeing, reputation, or survival of the firm or some portion thereof" (James & Wooten, 2005).

Effectively managing crises is essential for healthcare leaders. As natural disasters increase in both frequency and intensity and as the COVID-19 **pandemic** demonstrated, urgent threats confront healthcare organizations on a regular basis. Managing the impact of a catastrophic weather occurrence or a mass casualty event is a complicated task, but there are actions that can be taken to be better prepared for the significant impacts that such events create.

The basic assumption of crisis management is that normal, day-to-day operations are not suited to managing a crisis. Instead, the organization's resources must focus on the crisis. Among the tasks that make **crisis leadership** challenging during a severe crisis is that impacted individuals may process and act on information differently than during noncrisis situations (Quarantelli, 1989). Moreover, both impacted individuals and the public may be more vigilant observers of both your words and body language.

Maintaining continuity of access to and the delivery of healthcare services requires a certain minimal level of preparedness. This requires considering the impact of staffing, funding, leadership, committees, plans, training, and exercises, among other factors. These activities require financial and staffing resources. Studies on the return on investments in healthcare system preparedness should be recognized, as they have shown clear benefits (Stryckman et al., 2015).

## AREAS AND TYPES OF CRISIS MANAGEMENTS

**Crisis management** may be defined as the method an organization uses to address disruptive incidents that may cause harm to the entity. During a crisis, organizational leadership must focus on taking appropriate actions to resolve the crisis. This requires teamwork, communication with all stakeholders affected by the crisis, helping staff and others cope with the crisis, assuring that unaffected operations continue to function, working through the crisis until operations return to normal, and finally rebuilding the organization and its people.

Leadership and governance play a critical role in the healthcare crisis management field (Morris et al., 2016; Ricci et al., 2015) as managers seek to blend the contributions from related disciplines at work within the organization (Box 24.1) to realize a comprehensive approach to crisis management, the ultimate goals of which are increased readiness and resilience (Son et al., 2020). In turn, these are the products of effective preparedness and mitigation activities.

Many healthcare administrators rely on compliance with accreditation (e.g., The Joint Commission, Commission on the Accreditation of Rehabilitation Facilities), regulatory (e.g., Centers for Medicare & Medicaid Services [CMS]), and grant (e.g., Administration for Strategic Preparedness and Response's [ASPR] Hospital Preparedness Program) requirements to ensure the capability exists to manage crises that may impact the organization. For example, the CMS Emergency Preparedness Rule (CMS 2016) requires 17 provider and supplier types that wish to participate in the Medicare or Medicaid

> **BOX 24.1: INTERDISCIPLINARY APPROACH TO A COMPREHENSIVE HEALTHCARE SYSTEM CRISIS MANAGEMENT CAPABILITY**
>
> - CEM
> - Information system contingency planning
> - ICA and ERM
> - COOP/business continuity
> - ICS
> - Crisis management

program to comply with specified emergency preparedness regulations. The Rule requires four core elements: risk assessment and emergency planning, a communication plan, policies and procedures, and training and testing that is maintained and updated at least annually.

> **CASE STUDY 24.1: HURRICANE SANDY AND VETERANS AFFAIRS NEW YORK HARBOR HEALTHCARE SYSTEM MANHATTAN CAMPUS**
>
> On October 29, 2012, Hurricane Sandy made landfall in New York. Two days earlier, the Director of the U.S. Department of Veterans Affairs (VA) New York Harbor Healthcare System, Martina Parauda, decided to evacuate the Manhattan VA Medical Center (VAMC) campus. New York University Langone Medical Center and Bellevue Hospital, both located near the Manhattan VAMC, decided not to evacuate before the storm. Director Parauda indicated that her prior experience with storm-related flooding at the facility with a nor'easter in 1992 with similar weather conditions, including a full moon and high tide, led to her decision (Ricci et al., 2015).
>
> Prior to Hurricane Katrina, few hospitals had evacuation plans in place, and evacuation in advance of a major storm was rarely a consideration (Ricci et al., 2015). The decision to evacuate a hospital or shelter in place is challenging because of the health risks and complex logistics required to evacuate medically frail inpatients as well as the uncertainty inherent in a storm's path.
>
> About 14 months prior to Hurricane Sandy, another storm, Hurricane Irene, struck New York City in August 2011. The Manhattan VAMC also evacuated during Hurricane Irene, as did other hospitals in the storm's path, following a mandatory evacuation order from the Mayor of New York for hospitals in the path of the storm. As a federal facility, the Manhattan VAMC campus was exempt from the city's evacuation mandate. Nonetheless, the Mayor's order was viewed as the most influential factor in the Manhattan VAMC's decision to evacuate, despite senior executives at the facility expressing a belief that the facility could withstand Irene's impact (Ricci et al., 2015). Ultimately, Irene's impact on New York City was much less severe than expected and the Manhattan VAMC was able to fully reopen within a few days.
>
> Flooding from Hurricane Sandy led to the failure of the Manhattan VAMC's major utility systems, including electrical, elevator, fire protection, heating, information technology, and water systems. The flooding destroyed more than 150,000 square feet of ambulatory care and related support areas, as well as clinical supplies and equipment, including the MRI unit. Some ambulatory services resumed at the Manhattan VAMC about 5 months after the storm, while full inpatient services restarted after about 7 months.
>
> The storm displaced many vulnerable Veteran patients, and older adults, disabled, home care dependents, or those with severe mental illness were placed at particular risk as a consequence

(Griffin et al., 2019). To find their displaced patients, the facility called on other federal and community partners to help find and care for their patients. For example, Manhattan VAMC end-stage renal disease patients used nearby VA sites and non-VA clinics for their care during the closure of the Manhattan VAMC dialysis unit (Lukowsky et al., 2019). VA home care, social work, and mental health staff traveled to sites in the community.

To help meet the healthcare needs of former Manhattan VAMC patients in the months after the storm and while the Manhattan VAMC campus was being restored, many staff operated out of the Brooklyn VAMC campus, and some worked out of the Bronx VAMC (Morris et al., 2016). Integrating the staff of the two facilities created a "clash" of organizational cultures. Staff feared the loss of their jobs and worried about whether the Manhattan VAMC campus would permanently close. Moreover, the commute to the Brooklyn VAMC campus was a long one for many staff, and it complicated childcare issues for many employees. In addition, many staff were also victims of the storm itself. One staff member stated "There was [one staff member] who couldn't find her parents for a long time, but she was here. There's another story about a nursing assistant saying, 'all the clothes I own, I'm wearing,' but she was here." To help staff cope with these challenges, senior facility leaders sought to recognize the basic needs of staff and accommodate their needs and requests as equitably as possible. Vans were made available to transport staff between facilities. In particular, frequent, open forums were held to answer questions and share recovery progress.

Enterprise risk management (ERM; Martin, 2020), including internal controls assessment (ICA) or evaluation, is a major component of an effective governance approach. ERM provides a framework that addresses identifying threats, assessing their impact in both likelihood and magnitude, and managing those risks, allowing organizations to concentrate efforts toward key points of potential failure. ERM clarifies the broad array of risks confronting complex organizations to ensure that they are appropriately managed. ICA, in turn, delineates a process for directing, monitoring, and measuring an organization's resources to assure its operational effectiveness, efficiency, and compliance with laws. It includes the reliability of financial reporting through mechanisms such as audits and timely feedback on achieving goals.

Comprehensive emergency management (CEM) was conceptualized by the National Governors Association in 1979 (National Governors Association [U.S.]. Center for Policy Research, 1979) and was embraced as the primary policy framework by the Federal Emergency Management Agency upon its creation in 1980. CEM addresses all hazards through activities across four phases—mitigation, preparedness, response, and recovery—that occur in a cycle. For example, areas for improvement identified in response and recovery to an **emergency** are addressed in future mitigation and preparedness activities.

The first phase, mitigation, should begin before the crisis occurs and include activities that prevent a crisis, reduce its likelihood, or reduce the impact of unavoidable or accidental hazards. For example, building safety codes help mitigate the likelihood of a fire occurring, but should one occur by accident, the financial impact of the fire can be mitigated by purchasing fire insurance beforehand.

Next, **preparedness** includes the development of crisis plans that describe what to do when an event occurs. For example, training and exercises help organizations improve their preparedness, and individuals may create disaster preparedness kits for their households. Business continuity planning is part of this phase. It includes setting up a plan to ensure the organization's own survival.

The response phase concerns activities that take place during the crisis, such as sheltering in place because of a tornado or active shooter. Finally, after the immediate threat has receded, the recovery phase begins. During this phase, individuals and organizations should consider how to protect their health or continued viability. In addition, it is important to start to consider efforts to mitigate the effects of future crises.

A key component of the CEM process is the hazard vulnerability analysis (HVA; Kappy et al., 2022). The HVA is used to identify hazards that are likely to impact the organization's operations and prioritize them through a scoring process. Consequently, in most organizations, standard operating procedures or preplans are developed to address mitigation, preparedness, response, and recovery from these hazards. One "all-hazards" approach to analyzing what those impacts would be is to use mission critical systems (Table 24.1).

Contingency planning could be considered the initial step in being prepared for a crisis. It includes simulated scenarios that are developed to prepare for any eventuality. These scenarios are used as drills whereby crisis management teams rehearse a crisis plan. The National Institute of Standards and Technology provides a contingency planning guide for information technology systems (Swanson et al., 2010). It includes "information system contingency planning," or plans and procedures to enable the recovery of information systems, operations, and data, including contingencies for using alternate processes to restore operations.

Continuity of Operations (COOP) and business continuity both focus on the identification of an organization's critical business functions; the impacts on these functions from likely hazards; and strategies for reducing those impacts, maintaining the organization's viability, and timely restoring its functions. Each critical function should have its own contingency plan and be tested through drills and exercises.

One component of COOP/business continuity planning is the business process analysis or BPA. The BPA is used to analyze each critical business function to determine outputs and inputs, dependencies, and to identify leadership and required staff, communications and information systems, alternate location requirements, and resources and funding. Of note are the dependencies, as they may involve external entities, including parts of the supply chain that allow the organization to perform its essential functions.

The incident command system (ICS; U.S. Department of Homeland Security, 2011) is a standardized approach to the command, control, and coordination of on-scene incident management that provides a common hierarchy within which personnel from multiple organizations can be effective during an emergency response. ICS was initially developed to address interagency response problems fighting wildfires in California and Arizona. Now, ICS is used by both public and private organizations. It includes an action planning process whereby incidents are managed by addressing specific prioritized objectives to resolve issues created by the impact of hazards.

ICS typically includes a single incident commander who oversees the response and is the final decision-maker. It includes a command staff consisting of a safety officer tasked with assuring the safety of all assigned personnel, a public information officer who serves

**TABLE 24.1. HEALTHCARE FACILITY MISSION CRITICAL SYSTEMS**

| LIGHTING | COMMUNICATIONS |
| --- | --- |
| Electrical power | Computer applications (see additional information) |
| Steam distribution | Alarms |
| Heating, ventilation, and air conditioning | Vertical transportation (elevators) |
| Water delivery | Central medical gases |
| Water conditioning | Staff |
| Waste system | Critical supplies and supply chain |

as the information conduit to and from internal and external stakeholders such as the media, and a liaison officer who serves as the primary contact for agencies assisting during an incident. ICS also incorporates a general staff consisting of an operations section chief who directs actions to meet the incident objectives, a planning section chief tasked with collecting information about the incident, a finance/administration section chief, and a logistics section chief who is responsible for providing required resources and services. The hospital ICS is a modified ICS structure specifically designed for hospitals that might, for example, include a medical or technical specialist.

## ANALYZE STRATEGIC FAILURES LEADING TO A CRISIS

Various approaches exist to analyze failures that lead to crises. It is essential to recognize that opportunities to learn from crises are not specific to any individual organization. Reviewing reports from "proxy" events that impacted other entities may shed light on the causative factors that led to strategic failures and crises and provide lessons to make other unimpacted organizations more resilient.

**After-action reviews** (AAR) and reports (Davies et al., 2019), originally developed by the U.S. Army, document the feedback received from participants involved with an incident or exercise. The AAR process is focused on collecting information about what went well and what areas may be improved. It helps the emergency manager program determine the program improvements needed in a changing organizational environment.

Root cause analysis (Wilson et al., 1993) is similar to the AAR process. However, it may be used to further investigate the underlying reasons for recurring issues. Root cause analysis involves identifying and describing the problem, establishing a timeline from the normal situation until the problem occurs, distinguishing between the root cause and other causal factors, and creating a causal graph between the root cause and the problem. High-reliability organizations are entities that avoid catastrophes in situations where accidents are expected to occur because of inherent complexity (Tolk et al., 2015). It asserts that catastrophic failures result from the combination of organizational cultures and system failures and was derived from studies of disasters such as the Three Mile Island nuclear incident and studies of the air traffic control system. High-reliability organizations incorporate five principles: sensitivity to operations and a focus on situational awareness; preoccupation with failure, leading to prompt error reporting; a reluctance to simplify understanding of the work environment; a commitment to resilience that recognizes that errors will occur; and deference to expertise rather than hierarchy where crisis decisions are made (Weick & Sutcliffe, 2015).

The concept of a learning organization is relevant to crisis management (Laitinen & Ihalainen, 2022). A learning organization may be conceptualized as a company that facilitates the learning of its members and continuously transforms itself (Akhnif et al., 2017; Anderson et al., 2022). Crises often lead to organizational change as such events challenge how people think and learn. Learning organizations require personal mastery (i.e., the capacity to accomplish personal goals; shared vision, which requires trust and collaboration; mental models) which challenge assumptions; team learning in order to work collaboratively; and systems thinking, which recognizes how components form an interrelated system.

## AN ORGANIZATION'S PUBLIC COMMUNICATIONS REGARDING A CRISIS

Crises can lead to fear and confusion. Consequently, individuals may turn to unreliable or incomplete sources of information. Clear, factual, and timely communication is needed during crises to counter these sources (Reynolds & Seeger, 2005).

Communication during a crisis involves alerts, warnings, and messages related to the organization's response and guidance to its constituents. Crisis communications plans should address the needs of patients, survivors and their families, employees and their families, news media, the broader community, management, directors and investors, elected officials, regulators, and suppliers (Benoit, 2015).

**Crisis communications** may be divided into five phases: precrisis, initial, maintenance, resolution, and evaluation (Centers for Disease Control and Prevention, 2014). The precrisis phase includes planning to establish relationships with other organizations, develop recommendations, and test messaging. The initial phase of a crisis is typically marked by confusion and media interest. Accordingly, it is vital to learn the facts about what occurred and determine your organization's response as rapidly as possible. It is also important to provide accurate, consistent messaging in the initial phases of an emergency. During the maintenance phase, the public should be helped to understand its own risks. To limit public concern, it is helpful to be able to answer questions regarding how the crisis happened, whether it has happened before, how it can be prevented from recurring, and whether there will be long-term public impacts. During the resolution phase, communications should focus on educating the public about future crises and obtaining support for policy changes. Finally, the evaluation phase examines lessons learned.

Various crisis communication strategies have been proposed (Glik, 2007; Su et al., 2022). It is generally accepted that messages should be delivered by an identified spokesperson, highlight information for which there is a need to know, and avoid technical jargon. In addition, the widespread use of social media necessitates that crisis management officials use and monitor social media platforms to understand needs and counter misinformation (Himelein-Wachowiak et al., 2021). Finally, messages should be adapted to different audiences and incorporate the diverse languages represented in their communities (Anakwe et al., 2022).

# METHODS TO ANALYZE THE STRENGTHS AND WEAKNESSES OF A CRISIS RESPONSE AND MITIGATE FUTURE CRISIS

A focus on preparedness helps reduce the time, financial costs, and other negative impacts associated with crises. Nevertheless, planning for crises requires both time and resources, as well as ongoing efforts to help ensure that individuals properly execute the plans.

Belardo and Harrald (1992) argued, "ineffective precrisis planning was, according to most observers, a primary factor contributing to the failure of these response efforts." They proposed using decision analysis methods and decision support tools to develop a scenario-driven planning process to improve the contingency planning process.

Common weaknesses of crisis plans include failing to determine certain potential hazards or inadequately designed responses to address them. Establishing an appropriate plan specific to that organization is also essential. For example, a response plan for a rural hospital should differ from that of an urban, academic medical center or a skilled nursing facility. Having clear procedures regarding specific duties in a crisis helps to avoid indecision and confusion. Accordingly, drills and exercises are important to ensure that employees understand their responsibilities during a crisis. Finally, organizations do not operate in isolation. As such, an effective emergency plan requires communication with outside entities.

Various strategies exist to gather feedback and understand the strengths and weaknesses of a crisis response. For example, a commonly used model for AARs is the Homeland Security Exercise and Evaluation Program, which proposes principles for exercise programs and an approach to evaluation and improvement planning (U.S. Department of Homeland Security, 2020). Another approach is the use of process evaluations that examine whether program activities have been implemented as intended during the crisis response.

Metrics have been developed to measure healthcare preparedness. For example, ASPR developed the Healthcare Preparedness and Response Capabilities to describe objectives for the healthcare delivery system to prepare for, respond to, and recover from emergencies. Furthermore, the U.S. VA has developed comprehensive measures of hospital readiness (Der-Martirosian et al., 2017). These measures provide a consistent but flexible approach for ascertaining health system preparedness and clarify areas for needed improvement (Dobalian et al., 2016). This all-hazards-based tool has also been adapted for use outside the VA.

## COVID-19 AND IMPLICATIONS FOR HEALTHCARE SYSTEMS

The COVID-19 pandemic led to numerous changes in how healthcare systems operate. It has impacted staffing (Sirkin et al., 2023), led to increased practitioner burnout (Alanazy and Alruwaili, 2023), and highlighted supply chain concerns, particularly with respect to personal protective equipment (PPE).

### WIDESPREAD USE OF POLICIES FOR SCARCE RESOURCE ALLOCATION

Standards of care may be considered to fall within three groups, with the most common being conventional care (Institute of Medicine, 2012; National Academies of Sciences, Engineering, and Medicine, 2020). In contrast, when the demand for medical professionals, equipment, or pharmaceuticals begins to exceed the available supply, contingency care recognizes that usual care practices should be modified. Organizations may determine that crisis standards of care should apply during large-scale crises when resources are scarcer or unavailable. Crisis standards of care permit healthcare practitioners to triage patients and direct scarce resources toward patients they believe are most in need. This occurred during the COVID-19 pandemic in Arizona, Idaho, New Hampshire, and New Mexico (Hodge & Piatt, 2022; Romney et al., 2020).

### USE OF TECHNOLOGY TO SHIFT WORK AND PROVIDE VIRTUAL CARE

Telehealth was employed during crises before the COVID-19 pandemic, but such events did not lead to long-term changes in delivery modalities (Der-Martirosian et al., 2019; Der-Martirosian et al., 2020; Der-Martirosian et al., 2022). In contrast, COVID-19 led to an unprecedented explosion of telehealth that seems likely to persist (Der-Martirosian et al., 2021, Der-Martirosian et al., 2022; Sirkin et al., 2023).

### LEARNING HOW TO BEST MANAGE PERSONAL PROTECTIVE EQUIPMENT

During the early stages of the pandemic, it was recognized that understanding available PPE was insufficient to address supply needs (Best & Williams, 2021). More important was understanding the rate at which that PPE was being utilized (Raja et al., 2020). In addition, counterfeit PPE became a significant concern. Even among healthcare personnel, there was confusion regarding the difference between a face mask, a respirator, and later face shields and how to put them appropriately. Moreover, shifting guidance from the U.S. Centers for Disease Control and Prevention and the World Health Organization regarding when each was appropriate and in what setting proved challenging (Bajaj & Stanford, 2021; Larkin, 2021).

## CONCLUSION

When confronted with a large-scale emergency, there are a few key considerations. First, by their very nature, no agency will be able to address such events. Second, crisis management requires flexibility and improvisation. Third, the numerous organizations that respond to disasters work together infrequently, and after often unaware of conflicting capabilities, limitations, and under some circumstances, do not even know that each other exists. Thus, participating in local emergency management groups and healthcare coalitions before the event occurs is beneficial. Fourth, standard management approaches often are not applicable or may even be detrimental during a response. Finally, evaluating the effectiveness of a response requires a focus on the system, not merely the organization or individual.

Crises may derive from many causes, whether from increasingly common natural disasters, human-caused events, or political factors. As such, effectively managing crises is essential for healthcare leaders and any organization's long-term survival. Moreover, maintaining continuity of access to and the ability to deliver healthcare services requires at least a certain minimal level of preparedness if we are to ensure the health of the populations that each healthcare organization serves.

# END-OF-CHAPTER RESOURCES

## CRITICAL THINKING QUESTIONS

- Hospitals serve a critical role in local disaster response. During a financially challenging time for hospitals, should they be required to entail the financial challenges associated with being fully prepared for disasters?
- What actions can organizations take to ensure effective communication and engagement of diverse patient populations during an emergency?
- Disasters provide an opportunity for enhancing or damaging the reputation of an organization. Provide two recent examples of natural, human-caused, or other crises where the organization's reputation was impacted.
- What are the appropriate roles and responsibilities for health system administrators in preparing for and responding to pandemics of novel viruses such as COVID-19?
- During a disaster response, it is generally rare to refer to detailed preparedness plans. Why do you think this is the case? Given this, why spend time planning for such crises?
- The ability of the organization to remain operational during emergencies is the focus of COOP planning, physical security, and engineering design and construction. What are some low-cost examples of nonstructural mitigation approaches hospitals could employ to improve their resiliency?
- One method for effective risk mitigation is the use of ERM and internal controls analysis. Reflecting on the various components of a hospital or health system, how could such an organization employ this method to identify and manage risk?
- The ICS uses a standard organizational structure and management-by-objectives approach to address impacts caused by emergencies on the organization's functioning. How could a hospital balance the ICS structure with its everyday organizational structure?
- Based on the case study, what factors would you consider in deciding whether to evacuate a hospital before a storm? What would you need to know and when?
- As illustrated by the case study, disaster response requires a focus on the longer term as well as the shorter term effects of such crises on patients and staff. Failure to do so can impact the financial health and viability of an organization. How would you help staff cope with the effects of crises?

## LEARNING ACTIVITIES

**CourseConnect >**

To access self-assessment questions and interactive, competency-based learning activities for this chapter, visit www.springerpub.com/courseconnect. See inside front cover and tear-out card for CourseConnect details.

## REFERENCES

Akhnif, E., Macq, J., Idrissi Fakhreddine, M. O., & Meessen, B. (2017). Scoping literature review on the Learning Organisation concept as applied to the health system. *Health Research Policy and Systems*, 15(1), 16. https://doi.org/10.1186/s12961-017-0176-x

Alanazy, A. R. M., & Alruwaili, A. (2023). The global prevalence and associated factors of burnout among emergency department healthcare workers and the impact of the COVID-19 pandemic:

A systematic review and meta-analysis. *Healthcare (Basel, Switzerland), 11*(15), 2220. https://doi.org/10.3390/healthcare11152220

Anakwe, A., Majee, W., Ponder, M., & BeLue, R. (2022). COVID-19 and crisis communication among African American households. *Families Systems & Health, 40*(3), 408–412. https://doi.org/10.1037/fsh0000705

Anderson, J. L., Mugavero, M. J., Ivankova, N. V., Reamey, R. A., Varley, A. L., Samuel, S. E., & Cherrington, A. L. (2022). Adapting an interdisciplinary learning health system framework for academic health centers: A scoping review. *Academic Medicine, 97*(10), 1564–1572. https://doi.org/10.1097/acm.0000000000004712

Bajaj, S. S., & Stanford, F. C. (2021). The new CDC mask guidance: A catastrophe for health equity. *Journal of General Internal Medicine, 36*(10), 3217–3218. https://doi.org/10.1007/s11606-021-07026-7

Belardo, S., & Harrald, J. (1992). A framework for the application of group decision support systems to the problem of planning for catastrophic events. *IEEE Transactions on Engineering Management, 39*(4), 400–411. https://doi.org/10.1109/17.165425

Benoit, W. L. (2015). *Accounts, excuses, and apologies: Image repair theory and research.* SUNY Press.

Best, S., & Williams, S. J. (2021). What have we learnt about the sourcing of personal protective equipment during pandemics? Leadership and management in healthcare supply chain management: A scoping review. *Frontiers in Public Health, 9,* 765501. https://doi.org/10.3389/fpubh.2021.765501

Centers for Disease Control and Prevention. (2014). *Crisis and emergency risk communication.* Department of Health and Human Services.

Centers for Medicare &Medicaid Services. (2016). Medicare and Medicaid Programs; emergency preparedness requirements for Medicare and Medicaid participating providers and suppliers. Final rule. *Federal Register, 81*(180), 63859–64044. https://www.federalregister.gov/documents/2016/09/16/2016-21404/medicare-and-medicaid-programs-emergency-preparedness-requirements-for-medicare-and-medicaid

Davies, R., Vaughan, E., Fraser, G., Cook, R., Ciotti, M., & Suk, J. E. (2019). Enhancing reporting of after action reviews of public health emergencies to strengthen preparedness: A literature review and methodology appraisal. *Disaster Medicine and Public Health Preparedness, 13*(3), 618–625. https://doi.org/10.1017/dmp.2018.82

Der-Martirosian, C., Chu, K., & Dobalian, A. (2020). Use of telehealth to improve access to care at the United States Department of Veterans Affairs during the 2017 Atlantic Hurricane season. *Disaster Medicine and Public Health Preparedness, 17,* e6. https://doi.org/10.1017/dmp.2020.88

Der-Martirosian, C., Chu, K., Steers, W. N., Wyte-Lake, T., Balut, M. D., Dobalian, A., Heyworth, L., Paige, N. M., & Leung, L. (2022). Examining telehealth use among primary care patients, providers, and clinics during the COVID-19 pandemic. *BMC Primary Care, 23*(1), 155. https://doi.org/10.1186/s12875-022-01738-3

Der-Martirosian, C., Griffin, A. R., Chu, K., & Dobalian, A. (2019). Telehealth at the US Department of Veterans Affairs after Hurricane Sandy. *Journal of Telemedicine and Telecare, 25*(5), 310–317. https://doi.org/10.1177/1357633X17751005

Der-Martirosian, C., Heyworth, L., Chu, K., Mudoh, Y., & Dobalian, A. (2020). Patient characteristics of VA telehealth users during Hurricane Harvey. *Journal of Primary Care & Community Health, 11,* 2150132720931715. https://doi.org/10.1177/2150132720931715

Der-Martirosian, C., Radcliff, T. A., Gable, A. R., Riopelle, D., Hagigi, F. A., Brewster, P., & Dobalian, A. (2017). Assessing hospital disaster readiness over time at the US Department of Veterans Affairs. *Prehospital and Disaster Medicine, 32*(1), 46–57. https://doi.org/10.1017/S1049023X16001266

Der-Martirosian, C., Wyte-Lake, T., Balut, M., Chu, K., Heyworth, L., Leung, L. Ziaeian, B., Tubbesing, S., Mullur, R., & Dobalian, A. (2021). Implementation of telehealth services at the US Department of Veterans Affairs during the COVID-19 pandemic: Mixed methods study. *JMIR Formative Research, 5*(9), e29429. https://doi.org/10.2196/29429

Dobalian, A., Stein, J. A., Radcliff, T. A., Riopelle, D., Brewster, P., Hagigi, F., & Der-Martirosian, C. (2016). Developing valid measures of emergency management capabilities within US Department of Veterans Affairs Hospitals. *Prehospital and Disaster Medicine, 31*(5), 475–484. https://doi.org/10.1017/S1049023X16000625

Glik, D. C. (2007). Risk communication for public health emergencies. *Annual Review of Public Health, 28*, 33–54. https://doi.org/10.1146/annurev.publhealth.28.021406.144123

Griffin, A. R., Gable, A. R., Der-Martirosian, C., & Dobalian, A. (2019). Hospitals providing temporary emergency department services in alternative care settings after Hurricane Sandy. *Critical Care Nursing Clinics of North America, 31*(2), 249–256. https://doi.org/10.1016/j.cnc.2019.02.011

Himelein-Wachowiak, M., Giorgi, S., Devoto, A., Rahman, M., Ungar, L., Schwartz, H. A., Epstein, D. H., Leggio, L., & Curtis, B. (2021). Bots and misinformation spread on social media: implications for COVID-19. *Journal of Medical Internet Research, 23*(5), e26933. https://doi.org/10.2196/26933

Hodge, J. G., Jr., & Piatt, J. L. (2022). Legal decision-making and crisis standards of care: Tiebreaking during the COVID-19 pandemic and in other public health emergencies." *JAMA Health Forum, 3*(1), e214799. https://doi.org/10.1001/jamahealthforum.2021.4799

Institute of Medicine. (2012). *Crisis standards of care: A systems framework for catastrophic disaster response. Introduction and CSC framework.* (Vol. 1). The National Academies Press.

James, E. H., & Wooten, L. P. (2005). Leadership as (Un)usual: How to display competence in times of crisis. *Organizational Dynamics, 34*(2), 141–152. http://doi.org/10.1016/j.orgdyn.2005.03.005

Kappy, B., Parish, A., Barda, A., Frost, P., & Timm, N. (2022). Pediatric-specific hazard vulnerability analysis: The missing component of regional and hospital-based preparedness. *Disaster Medicine and Public Health Preparedness, 17*, e199. https://doi.org/10.1017/dmp.2022.90

Laitinen, I., & Ihalainen, J. (2022). Organisational learning during the coronavirus pandemic: A case study on models for extended learning and complexity management. *Journal of Adult and Continuing Education, 28*(2), 378–396. https://doi.org/10.1177/14779714221079367

Larkin, M. (2021). Mask confusion in NYC with abrupt CDC guidance changes. *Lancet Infectious Diseases, 21*(7), 921. https://doi.org/10.1016/S1473-3099(21)00343-1

Lerbinger, O. (2012). *The crisis manager.* Routledge.

Lukowsky, L. R., Dobalian, A., Goldfarb, D. S., Kalantar-Zadeh, K., & Der-Martirosian, C. (2019). Access to care for VA dialysis patients during Superstorm Sandy. *Journal of Primary Care & Community Health, 10*, 2150132719863599. https://doi.org/10.1177/2150132719863599

Martin, N. (2020). Enabling effective oversight: Enterprise risk management and board governance in healthcare. *Healthcare Management Forum, 33*(4), 182–185. https://doi.org/10.1177/0840470420907260

Morris, A. M., Ricci, K. A., Griffin, A. R., Heslin, K. C., & Dobalian, A. (2016). Personal and professional challenges confronted by hospital staff following hurricane sandy: a qualitative assessment of management perspectives. *BMC Emergency Medicine, 16*(1), 18. https://doi.org/10.1186/s12873-016-0082-5

National Academies of Sciences, Engineering and Medicine. (2020, July 28). *Rapid expert consultation on staffing considerations for crisis standards of care for the COVID-19 pandemic.* The National Academies Press.

National Governors' Association (U.S.). Center for Policy Research. (1979). *Comprehensive emergency management: A Governor's guide.* Washington: [Dept. of Defense], Defense Civil Preparedness Agency: for sale by the Supt. of Docs., U.S. Govt. Print. Off.

Quarantelli, E. L. (1989). *How individuals and groups react during disasters: Planning and managing implications for EMS delivery.* http://udspace.udel.edu/handle/19716/510

Raja, S., Patolia, H. H., & Baffoe-Bonnie, A. W. (2020). Calculating an institutional personal protective equipment (PPE) burn rate to project future usage patterns during the 2020 COVID-19 pandemic. *Infection Control and Hospital Epidemiology, 41*(12), 1474–1475. https://doi.org/10.1017/ice.2020.190

Reynolds, B., & Seeger, M. W. (2005). Crisis and emergency risk communication as an integrative model. *Journal of Health Communication, 10*(1), 43–55. https://doi.org/10.1080/10810730590904571

Ricci, K. A., Griffin, A. R., Heslin, K. C., Kranke, D., & Dobalian, A. (2015). Evacuate or shelter-in-place? The role of corporate memory and political environment in hospital-evacuation decision making. *Prehospital and Disaster Medicine, 30*(3), 233–238. https://doi.org/10.1017/S1049023X15000229

Romney, D., Fox, H., Carlson, S., Bachmann, D., O'Mathuna, D., & Kman, N. (2020). Allocation of scarce resources in a pandemic: A systematic review of US state crisis standards of care documents. *Disaster Medicine and Public Health Preparedness, 14*(5), 677–683. https://doi.org/10.1017/dmp.2020.101

Sirkin, J. T., Flanagan, E., Tong, S. T., Coffman, M., McNellis, R. J., McPherson, T., & Bierman, A. S. (2023). Primary care's challenges and responses in the face of the COVID-19 pandemic: Insights from AHRQ's learning community. *Annals of Family Medicine, 21*(1), 76–82. https://doi.org/10.1370/afm.2904

Son, C., Sasangohar, F., Neville, T., Peres, S. C., & Moon, J. (2020). Investigating resilience in emergency management: An integrative review of literature. *Applied Ergonomics, 87*, 103114. https://doi.org/10.1016/j.apergo.2020.103114

Stryckman, B., Grace, T. L., Schwarz, P., & Marcozzi, D. (2015). An economic analysis and approach for health care preparedness in a substate region. *Disaster Medicine and Public Health Preparedness, 9*(4), 344–348. https://doi.org/10.1017/dmp.2015.37

Su, Z., Zhang, H., McDonnell, D., Ahmad, J., Cheshmehzangi, A., & Yuan, C. (2022). Crisis communication strategies for health officials. *Frontiers in Public Health, 10*, 796572. https://doi.org/10.3389/fpubh.2022.796572

Swanson, M., Bowen, P., Phillips, A., Gallup, D., & Lynes, D. (2010). *NIST Special Publication (SP) 800-34, Revision 1: Contingency planning guide for federal information systems*. National Institute of Standards and Technology (NIST).

Tolk, J. N., Cantu, J., & Beruvides, M. (2015). High reliability organization research: A literature review for health care. *Engineering Management Journal, 27*(4), 218–237. https://doi.org/10.1080/10429247.2015.1105087

U.S. Department of Homeland Security. (2011). *National Incident Management System training program*. Department of Homeland Security.

U.S. Department of Homeland Security. (2020). *Homeland Security Exercise and Evaluation Program*. https://www.fema.gov/sites/default/files/2020-04/Homeland-Security-Exercise-and-Evaluation-Program-Doctrine-2020-Revision-2-2-25.pdf

Weick, K. E., & Sutcliffe, K. M. (2015). *Managing the unexpected : sustained performance in a complex world*. John Wiley & Sons, Inc.

Wilson, P. F., Dell, L. D., & Anderson, G. F. (1993). *Root cause analysis: A tool for total quality management*. ASQC Quality Press.

CHAPTER 25

# DIVERSITY, EQUITY, AND INCLUSION IN HEALTHCARE MANAGEMENT

Ebbin Dotson, Darren Brownlee, and James E. Taylor

## LEARNING OBJECTIVES

- *Diversity mastery:* Define and apply key principles of diversity in healthcare management.
- *Equity implementation:* Possess the skills to foster equity in healthcare organizations.
- *Inclusion proficiency:* Create an inclusive healthcare environment by encouraging diverse perspectives.
- *Belonging and leadership development:* Comprehend the concept of belonging in healthcare management and how it extends beyond inclusion.
- *Diversity leadership framework application:* Be proficient in applying an emphasis on diversity leadership considering organizational best practices.

## KEY TERMS

- Affinity groups
- Belonging
- Cultural competency
- Diversity
- Equity
- Employee resource groups (ERGs)
- Inclusion
- Leadership skills
- Organizational culture
- Patient care

# INTRODUCTION—THE IMPORTANCE OF DIVERSITY, EQUITY, AND INCLUSION IN HEALTHCARE MANAGEMENT

In healthcare management, embracing **diversity, equity, and inclusion (DEI)** is crucial for fostering a thriving and inclusive **organizational culture** that positively impacts staff, learners, and patients. Many healthcare organizations root DEI within a broader principle of belonging, which is used as an umbrella term in this chapter. By implementing belonging-based best practices on diversity, equity, and inclusion, healthcare organizations can attract and retain a diverse talent pool, promote staff engagement, and ultimately provide higher quality and culturally competent care. This chapter highlights the significance of DEI in healthcare management and explores the management techniques and leadership skills necessary to cultivate an inclusive and equitable environment.

The healthcare management practices of DEI can be discussed in several ways. Leaders implement decisions using frameworks. DEI is no different than any other management maximization situation. Our framework for learning is termed "diversity leadership CORE." The CORE stands for **C**onsidering **O**rganizational best practices, **R**ecognizing equity and diversity management techniques, and **E**mphasizing leadership skills in navigating goals. This comprehensive approach ensures that DEI is not just an afterthought but is integrated into the very fabric of healthcare management.

The diversity leadership CORE framework emphasizes the importance of proactive rather than reactive measures in promoting DEI. By considering organizational best practices, healthcare leaders can ensure that DEI principles are embedded in every policy and procedure. Recognizing equity goes beyond just acknowledging differences; it is about ensuring that every individual has an equal opportunity to achieve the best health outcomes. Diversity management techniques are essential tools for leaders to ensure that the workforce reflects the diverse populations they serve. Emphasizing leadership skills in navigating DEI goals is crucial. Leaders must be equipped with the knowledge and skills to drive change, foster inclusive environments, and ensure that DEI principles are upheld at all levels of the organization.

Furthermore, the successful implementation of the diversity leadership CORE framework (Figure 25.1 and Box 25.1) requires continuous education, training, and evaluation.

**FIGURE 25.1.** Diversity leadership CORE framework.

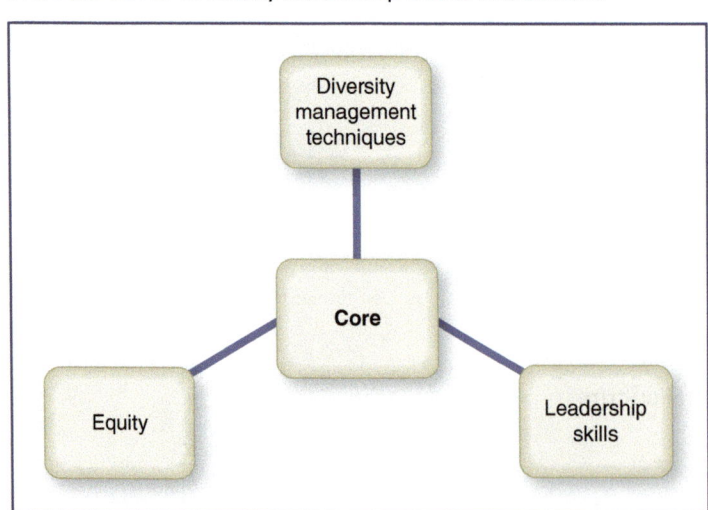

> **BOX 25.1: DIVERSITY LEADERSHIP CORE FRAMEWORK**
>
> The central word "CORE" is the foundation of the framework, representing the core principles of diversity leadership. Diversity management techniques emphasize the importance of strategies for managing and embracing diversity within healthcare organizations. Equity highlights the need for recognizing and promoting equity to ensure fair and just opportunities for all individuals. Leadership connection to the CORE indicates the significance of leadership skills in driving DEI initiatives.

Healthcare organizations should invest in DEI training programs for their staff and leadership. Regular evaluations and feedback mechanisms can help in identifying areas of improvement and ensuring that the organization is on the right track toward achieving its DEI goals. In the subsequent sections of this chapter, we delve deeper into each component of the diversity leadership CORE framework, providing actionable insights and best practices for healthcare leaders. Let us look at each component of the framework separately.

## ORGANIZATIONAL BEST PRACTICES ON DIVERSITY, EQUITY, AND INCLUSION

Organizations aiming to embrace DEI and **belonging** within healthcare management recognize the critical importance of cultivating a diverse workforce that reflects the diverse patient populations they serve (Smith et al., 2020). Implementing best practices in diversity involves the strategic recruitment and hiring of individuals from various backgrounds, cultures, and experiences (Jackson & Ruderman, 2019). Initiatives such as diverse hiring practices, diversity recruitment initiatives, and the establishment of measurable diversity goals are crucial (Johnson, 2021).

Equity in healthcare management entails actively involving all staff, learners, and patients in decision-making processes, ensuring equitable access to opportunities, and addressing systemic barriers that might impede staff growth (Hunt et al., 2023). Best practices on equity encompass transparent promotion and advancement criteria, providing training and resources for professional development, and offering mentorship programs (Loden & Rosener, 2020).

Creating an inclusive work environment is a cornerstone of DEI efforts. Best practices on inclusion involve fostering a welcoming and respectful atmosphere; encouraging diverse perspectives in discussions; and actively seeking input from all staff, learners, and patients in decision-making (Thomas & Ely, 1996). Research indicates that inclusive organizations have higher staff satisfaction and better innovation outcomes (Cox & Blake, 2021).

Organizations also recognize the concept of belonging, which goes beyond inclusion and fosters a deep emotional connection between staff and the organization. Best practices on belonging include developing succession planning programs to promote diverse leaders' growth, supporting underrepresented staff through **affinity groups** and **employee resource groups (ERGs)**, and cultivating an inclusive culture that celebrates diverse contributions (Holt & Washington, 2018).

## DIVERSITY MANAGEMENT TECHNIQUES

Healthcare organizations place great emphasis on attracting, engaging, and retaining diverse talent (Box 25.2). Attracting diverse talent involves actively sourcing candidates from underrepresented communities and partnering with organizations that promote

> **BOX 25.2: DIVERSITY MANAGEMENT TECHNIQUES**
>
> *Attract (recruit):* Healthcare organizations can attract diverse talent by actively sourcing candidates from underrepresented communities, partnering with organizations that promote diversity in the healthcare field, and using inclusive language in job postings to signal a commitment to diversity and inclusion.
>
> *Engage (train):* Once diverse talent is recruited, engagement can be fostered through comprehensive training programs that address cultural competency, unconscious bias, and communication skills. Offering ongoing professional development opportunities that cater to diverse needs and perspectives is also vital.
>
> *Retain (sustain):* Retaining diverse talent requires creating an inclusive work environment where employees feel valued and supported. Providing mentorship and sponsorship opportunities, recognizing and celebrating diverse achievements, and offering equitable compensation and benefits contribute to employee retention.

diversity in healthcare. Using inclusive language in job postings signal a commitment to diversity and inclusion. Engaging diverse talent is achieved through comprehensive training programs addressing **cultural competency**, unconscious bias, and communication skills. Ongoing professional development opportunities catering to diverse needs and perspectives are essential to keep talent engaged. To retain diverse talent, organizations create inclusive work environments that value and support all staff, learners, and patients. They provide mentorship and sponsorship opportunities, recognize and celebrate diverse achievements, and also commit to offering equitable compensation and benefits as a mechanism to ensure staff retention.

## LEADERSHIP SKILLS AND CULTURAL COMPETENCIES

Effective healthcare leaders in DEI management possess key attributes such as empathy, active listening, and a steadfast commitment to inclusivity. They value diverse perspectives and actively create a culture of respect and belonging for all team members. Leading by example, these leaders demonstrate a strong dedication to fairness and equity, ensuring that all individuals are treated with dignity and respect. Moreover, culturally competent leaders in healthcare management exhibit behaviors that foster understanding and effective communication across diverse cultures. They adapt their leadership styles to accommodate the unique needs and backgrounds of team members. Recognizing the impact of culture on healthcare delivery, these leaders proactively seek to learn about different cultures and incorporate culturally appropriate practices in their leadership approach. By embodying these **leadership skills** and cultural competencies, healthcare leaders can create inclusive and equitable environments that empower their workforce and enhance **patient care** (Box 25.3).

By embracing DEI principles and implementing best practices in healthcare management, organizations can create a culture of respect, fairness, and belonging that positively impacts staff, learners, and patients. Leaders who cultivate diversity, equity, inclusion, and belonging contribute to a more engaged and motivated workforce, leading to improved healthcare outcomes and patient satisfaction. Additionally, healthcare organizations that prioritize DEI are better equipped to address health disparities and deliver culturally competent care that meets the diverse needs of their communities. As healthcare management continues to evolve, an unwavering commitment to DEI remains vital in creating a more equitable and inclusive healthcare system for all.

> **BOX 25.3: POSITIVE LEADERSHIP ATTRIBUTES AND BEHAVIORS**
>
> - *Leadership skills (attributes):* Effective healthcare leaders in DEI management exhibit empathy, active listening, and a commitment to inclusivity. They value diverse perspectives and actively seek to create a culture of respect and belonging. Effective leaders lead by example and demonstrate a commitment to fairness and equity.
> - *Cultural competencies (behaviors):* Culturally competent leaders in healthcare management possess the ability to communicate effectively across cultures, adapt their leadership styles to accommodate diverse team members, and understand the impact of culture on healthcare delivery. They actively seek to learn about different cultures and incorporate culturally appropriate practices in their leadership.

# DIVERSITY, EQUITY, AND INCLUSION DEFINITIONS IN HEALTHCARE

In today's diverse and interconnected world, the importance of DEI cannot be overstated. Understanding the various terms and concepts related to DEI is essential for creating an equitable and inclusive workplace and society. In healthcare, DEI are essential principles that drive the pursuit of equitable access to quality care and positive health outcomes for all individuals, regardless of their background or identity. Understanding the key DEI concepts and their application in healthcare settings is crucial for creating a more inclusive and culturally sensitive environment that meets the diverse needs of patients and healthcare professionals.

## DIVERSITY IN HEALTHCARE

Diversity in healthcare refers to the presence of a wide range of individuals from different backgrounds, cultures, races, ethnicities, genders, sexual orientations, and other identities within the healthcare workforce (organization). Embracing diversity in healthcare is vital for several reasons:

- *Cultural competency:* A diverse healthcare workforce enhances cultural competency, allowing healthcare providers to understand and respect the unique beliefs, values, and practices of patients from various backgrounds.
- *Addressing health disparities:* Certain populations, such as racial and ethnic minorities, face disproportionate health disparities due to historical and systemic factors. A diverse healthcare workforce is better equipped to address these disparities and advocate for equitable healthcare policies and practices.
- *Improved patient outcomes:* Research has shown that diverse healthcare teams are associated with improved patient outcomes. Diverse perspectives and experiences lead to better problem-solving, decision-making, and innovation in patient care.
- *Enhanced patient trust:* Patients tend to feel more comfortable and trusting when they can relate to their healthcare providers on a personal level.

## EQUITY IN HEALTHCARE

Equity in healthcare refers to the fair distribution of resources, opportunities, and services to ensure that all individuals have an equal chance of achieving optimal health outcomes.

Achieving health equity is a multifaceted approach that involves addressing **social determinants of health (SDOH)**, eliminating disparities, and providing targeted support to vulnerable populations. Key aspects of equity in healthcare include the following:

- *SDOH:* SDOH, such as income, education, housing, and access to healthcare, significantly influence health outcomes. Addressing these factors is critical for achieving health equity.
- *Reducing health disparities:* Health disparities occur when certain groups experience higher rates of illness, disability, or death compared to others. Equity-focused interventions aim to reduce these disparities and level the healthcare playing field.
- *Language services:* Providing language services, such as interpretation and translation, is essential for overcoming language barriers and ensuring that individuals with limited English proficiency can access healthcare information and services effectively.
- *Culturally and linguistically appropriate services (CLAS):* CLAS in healthcare involves tailoring care to meet the cultural, linguistic, and health literacy needs of diverse patient populations. This approach improves patient satisfaction and health outcomes.

## INCLUSION IN HEALTHCARE

Inclusion in healthcare involves creating an environment where all individuals feel valued, respected, and welcomed. It goes beyond diversity and ensures that diverse voices are heard, considered, and integrated into decision-making processes. The significance of inclusion in healthcare includes the following:

- *Promoting psychological safety:* Inclusive healthcare settings foster psychological safety, where healthcare professionals and patients feel comfortable expressing their opinions, concerns, and needs without fear of judgment or discrimination.
- *Diverse leadership representation:* Inclusive healthcare organizations prioritize diverse leadership representation, ensuring that decision-making reflects the perspectives and experiences of all stakeholders.
- *ERGs and affinity groups:* ERGs and affinity groups provide a platform for individuals with shared backgrounds or identities to connect, advocate for inclusive practices, and contribute to a supportive workplace culture.
- *Support for healthcare professionals:* Inclusive healthcare settings offer support, mentorship, and professional development opportunities for underrepresented healthcare professionals, promoting career advancement and retention.

## COMMUNITY AND SOCIAL DETERMINANTS OF HEALTH

SDOH are the conditions in which people are born, grow, live, work, and age (WHO, 2021). The studies evaluated SDOH, with a general belief that clinical or healthcare contributes to only 10% to 20% of a population's health outcomes (Hood et al., 2016) and that socioeconomic factors, the physical environment, and health behaviors are associated with the remaining 80% to 90% of health outcomes (Figure 25.2).

These nonclinical factors, popularized as SDOH, have mainly been defined as conditions affecting an individual's health outside of the hospital walls. The six determinant domains of health, economic stability, neighborhood and physical environment, education, food, community, and social context, and health care systems, are all variables that influence the health outcomes of mortality, morbidity, life expectancy, health care expenditures, health status and functional limitations (Table 25.1).

**FIGURE 25.2.** The impact of social determinants of health.

- Socioeconomic factors (40%): Education, Job status, Family/social support, Income, Community safety
- Physical Environment (10%)
- Health Behaviors (30%): Tobacco use, Diet and exercise, Alcohol use, Sexual activity
- Healthcare (20%): Access to care, Quality of care

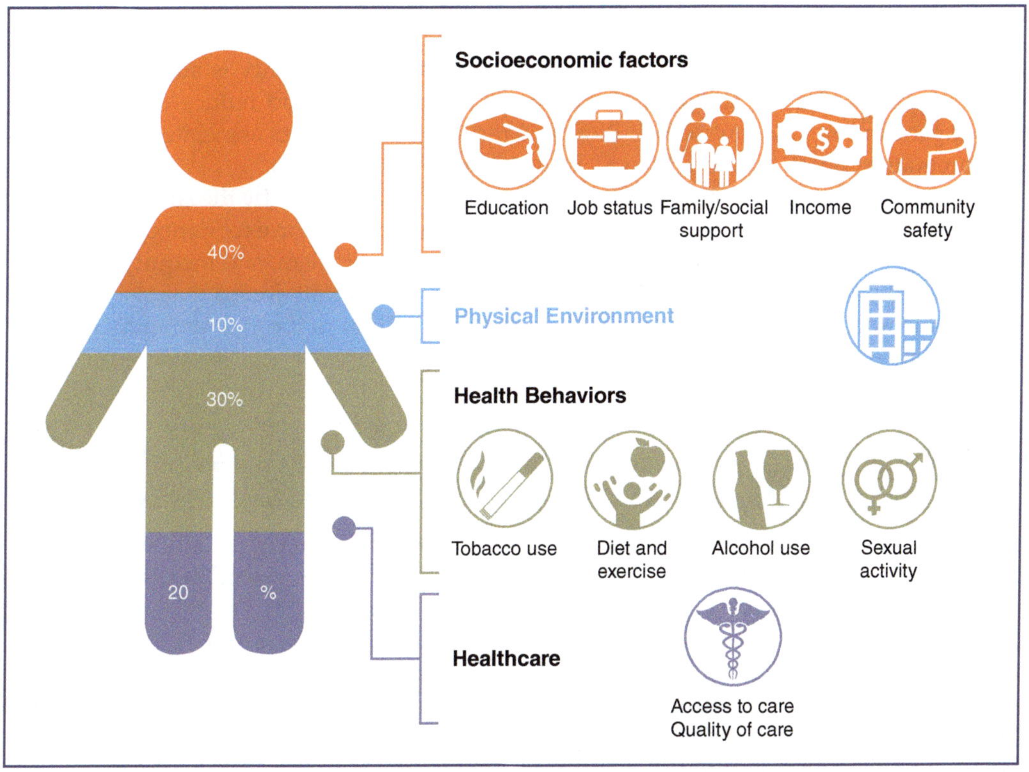

*Source:* Adapted from Institute for Clinical Systems Improvement. (2014). *Going beyond clinical walls: Solving complex problems.* Retrieved from https://www.ncbi.nlm.nih.gov/pmc/articles/PMC4282514/.

### TABLE 25.1. SOCIAL DETERMINANTS OF HEALTH

| ECONOMIC STABILITY | | | | | |
|---|---|---|---|---|---|
| Debt | Employment | Expenses | Income | Medical Bills | Support |
| **Neighborhood and Physical Environment** | | | | | |
| Housing | Parks/Playgrounds | Safety | Transportation | Walkability | Zip Code/Geography |
| **Education** | | | | | |
| Early Childhood Education | Higher Education | Language | Literacy | Vocational Training | |
| **Food** | | | | | |
| Access to Healthy Options | Hunger | | | | |
| **Community and Social Context** | | | | | |
| Community Engagement | Discrimination | Social Integration | Support Systems | Stress | |
| **Healthcare System** | | | | | |
| Health Coverage | Provider Availability | Provider Linguistic and Cultural Competency | Quality of Care | | |
| **Health Outcomes:** Mortality, Morbidity, Life Expectancy, Healthcare Expenditures, Health Status, Functional Limitations. | | | | | |

As SDOH impacts more than that of provisional clinical care ("health is more than healthcare"), addressing SDOH is important to improving an individual's health regardless of age, sex, race, or ethnicity. Additionally, in addressing SDOH, it is the general belief that longstanding disparities of care are reduced and health equity is advanced. Moreover, research estimates that eliminating health inequities would reduce direct medical care expenditures by about $230 billion and reduce indirect costs associated with illness and premature death by more than $1 trillion (LaVeist et al., 2011).

In 2021, racism was elevated to the level of a public health crisis by the American Public Health Association. The organization noted that people of color experience more direct negative consequences on their health and wellness due to racism, and inequity driven by racism affects society as a whole (APHA, 2021). A 2020 estimate found that closing racial gaps in income, wealth, and education could add $5 trillion to the U.S. economy over the next 5 years (Peterson & Mann, 2020).

## EMPHASIZING LEADERSHIP SKILLS—APPLICATION OF DIVERSITY, EQUITY, AND INCLUSION IN HEALTHCARE

In healthcare, the application of DEI principles is vital for creating an equitable and culturally competent healthcare system. To achieve this, organizations and healthcare professionals can take concrete steps toward achieving health equity.

Managerially, there are several practical applications leaders assess in their decision-making (Table 25.2). For workforce readiness, providing cultural competency training enhances cross-cultural communication in addition to understanding diverse patient populations' needs. Actively recruiting individuals from diverse backgrounds helps increase representation within the healthcare workforce. Adopting a patient-centered approach that respects patients' cultural beliefs and preferences ensures personalized and effective care. Language access services, such as interpreters and translated materials, accommodate patients with limited English proficiency. Targeted interventions and programs are developed to address health disparities in underserved communities. Creating

**TABLE 25.2. APPLICATION OF DEI DEFINITIONS IN HEALTHCARE**

| DEI ASPECT | ACTION |
|---|---|
| Cultural competency training | Provide training to enhance cross-cultural communication and understand diverse patient populations' needs. |
| Diverse hiring practices | Actively recruit individuals from diverse backgrounds to increase workforce representation. |
| Patient-centered care | Adopt a patient-centered approach that incorporates patients' cultural beliefs and preferences into treatment plans. |
| Language access services | Ensure availability of language access services (interpreters, translated materials) for patients with limited English proficiency. |
| Addressing health disparities | Develop targeted interventions and programs to improve health outcomes in underserved communities. |
| Promoting inclusive policies | Create and implement policies that support diversity, equity, and inclusion within the organization and healthcare delivery. |
| Partnerships with diverse communities | Collaborate with community-based organizations and leaders to understand unique healthcare needs of diverse populations and develop culturally relevant solutions. |

DEI, diversity, equity, and inclusion.

inclusive policies and fostering partnerships with diverse communities further support DEI implementation. By integrating DEI principles into healthcare, organizations foster an environment where individuals feel valued, respected, and empowered, ultimately leading to improved health outcomes for everyone.

By integrating DEI principles into every aspect of healthcare, organizations can build a more equitable and inclusive healthcare system that meets the needs of all individuals and contributes to improved health outcomes for everyone. Embracing diversity, ensuring equity, and promoting inclusion will lead to a healthcare environment where every individual feels valued, respected, and empowered. By implementing these actions, healthcare organizations can work toward building a more equitable and inclusive healthcare system that caters to the diverse needs of patients and supports an inclusive and empowered workforce.

Several key organizations in the healthcare and medical fields are committed to promoting diversity, equity, and inclusion within their respective domains. These organizations recognize the importance of cultivating an inclusive culture and acknowledging the value of diverse perspectives. Table 25.3 highlights some of their DEI commitments.

Politically, the perspective of professional organizations on DEI reflects a growing recognition of the importance of promoting diversity and inclusion within the healthcare industry. Several prominent organizations, including the American College of Healthcare Executives (ACHE), Healthcare Information and Management Systems Society (HIMSS), Medical Group Management Association (MGMA), National Association of Health Services Executives (NAHSE), and the National Association of Latino Healthcare Executives

### TABLE 25.3. KEY HEALTHCARE MANAGEMENT ORGANIZATIONS' DEI COMMITMENTS

| AAMC | The AAMC values the diversity of identities and experiences among medical students, physicians, and their patients. It understands that diverse expertise, ideas, and strengths are essential for advocating for equity and justice in healthcare policies, products, and services. The AAMC aims to attract and retain the best talent, providing opportunities for personal and professional development while fostering an equitable and inclusive workplace. |
|---|---|
| AHA | The AHA believes in the fair and equitable treatment of all individuals and recognizes diversity, equity, and inclusion as ethical and business imperatives. It views diversity in its leaders, members, and staff as a catalyst for a stronger healthcare workforce, better decision-making, and improved outcomes. AHA fosters an inclusive and equitable culture that values the contributions of all individuals, regardless of their race, ethnicity, gender, religion, age, marital status, sexual orientation, gender identity, or disability. |
| NALHE | NALHE is committed to increasing senior-level Latinx representation in hospitals and health systems in the United States. It recognizes that diversity within healthcare leadership is essential for promoting health equity and aims to transform the Latinx leadership experience. NALHE is dedicated to creating an inclusive culture that respects and values all people, irrespective of their backgrounds or identities. |
| ACHE | ACHE encourages diversity within healthcare leadership and believes in fair and equitable treatment for all individuals. It recognizes that diversity, equity, and inclusion are not only ethical imperatives but also vital for achieving better outcomes and gaining a competitive advantage. ACHE fosters an inclusive environment that supports the advancement of all individuals, regardless of their race, ethnicity, national origin, gender, religion, age, marital status, sexual orientation, gender identity, or disability. |

AAMC, American Association of Medical Colleges; ACHE, American College of Healthcare Executives; AHA, American Hospital Association; DEI, diversity, equity, and inclusion; NALHE, National Association of Latino Healthcare Executives.

(NALHE), have made significant strides in advocating for and implementing DEI initiatives in healthcare management.

These organizations acknowledge that embracing DEI principles in the healthcare sector is not only an ethical imperative but also a strategic approach to achieving better patient outcomes and organizational success. They have created platforms, communities, and networks to foster collaboration and knowledge-sharing among healthcare leaders and professionals interested in advancing DEI.

ACHE, HIMSS, MGMA, NAHSE, and NALHE are at the forefront of promoting DEI in the C-suite of healthcare organizations. They advocate for the appointment of chief diversity officers (CDOs) or chief equity officers to oversee DEI initiatives at the executive level. This demonstrates the organizations' commitment to making DEI a strategic priority by integrating it into top leadership positions.

The organizations emphasize the importance of defining clear roles and responsibilities for CDOs and other DEI leaders, establishing specific organizational targets for DEI, and incorporating DEI considerations into succession planning. By doing so, they aim to create a culture that values diversity and actively promotes opportunities for underrepresented individuals to advance within the healthcare industry.

Moreover, these professional organizations highlight the significance of incorporating DEI principles into various aspects of healthcare management, including reporting structures and span of control. This ensures that DEI considerations are integrated throughout the organizational structure, promoting a more inclusive and equitable environment for all staff and patients.

Overall, the perspective of these professional organizations on DEI and JEDI (Justice, Equity, Diversity, and Inclusion) is a commitment to transforming the healthcare industry into one that embraces diversity, fosters inclusion, and advocates for equity. By working together and sharing best practices, they strive to create a future where healthcare organizations are better equipped to meet the needs of diverse patient populations, improve health outcomes, and create a more inclusive and equitable healthcare landscape for all.

## QUANTITATIVE: BY THE NUMBERS

The quantitative DEI implications of C-suite leaders in healthcare organizations are crucial to understanding the representation and impact of underrepresented minorities (URMs), the appointment of CDOs or chief equity officers, and the presence of medical doctors (MDs) in leadership positions. These aspects play a significant role in shaping diversity, inclusion, and decision-making processes within the healthcare industry.

*Representation of URMs:* The representation of URMs in C-suite leadership positions has historically been low in healthcare organizations. Numerous studies and reports have indicated a plateaued low percentage of underrepresentation of URMs at the executive level in healthcare. The American Hospital Association (AHA) found that only 16% of surveyed healthcare organizations had chief executive officers (CEOs) of color, indicating a lack of diversity in top leadership roles (AHA, 2021). Periodic surveys from ACHE show trend lines in 2008, 2012, and 2016 in which leadership diversity has not made significant strides. As organizations continue to prioritize diversity and inclusion, efforts to increase URM representation in C-suite positions are gaining momentum.

The rise of CDOs or chief equity officers signaled a change in how healthcare organizations structured DEI commitments. These roles gained national prominence in healthcare organizations between 2000 and 2020. Several reports and surveys have indicated a legitimization trend within health systems and other healthcare organizations. According to a 2020 survey by the AHA, 65% of surveyed hospitals and health systems had a designated diversity and inclusion officer, representing a significant increase compared to previous years. This trend highlights the recognition of the importance of DEI initiatives and the role of dedicated leaders in driving change.

There has always been a recognition of the value of having MDs in leadership positions within healthcare organizations. As healthcare systems become more complex and patient centered, having MDs in executive roles brings unique insights into clinical care, patient outcomes, and medical expertise. A study by the American Association of Medical Colleges (AAMC) in 2019 found that 13% of healthcare CEOs had medical degrees, showcasing the growing importance of clinical expertise at the leadership level.

To understand the DEI implications, it is worth noting the diversity within clinical enterprise as a whole (Saizan et al., 2021). In 2018, <12% of physicians were from underrepresented backgrounds in medicine (Laurencin & Murray, 2017; LaVeist et al., 2003; Merchant & Omary, 2010). Healthcare leadership was predominantly composed of White individuals, comprising 98%. Racial and ethnic minorities constituted around 19.2% of registered nurses and 8% of PhD investigators in other medical sectors (American Association of Critical-Care Nurses [AACN] Fact Sheet, n.d.; Blanchard et al., 2021). These statistics highlight the pressing need to address the lack of diversity in the medical workforce, as it negatively affects health outcomes, especially for underserved backgrounds and minorities. Inclusive leadership and diverse interprofessional healthcare teams are crucial for bridging cultural gaps, enhancing collaborations, and providing comprehensive care to underserved populations. This approach can help reduce health disparities, lower healthcare costs, and optimize healthcare system utilization.

## CASE STUDY 25.1: NAVIGATING DIVERSITY IN HEALTHCARE LEADERSHIP—DIVERSIFYING CLINICAL LEADERSHIP

In a bustling urban hospital, the leadership team aspires to provide the highest quality of patient care while fostering an inclusive and diverse environment. However, the lack of racial and ethnic diversity within the leadership ranks is a challenge that cannot be ignored. This case study delves into the experiences of Dr. Rodriguez, a dedicated physician who is eager to break through the glass ceiling and become a healthcare leader.

Dr. Rodriguez, a highly skilled cardiologist, has been serving the hospital for over a decade. Her commitment to patient care and her expertise are well recognized by her colleagues and patients alike. Over the years, Dr. Rodriguez has expressed interest in taking on leadership roles, envisioning herself contributing to hospital-wide decisions and strategies. However, she has noticed that leadership positions within the hospital tend to be predominantly occupied by individuals who do not reflect the diverse patient population they serve.

Despite her aspirations, Dr. Rodriguez faces challenges that are all too familiar to many healthcare professionals of color. She has observed that opportunities for mentorship and career development are not equally accessible to individuals like her. Limited exposure and visibility at networking events often leave her feeling isolated in her pursuit of advancement. She recognizes that her unique insights, grounded in her cultural background, could greatly benefit the hospital's decision-making processes and patient care strategies.

As Dr. Rodriguez contemplates her next steps, she stumbles upon the article "Exploring the Current State of Racial and Ethnic Minorities in Healthcare Leadership" by Poole and Brownlee (2023). This article sheds light on the underrepresentation of individuals like her in healthcare leadership positions. It delves into the barriers faced by minority leaders, including systemic biases, lack of mentorship, and limited access to advancement opportunities.

The article presents a series of recommendations that resonate with Dr. Rodriguez's own aspirations. It suggests implementing targeted mentorship and professional development programs for minority leaders, creating a more inclusive recruitment process, and fostering a culturally competent leadership culture. Dr. Rodriguez feels inspired by these recommendations and is determined to advocate for change within her organization.

## CASE STUDY DISCUSSION QUESTIONS

- How does the underrepresentation of racial and ethnic minorities in healthcare leadership impact patient care outcomes and the overall hospital environment?
- What are some of the systemic barriers that Dr. Rodriguez and other minority healthcare professionals might face in their journey toward leadership roles?
- How can healthcare organizations benefit from the diverse perspectives that minority leaders bring to decision-making processes?
- What strategies can healthcare organizations implement to provide equal access to mentorship and career development opportunities for all professionals, regardless of their background?
- In what ways can the recommendations presented in the article by Poole and Brownlee be tailored to Dr. Rodriguez's hospital to promote diversity and inclusion in leadership?

## CASE STUDY CONCLUSION

Dr. Rodriguez's journey represents the experiences of countless minority healthcare professionals who aspire to lead and make meaningful contributions to their organizations. By addressing the challenges highlighted in the article and adopting the recommended strategies, healthcare institutions can pave the way for a more inclusive and diverse leadership landscape.

Link to the article: https://www.proquest.com/openview/ffbf2c3052ce17576d4dcbde28d98351/1?pq-origsite= gscholar&cbl=2037550

Overall, the quantitative data and trends suggest that healthcare organizations are increasingly recognizing the importance of diversity, equity, and inclusion in their leadership teams. The efforts to increase URM representation, appoint CDOs or chief equity officers, and recognize the value of MDs in leadership positions reflect a commitment to creating an inclusive and patient-centered healthcare system. Ongoing efforts and data monitoring are essential to continue advancing DEI in C-suite leadership and driving positive change within the healthcare industry.

## CONCLUSION

In conclusion, the pursuit of diversity, equity, and inclusion is an ongoing journey that requires the collective effort of individuals, organizations, and societies. Understanding the various terms and concepts related to DEI is crucial for creating a more equitable and inclusive world where everyone's unique backgrounds and experiences are respected and celebrated. Organizations that embrace DEI principles stand to benefit from a diverse and engaged workforce, improved decision-making, and better outcomes in their respective fields. By actively promoting diversity, equity, and inclusion, we can create a more just and compassionate society for everyone.

# END-OF-CHAPTER RESOURCES

## CRITICAL THINKING QUESTIONS

- How does embracing DEI in healthcare management positively impact staff, learners, and patients?
- What is the significance of the concept of belonging in fostering an inclusive organizational culture in healthcare management?
- Discuss the diversity leadership CORE framework and its components. How does it contribute to effective DEI management?
- Why is it essential for healthcare organizations to adopt proactive measures rather than reactive ones in promoting DEI?
- In what ways can leaders emphasize diversity management techniques to ensure that the workforce reflects the diverse populations they serve?
- What role does continuous education, training, and evaluation play in the successful implementation of DEI initiatives in healthcare organizations?
- How does diversity contribute to cultural competency in healthcare, and why is cultural competency important for providing quality care?
- Discuss the role of a diverse healthcare workforce in addressing health disparities. How can diversity in leadership influence healthcare policies and practices to reduce disparities?
- Why is inclusion important in healthcare settings, and how does it differ from diversity? How can inclusive practices enhance patient trust and healthcare outcomes?
- What steps can healthcare organizations take to integrate DEI principles into their operations, and why is this integration important?

## LEARNING ACTIVITIES

### CourseConnect ▶

To access self-assessment questions and interactive, competency-based learning activities for this chapter, visit www.springerpub.com/courseconnect. See inside front cover and tear-out card for CourseConnect details.

## REFERENCES

AACN Fact Sheet. (n.d.). *Enhancing diversity in the nursing workforce.* https://www.aacnnursing.org/News-Information/Fact-Sheets/Enhancing-Diversity

Abe-Jones, Y., Rambachan, A., Fernandez, A., & Shahram, Y. (2021). Racial disparities in 7-day readmissions from an adult hospital medicine service. *Journal of Racial and Ethnic Health Disparities, 9*(4), 1500–1505. https://doi.org/10.1007/s40615-021-01088-3

American Hospital Association. (2021). *Health equity resource series: Equity of care.* https://www.aha.org

American Public Health Association. (2021). *Racism is a public health crisis.* https://www.apha.org/topics-and-issues/health-equity/racism-and-health

Association of American Medical Colleges. (2019). *Figure 18: Percentage of all active physicians by race/ethnicity, 2018.* Retrieved December 31, 2020, from https://www.aamc.org/data-reports/workforce/interactive-data/figure-18-percentage-all-active-physicians-race/ethnicity-2018

Bibbins-Domingo, K. (2019). Integrating social care into the delivery of health care. *Journal of the American Medical Association, 322*(18), 1763–1764. https://doi.org/10.1001/jama.2019.15603

Blanchard, S. A., Rivers, R., Martinez, W., & Agodoa, L. (2021). Building the network of minority health research investigators: A novel program to enhance leadership and success of underrepresented minorities in biomedical research. *Ethnicity & Disease, 29*(Suppl. 1), 119–122. https://doi.org/10.18865/ed.29.S1.119

Bruce, M. M., Hogue, C. A., & Johnson, E. L. (2021). A national dental hygiene faculty development program to promote diversity, equity, and inclusion. *Journal of Dental Hygiene, 95*(6), 56–61. https://doi.org/10.1002/jdh.12559

Clark, S. G., Cohen, A., & Heard-Garris, N. J. (2022). Moving beyond words: Leveraging financial resources to improve diversity, equity, and inclusion in academic medical centers. *Journal of Racial and Ethnic Health Disparities, 9*(6), 1519–1524. https://doi.org/10.1007/s40615-021-01088-3

Cox, T. H., & Blake, S. (1991). Managing cultural diversity: Implications for organizational competitiveness. *Academy of Management Executive, 5*(3), 45–56. https://doi.org/10.5465/ame.1991.4274465

DeVoe, J. E., Bazemore, A. W., Cottrell, E. K., Likumahuwa-Ackman, S., Grandmont, J., Spach, N., & Gold, R. (2016). Perspectives in primary care: A conceptual framework and path for integrating social determinants of health into primary care practice. *Annals of Family Medicine, 14*(2), 104–108. https://doi.org/10.1370/afm.1903

Gaffney, A. W., Himmelstein, D. U., Christiani, D. C., & Woolhandler, S. (2021). Socioeconomic inequality in respiratory health in the US from 1959 to 2018. *JAMA Internal Medicine, 181*(7), 968–976. https://doi.org/10.1001/jamainternmed.2021.2441

Gershon, A. S., Dolmage, T. E., Stephenson, A., & Jackson, B. (2012). Chronic obstructive pulmonary disease and socioeconomic status: A systematic review. *Journal of Chronic Obstructive Pulmonary Disease, 9*(3), 216–226. https://doi.org/10.3109/15412555.2011.648030

George, A., Teelucksingh, K., & Fortune, K. (2023). Diversity, equity, and inclusion in the profession of pharmacy: The perspective of three pharmacy leaders. *International Journal of Applied Pharmacy, 15*(1), 12–19. https://doi.org/10.22159/ijap.2023v15i1.43459

Hadie, D. Y., Gruby, M. C., Wibowo, A. W., & Fox, H. M. (2022). Incorporating gender equity, diversity, and inclusion in the mainstreaming of fisheries: A study from Indonesia. *Fisheries, 47*(2), 101–107. https://doi.org/10.1002/fsh.10553

Holt, K., & Washington, M. (2018). The role of employee resource groups in fostering belonging and organizational success. *Journal of Diversity Management, 13*(1), 15–22.

Hood, C. M., Gennuso, K. P., Swain, G. R., & Catlin, B. B. (2016). County health rankings: Relationships between determinant factors and health outcomes. *American Journal of Preventive Medicine, 50*(2), 129–135. https://doi.org/10.1016/j.amepre.2015.08.024

Hunt, V., Dixon-Fyle, S., Huber, C., Martínez Márquez, M. del M., Prince, S., & Thomas, A. (2023). Diversity matters even more: The case for holistic impact. McKinsey & Company. https://www.mckinsey.com/featured-insights/diversity-and-inclusion/diversity-matters-even-more-the-case-for-holistic-impact

Jack, L. (2022). New for PCD in 2022: Increased impact factor, expanded expertise, first guest editorial board, and progress in diversity, equity, and inclusion goals. *Preventing Chronic Disease, 19*, 220197. https://doi.org/10.5888/pcd19.220197

Jackson, S. E., & Ruderman, M. N. (1995). Diversity in work teams: Research paradigms for a changing workplace. *American Psychological Association.* https://doi.org/10.1037/10101-000

Johnson, A. G. (2021). *Privilege, power, and difference* (3rd ed.). McGraw-Hill Education.

Laurencin, C., & Murray, M. (2017). An American crisis: The lack of black men in medicine. *Journal of Racial and Ethnic Health Disparities, 4*(3), 317–321. https://doi.org/10.1007/s40615-017-0380-y

LaVeist, T. A., Gaskin, D. J., & Richard, P. A. (2003). Racial segregation and longevity among African Americans: An individual-level analysis. *Health Services Research, 38*(6 Pt 2), 1715–1728. https://doi.org/10.1111/1475-6773.00199

LaVeist, T. A., Gaskin, D., & Richard, P. (2011). *The economic burden of health inequalities in the United States.* Joint Center for Political and Economic Studies.

LaVeist, T. A., Nuru-Jeter, A., & Jones, K. E. (2003). The association of doctor-patient race concordance with health services utilization. *Journal of Public Health Policy, 24*, 312–313. https://doi.org/10.2307/3343378

Loden, M., & Rosener, J. B. (1991). *Workforce America!: Managing employee diversity as a vital resource.* McGraw-Hill.

Manan, M. R., Nawaz, I., Rahman, S., Razzaq, A., Zafar, F., Qazi, A., & Liblik, K. (2023). Diversity, equity, and inclusion on editorial boards of global health journals. *Perspectives in Nursing Education, 26*(1), 74–84. https://doi.org/10.21522/TIJNR.2023.11.05.TI.019

Merchant, J. L., & Omary, M. B. (2010). Underrepresentation of underrepresented minorities in academic medicine: The need to enhance the pipeline and the pipe. *Gastroenterology, 138*(1), 19–26.e3. https://doi.org/10.1053/j.gastro.2009.11.017

Peterson, D. M., & Mann, C. L. (2020). *Closing the racial inequality gaps: The Economic Cost of Black Inequality in the U.S.* CitiGPS: Global Perspectives and Solutions. https://www.citivelocity.com/citigps/

Poole, D., & Brownlee, D. (2023). Exploring the current state of racial and ethnic minorities in healthcare leadership. *Journal of Health Disparities Research and Practice, 16*(2), 22–33. https://www.proquest.com/openview/ffbf2c3052ce17576d4dcbde28d98351/1

Powell, T., Bischoff, J., Reddy, K., Nagy, S. E., Lawrence, T. M., Bates, M., & McCright, M. (2023a). Achieving a diverse, equitable and inclusive environment using the Pathway to Excellence® framework as a model. *Journal of Nursing Administration, 53*(9), 474–480. https://doi.org/10.1097/NNA.0000000000001318

Powell, T., Bischoff, J., Reddy, K., Nagy, S. E., Lawrence, T. M., & Others. (2023b). The intersection of diversity, equity, and inclusion in management practices: A descriptive study. *Journal of Management in Medicine, 12*(1), 102–115. https://doi.org/10.1108/JMM-03-2022-0043

Powell, T., Bischoff, J., Reddy, K., Nagy, S. E., Lawrence, T. M., & Others. (2023c). Diversity, equity, and inclusion task force initiatives within the society for vascular medicine: Current status and future challenges. *Journal of Vascular Medicine, 5*(6), 474–480. https://doi.org/10.1038/s41584-022-01040-0

Rambachan, A., Abe-Jones, Y., Fernandez, A., & Shahram, Y. (2021). Racial disparities in 7-day readmissions from an Adult Hospital Medicine Service. *Journal of Racial and Ethnic Health Disparities, 9*(4), 1500–1505. https://doi.org/10.1007/s40615-021-01088-3

Saizan, A. L., Douglas, A., Elbuluk, N., & Taylor, S. (2021). A diverse nation calls for a diverse healthcare force. *EClinicalMedicine, 34*, 100846. https://doi.org/10.1016/j.eclinm.2021.100846

Smith, D. B., Feng, Z., Fennell, M. L., Zinn, J., & Mor, V. (2007). Racial disparities in access to long-term care: The illusive pursuit of equity. *Journal of Health Politics, Policy and Law, 32*(5), 781–808. https://doi.org/10.1215/03616878-2007-035

Thomas, D. A., & Ely, R. J. (1996). Making differences matter: A new paradigm for managing diversity. *Harvard Business Review, 74*(5), 79–90.

Tsui, E. K. (2010). Sectoral job training as an intervention to improve health equity. *American Journal of Public Health, 100*(Suppl. 1), S88–S94. https://doi.org/10.2105/AJPH.2009.181826

Williams, S., Eden, S., Megdal, S., & Joe-Gaddy, V. (2023). Diversity, equity, inclusion, and justice in water dialogues: A review and conceptualization. *Water Resources Research, 59*(2), e2022WR033864. https://doi.org/10.1029/2022WR033864

World Health Organization. (2021). *Social determinants of health.* https://www.who.int/health-topics/social-determinants-of-health

# CHAPTER 26

# LEADERSHIP AND PROFESSIONAL PERFORMANCE

Laurie Baedke and Natalie Lamberton

## LEARNING OBJECTIVES

- Examine the correlation between a focus on strengths and increased performance, engagement, and well-being.
- Leverage feedback as a tool to increase self-awareness and performance.
- Identify the four components of emotional intelligence: self-awareness, self-management, social awareness, and relationship management.
- Employ lifelong learning as an approach to continuous professional growth and development.
- Apply knowledge acquired in this chapter to develop an action plan for improving personal leadership skills and performance.

## KEY TERMS

- Accountability
- Emotional intelligence
- Followership
- Integrity
- Leadership
- Performance
- Professional development
- Self-awareness

## INTRODUCTION

From the outset, accomplished leaders seem to be the unicorns within their respective organizations and communities. *They have that "something special".* The qualities we associate with high-performance leadership appear elusive. The truth is our top leaders are very human and embrace that humanity. This notion is essential in healthcare, which demands competence, authenticity, compassion, and a commitment to leadership and professional performance.

The skills that inform a well-respected leader can be taught, earned, and are within one's reach. Furthermore, the preeminent leaders among us are not satisfied with anything less than continuous improvement. The rewards of a lifelong commitment to personal growth and **professional development** are akin to compound interest. Like savings, the knowledge and experiences we acquire build upon themselves with time. As investor giant Warren Buffett puts it:

*"If you are investing in your education and you are learning, you should do that as early as you possibly can, because then it will have time to compound over the longest period."*

In this chapter, we explore the following four tangible practices of leadership and leading *well* in a healthcare environment marked like never before by change and uncertainty:

- Leading self
- Leading others
- Leadership competencies
- Career path management

## LEADING SELF

To lead others well is to "lead" oneself well. And to "lead thyself" is to "know thyself." *Why so much "self" talk when leadership is about unifying and guiding others to the best versions of themselves and the "whole"?* An example of putting one's self first for the good of the whole, and that many of us can relate to, occurs as standard protocols during flights. What do the flight attendants tell us during the emergency briefing? They say, "Secure your oxygen mask first." Yes, before securing the masks of children or others with special needs, you must tend to your needs first.

While this behavior may seem *self-serving* at the outset, it is an essential condition of *serving others*, a demonstration of *care*. After all, how can you help your fellow passengers if you do not first ensure sufficient oxygen to effectively support them? *Performance* leadership is like this; self-aware leaders are keenly aware of their and other's needs, strengths, weaknesses, and complementarities. Like the frequent flyer who keeps cool under pressure and calmly applies their mask, the wise leader identifies and monitors respective personal attributes and evolving skills first, knowing this step is critical to provide the support (or "oxygen") that fuels, lifts, and serves others.

Consider the first decade of one's career as a "proving ground." Think of how far ahead one could be by intentionally practicing behaviors that garner insights into the self, which can then be applied to cultivate strong leadership skills. At heart, the "self" is a sum of many parts. In the context of healthcare management and administration, we are referring to an awareness of the following parts:

- Temperament
- Character
- Habits
- Biases
- Strengths
- Weaknesses

- Skills
- Knowledge

The more oneself is explored and known, the better. Self-aware leaders are well equipped to fix stagnation or failures. Moreover, they buoy promising areas, so teams rise to new heights of excellence. The practices and concepts associated with leadership and **self-awareness** are not about seeking perfection. This is an exercise in futility. The leaders we admire pursue progress.

Furthermore, ample rewards are to be reaped by embracing the "imperfect," gleaning from failures to continuously learn and improve in ways that would have been unthinkable without the less-than-perfect experience. Closely related to self-awareness is "self-management," the actionable items or behaviors that contribute to the qualities of being self-aware. In Drucker's (1977) classic *People and Performance*, the late management guru stated: "Unless we determine what shall be measured and what the yardstick of measurement in an area will be, the area itself will not be seen." Or, to distill it another way, *what gets measured, gets managed*.

Often, the dots between performance and metrics are connected at an organizational level; however, these intentional practices should be applied to quantify progress at a personal level, too. It is healthy and indeed essential to create structures, be it informal or formal, to assess ourselves. Only then can we best gauge our abilities in given areas, which can then inform our next steps toward building upon successes or adjusting to improve lackluster performance.

One other caveat: Self-awareness is essential for effective leaders, but this attribute alone does not catapult emerging leaders into the C-suite. No single characteristic or success will accomplish such dramatic leaps. The opportunity to lead results from a combination of education, training, technical skills, and behavioral competencies (i.e., communication and negotiation prowess). Plus, leaders are *made* over several years or decades. Apply the concept of compound interest to lifelong learning to, similarly, grow as an individual and in leadership.

On a solid foundation of self-awareness, the aspiring healthcare leader measures progress and recalibrates as needed to achieve short- and long-term goals. This leader has the know-how to repair what is not working and to elevate what is working *without regret*.

## ACTION STEPS TO SELF-AWARENESS

In *Heart, Smarts, Guts, and Luck*, Tjan et al. (2012) set out to quantify and objectively determine the qualities that separate a middling (or worse) manager or leader from a great one. As Tjan (2012) shares in *Harvard Business Review*, the research trio identified a single quality that trumps all and is evident in pretty much every standout exec or leader. It is the focus of this section. As Tjan notes, "The best thing leaders can do to improve their effectiveness is to become more aware of what motivates them and their decision-making. Without self-awareness, you cannot understand your strengths and weakness, your 'super powers' versus your 'kryptonite.'"

Helpfully, Tjan took this foundational concept a big leap forward by providing defined recommendations to become a self-aware leader. His three-pronged strategy boils down to the following:

- *Testing:* A seemingly endless array of tests are available to buttress a framework for knowing oneself better. Notables include CliftonStrengths and personality test staple Myers-Briggs Type Indicator (MBTI). Formal assessments facilitate highly beneficial self-reflection, which lends itself to improved personal awareness.

- *Map it and measure it:* Put the expectations for results from pivotal decisions "in writing." Review those expectations quarterly or semiannually. How do they line up with what transpired? Such analysis codifies one's reasoning and motivation for certain decisions and stimulates active, ongoing reflection and outcome assessment.
- *Put it in motion:* Self-awareness enables collaboration. By understanding one's bright spots and potential blind spots, leadership is in the ideal position to enlist and elevate talent that complements given divisions, units, and institutions.

Building upon the approaches celebrated by Tjan and his fellow researchers, we encourage grassroots thinking and actions. The following recommendations exist outside of formal frameworks popularized by personality metrics like MBTI® and CliftonStrengths®:

- *Be humble:* Acknowledge the others who made successes possible. Exercise grace, be quick to compliment, and lift others.
- *Be a seeker:* Identify those individuals who are likely to provide frank feedback about performance, decision-making, and other attributes. *Value* such feedback.
- *Prioritize self-evaluation:* High-performing leaders create a habit of jotting down strengths, weaknesses, and key decisions on a project-by-project basis or within a set monthly or quarterly timeframe. Note both thoughts on *how* to build strengths and improve upon weaknesses or setbacks, as well as the *deadline* to reach those objectives, and revisit these notes often.
- *Nurture authenticity:* Being authentic and genuine is one of the surest ways to cultivate trust. As Covey (2006) writes, trust is more than mere "touchy-feely" or a "nice-to-have" quality. The sky is the limit when one blends authentic, trustworthy leadership with self-awareness. Then, this currency will be used for good.
- *Hone in on a trademark "style":* Consider one's unique "brand" of influencing others. We are not talking about winning them or "love bombing" with kindness. Good leaders know leadership is not about "being liked." Rather, the ability to lead and inspire healthy **followership** is shaped by an understanding of one's "interpersonal" style and, importantly, its effect on others.
- *Go forward with confidence:* The connection between a strong sense of self and confidence is undeniable. So much of our self-confidence grows out of the ability to know who we are and what we stand for, and this combination of confidence and self-awareness propels significant strides in leadership prowess and on-the-job performance. Self-assured leaders understand that true rewards are garnered from tangible outcomes and progress—*not* from fleeting, even insincere, praise.

## LEADING OTHERS

We submit to you that leadership is a capacity. It can be learned and improved upon. Once you have gotten to know yourself, start with a blank slate when pondering the attributes that favorably contribute to your (and other's) ability to *lead well*.

It is never too early to develop and refine one's leadership style; however, it can become too late. If one waits to behave like an effective leader until they are formally appointed, the "goal" position or dream leadership role may remain out of reach. With the passage of time, a personal brand that is incongruous with the dream job can become embedded in other's minds. Instead, behave like a great leader, no matter current titles or formal responsibilities.

## THE ART OF FOLLOWERSHIP

We typically think of followers as the exact opposite of leaders. By definition, both the noun and verb suggest trailing behind or otherwise resulting from the leader before them. In a seminal *Harvard Business Review* article, "In Praise of Followers," which later evolved into *The Power of Followership*, Kelley (1988) posited that leaders and followers are often the "same people." He noted most managers have subordinates. Moreover, they share many essential (and beneficial) leadership qualities not limited to managing themselves well; committing to an employer's purpose, principles, and people; a passion for building upon competencies; and courage, honesty, and credibility.

Since the ultimate validation of a good leader is good performance, Kelley provided compelling research to support the value of mastering the "art" of followership. Kelley attributed 80% of an organization's outcomes, successes, and contributions to followers. Comparatively, he asserted that no more than 20% of these same outcomes may be attributed to leaders. The power of followers is illustrated in two key ways:

- Their role in carrying out the vision and strategies as tasked by leadership
- The weight their feedback plays in leaders crafting strategies to ultimately boost an institution's success/progress

Good followers are on the leadership "fast track"; they can be counted on to spearhead meetings and action items when the formal leader is otherwise indisposed. Healthcare presents a seemingly endless series of sudden pivots, obligations, and crises, making it all the more important for leaders to have such a trusted "follower" to lean in on as a reliable second-in-command. Be graceful. Rise to the occasion. After all, no one starts off leading a division, department, unit, clinic, or hospital. Take great care and intentionally incorporate followership into developing interpersonal and leadership styles.

## SEEING THE POSITIVE IN MISTAKES

Disappointments or missteps are often a wake-up call, sounding the alarm to simmering problems that require attention or a new direction. There is an art to reaping positives from seemingly negative failures or errors. To get the most out of these inevitable momentary setbacks or gray areas:

- Identify and address the issue head on, as difficult as it may seem. Do not procrastinate.
- Be honest about potential weaknesses that may have been amplified in one's decision-making or actions.
- Benefit from others who have "been there, done that." Seek the counsel of more seasoned executives and, moreover, be appreciative and open to the considerable wisdom that may be culled from constructive criticism.
- Do not play the "blame game." Take responsibility. Apologize as needed and be sufficiently humble to express regret.
- Observe and learn from how admired supervisors, mentors, and their ilk handle and overcome setbacks. Apply what is observed and their experiences into current thinking and future decision-making.

## AMPLIFY THE "CARE" IN "HEALTHCARE"

Routinely get back to the basics. What motivated you to go down the path of healthcare in the first place? Early careerists and seasoned executives alike will inevitably embrace trying circumstances at every career phase and life stage. Take a deep breath and remember: Healthcare is way more than a "job." It is absolutely a calling. Extend the same care that is observed in the doctor-nurse-patient relationship to one's staff and teams. A few pointers:

- Be an active and full participant in culture.
- Observe and learn from the culture.
- Be hungry to get things done.
- Acknowledge the contributions of others.
- Have fun! Understand unique organizational cultures to appropriately flourish at work *and* at play.
- Exercise kindness, but be wary of others taking advantage of such goodwill.

In another nod to the surprising contributors to leadership, consider how true leaders or spheres of influence can be found in the most unlikely of places. There may be an adored dietary or beloved environmental services staffer who is the wise "Yoda" of the hospital or practice. These individuals carry considerable clout and often informal, unwritten, unspoken, and implicit knowledge. This knowledge accumulates with years or decades of contributing within the four walls of a hospital or institution. Befriend these individuals in the most authentic and selfless of ways, and they will be an unwavering champion and sounding board as difficult conversations arise.

## DO NOT IGNORE THE "SNAKE"

Snake wrangling is probably the furthest thing from emerging healthcare leaders' minds. As a metaphor for a problem that can turn into a destructive force if allowed to lurk in the brush, the "snake" must be definitively squashed.

In a concept advanced by former leadership with Cerner (now Oracle Cerner), the "snake" or problem is dealt with swiftly and decisively—no second guessing. Similarly, this notion speaks to a "culture of accountability," whereby everyone rises and falls together. No one exists on an island or feels alone, left to their own devices to fruitlessly paddle or sink. Even when one's "charge" initially addresses the "snake," an effective leader follows up. Leadership ensures the snake does not somehow rear its head again or slither through the cracks. There is considerable unity in this approach.

## EMBRACE THE AVERAGE OF FIVE

There is nothing average about you with one notable exception, courtesy of Jim Rohn and his "Rule of Five." The late, great motivational speaker asserted that each of us is the average of the five people with whom we spend the most time. To support personal and professional growth, the company we keep ideally aligns with the latter versus the former sentiments. Notably, one's sphere or the resulting "average" that adds up to their collective influence is more complex and nebulous at best.

Our family members, friends, and colleagues have the capacity to elevate or drag us down (with them). We tend to become like those individuals within our "five." They shape our thoughts, beliefs, and behaviors. Scrutinize. Ask the tough questions. "Does this person push me to be better?" "Does this individual tempt me to coast?" "How is this individual similar, compatible, or complementary to me?" From there, adjust the amount of time that is spent with a given person based on those answers and introspection. Inventory at regular intervals. Careers are not static. Likewise, one's circle should never stand still. It should grow and evolve.

## THE STRENGTHS VERSUS WEAKNESSES CONUNDRUM

Considerable research substantiates the optimal potential realized by focusing on our dominant strengths; notably, the "Speed Reading Study" represents a cornerstone of strengths-based and positive development psychology. In "Investing in Strengths," Clifton and Harter (2003) took a deep dive into a 1950s-era research project that explored speed-reading improvements among 6,000 10th graders in Nebraska. Importantly, there were no "statistically significant differences" between the methods that were used by educators to teach rapid reading rates. Yet, it was found that "those students who read the fastest at the study's outset made the greatest gains ... from approximately 300 to 2,900 words per minute." Now, the students who read more slowly from the get-go also made gains but *they were small in comparison*.

What did these results tell Clifton and Harter? Namely, that we should resist the human predisposition to find fault and focus on weak areas. They advanced the notion of understanding each other's differences to then optimally position individuals, so they can then make the most of who they actually are (those talents). Through measurement and feedback—the "organizing framework" around positive psychology and potential—these authors contended that people who are self-aware of their innate talents are in a favorable position to understand their potential. According to Clifton and Harter, "They can then begin to integrate their awareness of their talents with knowledge and skills to develop strengths."

Alternately, when the laser focus is on weaknesses and beating oneself up over perceived deficiencies, confidence erodes, mistakes increase, and gains languish or stagnate. Here again, a formal framework or tests are the launchpad to understand one's inherent positives. Then, one actively solicits feedback (do not wait for it) and regularly reviews observations from others or formal performance reviews to glean additional external insights.

## PLAYING TO STRENGTHS IN HEALTHCARE: THE LEADERSHIP DYAD

*Dyad* is a term that refers to two individuals in what is characterized as "sociologically significant" relationships. In healthcare, the leadership dyad is typically made up of two "copartners," a physician leader and administrative leader. The definitive characteristic here is *complementarity*, the idea that two heads are better than one.

While this model has been accelerated in healthcare over the past 12 years, the pandemic underscored the value of its attributes. Our enterprises, medical groups, service lines, and departments have never been faced with more changes and crises. The Medical Group Management Association (2020) found that 77% of the more than 1,300 healthcare leaders surveyed were using the physician-administrator dyad model to collaborate and colead in overcoming and getting ahead of challenges presented in the current care environment (Gumminger, 2020).

When enthusiastically embarking on a coleadership relationship, it is essential to assess for "fit," the same type of fit that may be scrutinized within one's own team, circle, or network. Furthermore, it is essential for the coleaders within the relationship to intentionally work on their communication and synergies. A good starting point to assess and understand one's traits and how they intersect with the coleader (and in other relationships) is the NEO PI-R™ (NEO Personality Inventory-Revised™).

This assessment tool evaluates the "big five"—those key facets of one's personality. These five facets are as follows:

- *Emotionality:* The need for stability and how we react to and understand anger, stress, worry, and other negative emotions

- *Extraversion:* How we respond to social interactions and our general disposition in social situations
- *Openness:* The proclivity toward exploring ideas and nurturing curiosity
- *Agreeableness:* Our level of self-interest or service to others
- *Conscientiousness:* The structure in which we work (i.e., orderliness, discipline)

When two leaders enter into the dyad, they must set common ground rules before their complementarity in the aforementioned areas can shine and thrive. The idea of building upon and celebrating synergies and complementary strengths should also filter down and through the rest of the organization. By its nature, the dyad plays up synergistic strengths. This approach helps to keep poisonous cultures at bay; when similarities instead of synergies are the focus, harmful ingroups and outgroups can arise. These disparate groups may be based on gender identity, religious beliefs, or race or ethnic identity. As one might surmise, these divisions neither facilitate healthy team-building nor do they drive progress and performance.

By starting with truly complementary physician-admin leader dyads who then work on fostering and sustaining trust and transparency, these copartners lead and keep teams moving forward, in sync and unified. Unity at the top very much trickles down to unity throughout the organization, as leadership really sets the tone. MedAxiom executives who use the dyad model suggested in the American College of Cardiology's *Cardiology Magazine* (2020) the following practical steps for the clinician embarking into a relationship with an admin:

- Agree with the vision.
- Work on communicating it effectively.
- Consider the administrator as a true partner or peer (not a subordinate).
- Lead by example.

Likewise, administrative dyad leaders can benefit from the following:

- Articulating the "why" (the importance of the vision)
- Making timely decisions
- Pushing past barriers
- Providing the flexibility to perform
- Staying highly organized and understanding clinical domains

See the give and take and how these clinical-administrative partners should fit together like jigsaw pieces in a puzzle? They may not be exactly the same and that notion is very much the point of the dyad model; however, they still fit together seamlessly to complete the whole.

## LEADERSHIP COMPETENCIES

There is no "silver bullet" to high-performance leadership. Moreover, the path toward a career that gets results is often littered with seeming contradictions; for instance, so-called "soft skills" provide a very solid foundation for performance. Savvy, people-oriented leaders inspire enthusiasm and trust in ways that cold, calculating, results-at-all-costs leaders cannot.

In fact, Flaum (2018) developed a research-based report in conjunction with Cornell University that summarizes the "heart" of what makes an effective leader tick in the aptly titled: "When It Comes to Business Leadership, Nice Guys Finish First." As they concluded from an assessment of 72 executives at companies cutting a wide swathe of industries, the conventional wisdom is wrong. It is those leaders with strengths in the "soft skills" who perform better at driving hard results. These leaders are not "doormats," researchers asserted, but they

- are self-aware;
- hold teams accountable;
- make and deliver tough decisions in ways that are inspirational and fair—*not* abusive or "take no prisoners";
- cultivate "productive" conflict versus snuffing out challenges to the status quo; and
- exercise humility.

Such characteristics are essential to healthcare environments, which by definition are centered on the health and well-being of the clinician, staff, and community stakeholders, and the delivery of care that serves and heals.

## TRANSCENDING SMARTS

Similarly, we tend to give outsized credit to intelligence (IQ), technical competencies, and hard skills when assessing top-performing leaders within institutions. We do not give adequate credit to **emotional intelligence** (EI or EQ). But the tide is turning, due in no small part to the work of Goleman (2005). In his definitive book on the subject, *Emotional Intelligence*, the psychologist stated that effective leaders are unified by one common element:

> "They all have a high degree of what has come to be known as emotional intelligence. It's not that IQ and technical skills are irrelevant. They do matter, but mainly as threshold capabilities; that is, they are entry-level requirements for executive positions. But my research, along with other recent studies, clearly shows that emotional intelligence is the sine qua non of leadership."

He concluded that this human quotient sets mere tacticians apart from true leaders. We urge intentionality in assessing and building upon the following attributes of the emotionally intelligent leader (as highlighted by Dr. Goleman):

- *Self-awareness:* Recognition and understanding of emotions, motivations, and impact
- *Self-management:* Emotional regulation, flexibility, striving, and positivity
- *Social awareness:* Empathy, relational and organizational awareness
- *Relationship management:* Influence, coaching, mentoring, conflict resolution, and teamwork

Carnegie Institute of Technology (1918) researchers reportedly determined that 85% of one's financial successes is due to "human engineering skills." These skills include communication, negotiation, and leadership competencies. IQ or technical knowledge only accounted for the balance of those successes (at 15%). Such research further supports the so-called "Peter principle." Developed by Peter (1984), the self-proclaimed "hierarchiologist" posited that individuals within a hierarchy tend to rise to their "respective level of incompetence"; individuals are continuously promoted based on performance in given roles rather than technical competency in specific positions or areas. This ascendancy in the hierarchy continues only until levels are reached in which they have *no competence* and their current knowledge and skills fall short of the demands and responsibilities placed on them in the higher, present role.

Readers can stand out favorably, regardless of levels within a hospital system, by continuously working on EQ proficiency. In analyzing over 1 million frontline staff to C-suite-level workers, clinical and organizational psychologist Bradberry (2015) found those employees with the highest EQ scores tended to be middle managers. Scores to measure or quantify EQ climbed from the bottom upward until a point; once middle management was reached, scores suddenly started to go south. As Bradberry contended:

> "Once leaders get promoted, they enter an environment that tends to erode their emotional intelligence. They spend less time in meaningful interactions with their staff and lose sight of how their emotional states affect those around them. It's so easy to get out of touch that leaders' EQ levels sink further. It truly is lonely at the top."

The best performers among those top executives resisted this plight and managed to maintain their people savvy. There is a direct and positive correlation between performance and EQ scores with the author saying that, for every title and position analyzed, peak performers "are those with the highest EQ scores." So, while readers may get their foot in the corner office, it is unlikely that they will outshine their emotionally intelligent competition in a top role. Furthermore, in a longitudinal study of the drivers for executive derailments, the Center for Creative Leadership (1996) noted how low EQ factors were referenced by 50% of senior executives surveyed from across Fortune 500 companies in North America (Leslie & Van Velsor, 1996). They cited the following damaging behaviors:

- Inflexible management styles
- Use of outdated management approaches
- Stubbornness to the point of completely resisting change
- Poor working relationships
- Poor communication skills
- Failure to listen
- A lack of trustworthiness
- Inability to play well in the sandbox

In fact, one failed or derailed executive was described as "leaving dead bodies everywhere." As an observer would put it, "He would have people hanging out to dry if they wouldn't do what he wanted. He would push them to do what he wanted and then deny any involvement."

Nowhere in these summaries of key reasons for executive failures do we see references to technical know-how, training, cognitive capacity, or IQ overshadowing the EI, EQ, or human quotient. Fortunately, careerists who begin early to make analyses and improvements in areas like self-awareness second nature will be well ahead of others who never quite mastered themselves and fundamental interpersonal skills. Building upon this excellent starting point:

- Continuous work on self-awareness overcomes the initially awkward process of engaging in inner dialogues and honest self-reflection.
- "Self-regulation" also becomes second nature, as one consistently catalogues circumstances, pinpoints patterns, and sets and moves goalposts (as needed).
- The art of identifying sources of meaningful and helpful criticism is refined. Furthermore, these valuable insights do not sit on a shelf but are accounted for in actions and decisions.

## CONCLUSION

In the dynamic realm of healthcare management, leadership stands as a linchpin for organizational success. The insights gleaned from this exploration underscore the indispensable role of self-awareness in guiding effective leadership. By embracing authenticity, humility, and a commitment to continuous improvement, healthcare managers can foster a culture of excellence within their organizations. Moreover, the significance of followership cannot be overstated, as engaged and empowered followers are the lifeblood of organizational progress. As leadership paradigms evolve, the adoption of dyad models presents exciting opportunities for collaboration and synergy. By honing emotional intelligence, healthcare managers can enhance their leadership efficacy and amplify their organizational impact. Ultimately, the journey toward effective leadership is a continuous process of self-discovery and refinement, with each step forward paving the way for transformative change within healthcare institutions.

## END-OF-CHAPTER RESOURCES

### CRITICAL THINKING QUESTIONS

- How does self-awareness contribute to a leader's ability to effectively lead themselves and others?
- In what ways can leadership or personality assessments be helpful for leaders, and what benefits does this habit offer?
- Discuss the correlation between poor self-awareness and an alienating interpersonal style. How does this impact individual performance, team dynamics, and organizational culture?
- What strategies can leaders employ to consistently demonstrate **integrity** in their leadership approach? Consider the downside(s) of lapses in integrity and what ways leaders can best proactively protect themselves from the resultant negative impact.
- Why is followership important in leadership, and how can leaders both demonstrate and cultivate healthy followership in their teams/organizations?
- Consider examples of how insecurity can hinder leadership effectiveness. How can leaders mitigate it through self-awareness, personal/professional development, and mentoring/coaching?
- Explore the benefits and challenges of the leadership dyad model, particularly in healthcare settings. What attributes and complementarities are crucial for success in this model?
- Discuss the role of emotional intelligence (EQ) in leadership performance and success, regardless of career stage or title. How can leaders bolster their EQ skills to excel in their roles?
- Explore the reciprocal nature of mentorship relationships and how they benefit both mentors and mentees. How can mentees actively engage in the mentorship process to ensure mutual growth and development?
- Discuss the importance of aligning personal values, strengths, and long-term goals in the process of career strategic planning. How can individuals identify and leverage their unique attributes to create a road map for career advancement and fulfillment?

### LEARNING ACTIVITIES

**CourseConnect ▶**

To access self-assessment questions and interactive, competency-based learning activities for this chapter, visit www.springerpub.com/courseconnect. See inside front cover and tear-out card for CourseConnect details.

### REFERENCES

Bradberry, T. (2015, March 17). Why leaders lack emotional intelligence. *Inc.* https://www.inc.com/travis-bradberry/why-leaders-lack-emotional-intelligence.html

Clifton, D., & Harter, J. (2003). *Investing in strengths.* http://media.gallup.com/documents/whitepaper--investinginstrengths.pdf

Covey, S. M. R. (2006). *The speed of trust: The one thing that changes everything.* Free Press.

Drucker, P. (1977). *People and performance.* William Heinemann Limited.

Flaum, J. (2018, September). *When it comes to business leadership, nice guys finish first*. Green Peak Partners.

Goleman, D. (2005). *Emotional intelligence: Why it can matter more than IQ* (10th Anniversary ed.). Random House Publishing Group.

Gumminger, G. (2020, December 15). *Advantages of the dyad leadership model for healthcare organizations*. Thrive Global.

Kelley, R. (1988, November–December). In praise of followers. *Harvard Business Review*. https://hbr.org/1988/11/in-praise-of-followers

Leslie, J., & Van Velsor, E. (1996). *A look at derailment today: North America and Europe*. Center for Creative Leadership.

Peter, L. (1984). *Why things go wrong or the peter principle revisited*. William Morrow & Company.

Tjan, A. (2012, July 19). How leaders become self-aware. *Harvard Business Review*. https://hbr.org/2012/07/how-leaders-become-self-aware

Tjan, A., Harrington, R., & Hsieh, T. (2012). *Heart, smarts, guts, and luck*. Harvard Business Review Press.

Toegel, G., Liu, F., Coughlan, S. L., & Perrinjaquet, M. (2012, May). *Leadership dyads: Playing to your strengths*. Insights@IMD.

CHAPTER 27

# CASE: A LEADERSHIP DILEMMA: NAVIGATING CULTURE CHANGE IN A SURGICAL DEPARTMENT

Tiara Walz, Tiara Owens, and Lina Maria Alfonso

## LEARNING OBJECTIVES

- Apply conceptual and theoretical learning to real-world examples through a case study.
- Analyze and address contextual factors leading to a leadership dilemma.
- Incorporate professional and ethical considerations while devising innovative solutions for conflict resolution.
- Consider diversity, equity, and inclusion principles in the workplace, while also cultivating a culture conducive to thriving within the healthcare environment.
- Identify relevant theories from the textbook to improve morale and culture in the workplace as a healthcare leader.

## KEY CONCEPTS

- Communication techniques
- Conflict prevention
- Emotional intelligence
- Employee satisfaction
- Leadership theories
- Organizational culture
- Patient experience

## INTRODUCTION

In the constantly evolving landscape of healthcare, hospitals face numerous challenges that require adept leadership and strategic planning. This case explores a healthcare management dilemma related to professionalism, interpersonal challenges, and a potentially toxic work environment.

## MAJOR CHALLENGES/DILEMMA

Jessica has recently been hired at Tri-Star Terrace Lakes Medical Center (TTLMC) as the Surgical Services Senior Administrator where she oversees a team of diverse and skilled nurses, surgeons, and support staff. In her initial month of employment, the leadership team emphasized the importance of culture and building a strong employee retention pipeline. She knows that the surgical department faces significant challenges due to previous leadership and staff changes, as well as what she has seen since being hired. Jessica's first priorities in her new role are to focus on improving the culture between medical and administrative personnel in her department and boosting overall employee morale.

Conflicts that have been noted in the department include strained relationships among surgical nurses and surgeons, discontent toward the previous administrator, and a lack of trust among support staff. These disputes risk impacting communication, teamwork, and ultimately, patient outcomes. Recently, a specific incident has resulted in tensions reaching a critical point, necessitating prompt intervention.

Reaching the end of a busy shift, a surgeon leaves the operating room after an extensive surgery. After the procedure, the surgeon walks into the recovery unit and makes a loud, unprofessional comment to the staff regarding the surgery taking longer than anticipated due to the patient being overweight, along with other risk-associated factors. Another patient in the recovery unit overhears the surgeon. The patient subsequently calls one of the charge nurses to voice their concerns regarding overhearing such a sensitive issue and the observed surgeon's behavior.

A hushed conversation unfolds between the lead charge nurse, Christina, and another agitated staff member regarding the recent incident. Christina, concerned about the situation, decides to bring it to the attention of Jessica. Sarah, another staff member, overheard the exchange and started sharing her opinions with colleagues. Word quickly spread, turning the incident into a topic of discussion among the department staff.

Jessica, now aware of the brewing discontent, knows she needs to act. She addresses the issue head-on, recognizing the importance of maintaining a positive and professional environment. As part of her initial investigation, Jessica approaches the patient involved and directly seeks their feedback. The patient, visibly affected by the incident, expresses that the comment made by the physician was unnecessary and unprofessional. The patient asks, "Why didn't my presence warrant more professional demeanor from the hospital staff?" The patient informs Jessica that they will be filling out a patient feedback survey to ensure their voice is heard.

This dilemma not only sheds light on the importance of maintaining a respectful and considerate environment in healthcare but also emphasizes the significance of patient perspectives in shaping the quality of care provided. The conflict is rooted in a combination of factors, including communication breakdowns, low employee morale, vocalized unprofessional behavior among the staff, and a spillover effect to patient care. This incident has further heightened the discomfort within the team, thus putting the reputation of the surgical department and TTLMC at risk.

## ORGANIZATIONAL OVERVIEW

TTLMC, a member of the Terrace Lakes Healthcare System, is a world-class, nonprofit, 647-bed multispecialty academic medical center in the urban, metropolitan healthcare landscape of New Orleans, Louisiana. Founded in 1951, Terrace Lakes Healthcare System comprises a network of 12 hospitals and 20 community clinics, staffing over 35,500 employees, including more than 5,200 dedicated physicians.

With a population estimate of 369,749, according to the 2022 data from the United States Census Bureau (n.d.), TTLMC is in the center of a diverse city in the United States with a racial composition breakdown of 58.1% Black or African American, 32.7% White, 5.6% Hispanic or Latinx, 2.7% Asian, and 4.1% two or more races. The communities TTLMC serves face many barriers to achieving health equity, including health disparities and food insecurity. In fact, according to an annual report by Feeding America, 13.8% of seniors living in New Orleans experience food insecurity, marking the lowest level of food security among seniors in the United States (Ziliak & Gundersen, 2023). As one of New Orleans' metropolitan hospitals, TTLMC caters predominantly to an uninsured and underinsured patient demographic, thus encountering a challenging patient-payer mix. TTLMC provides care to many rural, low-income patients, primarily serving Medicaid and Medicare enrollees, while a smaller segment of the population is insured by private/commercial payers. The facility is known for its diverse and skilled workforce, representing the community that it serves and has become a hub for collaboration and high-quality patient care.

TTLMC provides specialty services in emergency medicine, surgical services, neurology, obstetrics, nephrology, and cardiology but stands as a beacon of surgical excellence in Louisiana's southern region's only level 1 trauma center. In addition to scheduled surgical procedures, TTLMC has surgical critical care-trained surgeons in house 24/7, is a training site for robotic surgery, and has one of the busiest surgical departments in Louisiana, conducting about 5,000 to 6,500 surgeries each year.

The vision for TTLMC is to be the premier destination for surgical excellence, offering innovative, compassionate, and exceptional care to its diverse community. This academic medical center envisions a healthcare landscape where its surgical department sets the benchmark for precision, safety, and patient satisfaction. Patient safety is of the utmost priority. Their team of highly skilled surgeons, anesthetists, nurses, and support staff collaborates seamlessly to deliver comprehensive and personalized surgical solutions.

## STAKEHOLDERS

- *Senior administrator:* Jessica's main priority is improving workplace culture while maintaining a positive environment for her clinical providers, staff, and patients.
- *Surgeons:* Surgeons are responsible for performing successful surgeries and providing leadership to the nursing and support staff.
- *Nursing staff/anesthesiologists/technicians:* The clinical staff support surgeons in the operating room and recovery, coordinate patient care, and ensure hospital policies and procedures are followed while caring for their patients.
- *Department support staff:* The support staff handle daily administrative tasks, ensure standards and compliance, and serve as liaisons to the patients in their care.
- *Patients:* Arguably the most important stakeholders, patients are the recipients of the healthcare services provided by the surgical department. They deserve high-quality patient care from compassionate, qualified professionals.

Culture issues and toxicity in the workplace have the potential to adversely affect all stakeholders involved. Furthermore, every stakeholder in the surgical department shares a vested interest in ensuring the well-being of patients, maintaining the quality of care, and safeguarding the reputation and prestige of TTLMC.

## CONSIDERATIONS

Jessica must focus on the work culture issues within her department. Employee feedback and input must be actively sought to understand the root causes of conflict, and open communication channels should be established to foster a culture of transparency. Professional development and training programs can play a crucial role in enhancing team dynamics, providing team members with the skills needed to navigate conflicts and collaborate effectively. Leadership and role modeling become paramount in setting the tone for a cohesive and respectful work environment.

Simultaneously, a thorough policy review and enforcement mechanism should be implemented to ensure adherence to guidelines that promote teamwork and patient-centered care. Team building initiatives can help rebuild trust and collaboration among team members, and conflict resolution mechanisms should be in place to address issues promptly. Establishing clear performance metrics and accountability measures will encourage a sense of responsibility among team members, fostering a commitment to continuous monitoring and improvement.

Long-term sustainability requires collaboration not only within the surgical team but also with human resources (HR) and legal departments. By prioritizing patient-centered care and maintaining a focus on the hospital's reputation, the organization can work toward resolving the observed challenges and restoring a positive and efficient surgical environment.

## KEY DECISIONS

- Address overall environment in the surgical department.
- Investigate the reported incident thoroughly.
- Take appropriate actions to rectify the situation(s), considering the interests of all stakeholders.

## MAJOR OUTCOME

The priority in this case is to establish and implement a cohesive strategy aimed at fostering a psychologically safe and inclusive environment for both hospital employees and patients. In particular, the major outcome should focus on improving the team morale, addressing a negative culture/climate, and addressing the direct patient impact response. These outcomes collectively contribute to the improvement and creation of a healthy, supportive, and high-performing culture within the surgical department.

## DISCUSSION QUESTIONS

1. Could this situation in the surgical department have been avoided? If so, how?
2. How could Jessica use her leadership skills to help manage this conflict?

3. How should Jessica handle:
   a. The patient complaint?
   b. The surgeon involved?
   c. Other internal stakeholders?
4. Which leadership theory or theories could Jessica consider using to manage team conflict?
5. What principles of diversity, equity, and inclusion could Jessica incorporate as she develops her leadership and conflict resolution strategies?
6. What leadership competencies should Jessica demonstrate to her team members to bring about change in the culture of the surgical department?
7. What measures can Jessica put in place to prevent future conflict and promote a positive and productive work environment?
8. What additional consequences could the department and TTLMC face if this situation is not addressed and/or resolved in a timely manner?
9. Discuss policies or procedures that could be implemented at the department level to prevent this dilemma from recurring.

## RESOURCES

Bregman, P. (2016, January 11). The right way to hold people accountable. *Harvard Business Review*. https://hbr.org/2016/01/the-right-way-to-hold-people-accountable

Brett, J. M., & Goldberg, S. B. (2017, July 10). How to handle a disagreement on your team. *Harvard Business Review*. https://hbr.org/2017/07/how-to-handle-a-disagreement-on-your-team

McKinley, S., & Zielinski, L. (2019, July 15). *Turning conflict into collaboration: How to manage workplace disagreements*. Healthcare Financial Management Association. https://www.hfma.org/leadership/turning-conflict-into-collaboration-how-to-manage-workplace-dis/

Piryani, R. M., & Piryani, S. (2019). Conflict management in healthcare. *Journal of Nepal Health Research Council*, 16(41), 481–482.

Ronquillo, Y., Ellis, V. L., & Toney-Butler, T. J. (2023). Conflict management. In StatPearls [Internet]. StatPearls Publishing. https://www.ncbi.nlm.nih.gov/books/NBK470432/

The Economic Times. (2023, December 7). *Leadership and conflict resolution: Navigating challenges in the workplace*. https://economictimes.indiatimes.com/jobs/c-suite/leadership-and-conflict-resolution-navigating-challenges-in-the-workplace/articleshow/104647514.cms

## REFERENCES

United States Census Bureau. (n.d.). *QuickFacts: New Orleans City, Louisiana*. https://www.census.gov/quickfacts/fact/table/neworleanscitylouisiana/PST120222

Ziliak, J. P., & Gundersen, C. (2023, April 26). *The state of senior hunger in America in 2021: An annual report*. https://www.feedingamerica.org/sites/default/files/2023-04/State%20of%20Senior%20Hunger%20in%202021.pdf

# GLOSSARY

**Abuse**  Refers to payment for items or services when there is no legal entitlement to that payment, without the individual or entity knowingly or intentionally misrepresenting facts to obtain payment.

**Accountable care organizations (ACO)**  Groups of physicians, hospitals, and other healthcare providers who voluntarily come together to provide coordinated, high-quality care to Medicare patients.

**Actuarially fair premium**  The expected medical expenses associated with an individual or population, calculated as the product of health status risk and medical care risk, limited to medical expenses.

**Acute care**  Short-term medical services addressing acute illnesses or injuries requiring prompt medical attention, including emergency medicine, surgery, trauma care, critical care, and intensive care.

**Addressing health disparities**  Involves identifying and eliminating preventable differences in health outcomes among populations. Strategies include policy reform, targeted interventions, and community engagement to achieve equity.

**Advertising**  Paid promotions of healthcare services using traditional media (TV, radio, newspapers) and digital platforms.

**Affinity groups**  Provide platforms for individuals with shared backgrounds or identities to connect, advocate for inclusivity, and foster a supportive workplace culture. Alongside employee resource groups (ERGs), these groups offer support and advocacy.

**After-action reviews (AAR)**  Document feedback from participants involved in an incident or exercise. The process identifies successful actions and areas for improvement, helping organizations adapt to changing environments.

**Alternative payment models (APM)**  Value-based reimbursement models designed to promote high-quality, cost-efficient care through incentive payments.

**Alternative strategies**  Organizational approaches to achieving strategic goals. Each alternative has pros and cons, requiring careful analysis to select the most effective approach.

**Anti-racism**  An active commitment to challenging and dismantling racist beliefs, policies, and practices. It involves advocating for racial equity, actively opposing racism, and supporting initiatives aimed at creating an inclusive and just society for all.

**Artificial intelligence (AI)**  The capability of computers or machines to perform tasks requiring human intelligence, such as summarizing information, learning from experiences, identifying patterns, and recognizing speech.

**Assessment**  The systematic collection, analysis, and interpretation of data in order to understand the health of a community and identify factors that influence it.

**Asymmetric information**  A situation where one party in a negotiation has more relevant information than the other.

**Attract**  Refers to the proactive strategies used by healthcare organizations to draw in diverse talent. This includes recruiting candidates from underrepresented communities, forming partnerships with diversity-focused organizations, and using inclusive language in job descriptions and outreach materials. Attracting diverse candidates is the first step in building an inclusive workforce and signals a clear commitment to equity and belonging.

**Autonomy**  The right of individuals to make their own decisions, which may be limited in some instances, such as with infants or children who lack legal capacity.

**Belonging**  The emotional experience of being accepted, included, and valued in a group or environment. In healthcare, it reflects an inclusive culture where individuals feel connected, respected, and empowered to contribute authentically.

**Beneficence**  The obligation of healthcare managers to act for the benefit of their organization and patients by preventing, removing, or mitigating harm.

**Beneficiary**  In health insurance, the individual covered by the insurance.

**BIPOC (Black, Indigenous, and People of Color)**  An acronym that highlights the unique experiences and challenges faced by Black, Indigenous, and People of Color individuals. It acknowledges the shared struggles against racism and discrimination and emphasizes the need for support, understanding, and allyship among these diverse communities.

**Blockchain technology**  A digital ledger technology applied in healthcare to preserve and exchange patient data among hospitals, laboratories, pharmacies, and physicians, reducing errors and enhancing accuracy.

**Budgeting**  A managerial accounting process involving the planning and control of financial resources.

**Burnout**  A state characterized by emotional exhaustion, detachment, cynicism, and a diminished sense of personal accomplishment.

**Buyer behavior**  The process consumers use to make decisions, influenced by rational factors (e.g., wait times) and emotional aspects (e.g., reputations).

**Career framework**  A structured approach to understanding career progression and stages.

**Career Stages**  Distinct phases in a career that is marked by evolving roles, responsibilities, skills and goals.

**Case rate**  A flat reimbursement amount to a provider for all services during an episode of care, promoting value-based care.

**Causal loop diagram**  A tool to understand system behaviors by identifying feedback and behavior cycles within a system.

**Change acceleration process**  The process of moving from the current state to an improved state by expediting transitions and maintaining results.

**Change management**  Frameworks and methodologies to help stakeholders navigate transitions during projects, creating a safe and supportive environment.

**Chief financial officer (CFO)**  The top financial expert in an organization, responsible for managing financial resources, reporting financial health, and advising on strategic decisions.

**Civil laws**  Laws addressing disputes between private parties, aiming to compensate the injured party.

**Coinsurance**  The portion of medical costs the insured person must pay after meeting the annual deductible.

**Community rating**  A method of estimating medical expenses based on the average costs of all individuals.

**Community rating by class**  A method that groups individuals, stratifies the population, and calculates expenses based on group composition.

**Compensatory damages**  Monetary compensation for lost wages, medical bills, and pain and suffering awarded to the injured party.

**Competencies**  Required knowledge, behaviors, skills and abilities required to perform within a specific profession or job.

**Complex adaptive systems**  Systems characterized by self-organization, unpredictability, and interactions among individual parts, such as healthcare teams.
**Compliance**  Adherence to healthcare laws, regulations, and policies.
**Comprehensive emergency management**  A cycle addressing all hazards through mitigation, preparedness, response, and recovery.
**Conflict in values**  When personal values clash with organizational values or activities.
**Content marketing**  Publishing stories and statements to promote an organization's brand, products, or services.
**Contingency**  An approach leveraging leaders' experience to match actions with likely outcomes within an organizational context.
**Continuum of care**  The spectrum of healthcare services needed throughout a condition, injury, or lifetime.
**Copayment**  The out-of-pocket amount paid at the time of medical service.
**Core functions of public health**  Refers to the essential activities and responsibilities that public health systems undertake to protect and improve the health of populations. These functions typically include assessment, policy development, and assurance.
**Cost accounting**  A managerial accounting tool that helps organizations determine the cost of providing a good or service.
**Criminal law**  Sanctions individuals, organizations, and business entities for violating rules that the society has determined are necessary to protect the public.
**Crisis communications**  Involves alerts, warnings, and messages related to an organization's response and guidance to its constituents. These messages address the needs of patients, survivors, employees, media, and other stakeholders.
**Crisis leadership**  Denotes the capacity of an individual in a leadership role to navigate an organization, team, or community through periods characterized by significant adversity, uncertainty, or threat. It encompasses the ability to make high-stakes decisions under pressure, sustain clear and consistent communication, and foster trust, confidence, and resilience among stakeholders.
**Crisis management**  The method an organization uses to address disruptive incidents that may cause harm to the entity. The goal is increased readiness and resilience.
**Cultural competency (behaviors)**  Actions that demonstrate awareness, sensitivity, and responsiveness to the cultural identities and needs of others. These include effective communication, adaptation of care, and respectful engagement across cultural differences.
**Cultural competency**  The ability to understand, appreciate, and effectively interact with individuals from diverse cultural backgrounds. It involves knowledge of different cultures, respect for cultural differences, and the ability to adapt communication and practices to be inclusive and culturally sensitive.
**Cultural humility**  An ongoing process of self-reflection and self-critique that involves acknowledging one's cultural biases and limitations. It emphasizes a commitment to learning from and respecting diverse cultural perspectives and experiences.
**Culturally and Linguistically Appropriate Services (CLAS)**  Refers to services and practices in healthcare and other fields that consider and respect the cultural and linguistic diversity of the individuals being served. It aims to provide equitable and inclusive care and support for diverse populations, including those with limited English proficiency.
**Customer relations management (CRM)**  Technology-centric management of customer data at all levels of the business relationship. CRM connects providers and consumers in healthcare, analyzes customer needs, and delivers tailored services to enhance retention.

**Data analytics**  The science and art of using tools and processes to extract information, knowledge, and insight to drive operational decisions.

**Data cleaning**  Process of identifying and correcting errors, inconsistencies, or inaccuracies in data to improve its quality. This includes handling missing values, removing duplicates, and correcting formatting issues.

**Data life cycle**  The generation, collection, processing/validation, storage/management, analysis/visualization, and data tracking in a continuous cycle.

**Data preprocessing**  Broader step that prepares raw data for analysis or modeling. It includes data cleaning, as well as transforming, normalizing, encoding, and splitting data to make it suitable for machine learning or statistical analysis.

**Data visualization**  The presentation of data using visual elements such as colors, graphs, maps, and dashboards.

**Deductible**  The annual amount due for medical services before a health insurance company contributes its portion of the costs.

**Demand**  A model involving trade between individuals and/or firms who supply a good or service and those who demand and purchase it.

**Digital marketing**  A mix of strategies leveraging consumer data to deliver customized messaging through email, advertising, social media, and paid search.

**Direct marketing**  Sending messages directly to potential buyers, often personalized, through email, phone, or postal mail.

**Disaster**  Events damaging an organization's reputation and/or assets.

**Display ads**  Digital advertisements displayed on electronic devices, much like billboards or posters in outdoor advertising.

**Diverse leadership representation**  Ensures that decision-makers reflect the populations they serve. It supports inclusive policy development, equitable practices, and accountability for organizational DEI goals.

**Diversity**  A varied workforce that mirrors patient demographics, supported by inclusive hiring practices and measurable diversity goals.

**Diversity mastery**  Refers to the ability to recognize, understand, and apply diversity principles effectively within an organization. It involves intentional practice in fostering representation, equity, and inclusion across teams and decision-making processes.

**DMAIC**  A problem-solving structure—Define, Measure, Analyze, Improve, and Control—enhancing Lean and Six Sigma techniques for better outcomes.

**Dynamic complexity**  A concept in systems thinking where the effects of actions differ in the short term versus the long term.

**Early career**  Initial phase that is focused skill-building, gaining experience, learning by doing and establishing credibility.

**Email marketing**  Direct marketing outreach to a target audience via email, often using lists purchased or generated internally.

**Emergency**  A sudden, unforeseen event or situation that poses an immediate threat to life, property, the environment, or public health, and requires urgent intervention to prevent escalation into a full-scale disaster. It typically demands rapid decision-making, mobilization of resources, and coordinated response efforts to mitigate harm and restore stability. Employee Resource Groups (ERGs) and Affinity Groups are voluntary associations of employees who come together based on shared characteristics or experiences, such as race, ethnicity, gender, or sexual orientation. These groups provide support, networking opportunities, and a platform for discussing specific concerns and advocating for inclusive practices within organizations.

**Emotional intelligence**  The combined attributes of self-awareness, self-management, social awareness, and relationship management.

**Employee engagement**  The emotional commitment and involvement employees feel toward their organization and its goals.

**Employee relations**  The management of relationships between employees and their employer, impacting a positive work environment and ensuring compliance.

**Employee resource groups (ERGs)**  Platforms for individuals with shared identities to connect, advocate for inclusivity, and contribute to workplace culture.

**Employee retention**  Organizational policies and practices designed to encourage employees to remain with the company.

**Employer-sponsored insurance**  Health insurance fully or partially purchased by employers for eligible employees and their families.

**Employment law**  The set of legal rights belonging to employees, including protections against discrimination, harassment, and retaliation.

**Encore career**  A later-life culminating stage emphasizing legacy, service that involves a shift from professional success to creating lasting significance.

**Endemic**  A disease or agent that is present or usually prevalent in a geographic area or population.

**End-of-life services**  Care provided to individuals near the end of life, addressing physical, emotional, social, and spiritual needs of both patients and their families.

**Engage**  Involves cultivating an environment where diverse employees feel connected and equipped to succeed. Healthcare organizations support engagement by providing training in cultural competency, unconscious bias, and effective communication. These programs, alongside continuous learning opportunities tailored to diverse needs, build an inclusive culture of growth and respect.

**Enhanced patient trust**  Arises when individuals feel respected, heard, and safe in healthcare environments. Culturally responsive care, diverse staffing, and transparent communication are critical to building this trust.

**Epidemic**  An extensive outbreak of a disease affecting many people at the same time, usually spreading rapidly.

**Equilibrium**  A state of balance where supply and demand curves cross.

**Equity**  Actively involving staff, learners, and patients in decision-making; ensuring access to opportunities; and addressing systemic barriers to growth.

**Ethics**  The moral principles guiding healthcare professionals, researchers, and policymakers in their actions.

**Evaluation**  A reflective assessment to analyze project outcomes, identify successes and areas for improvement, and align results with objectives.

**Execution**  The transition of healthcare projects from planning to action, where concepts are realized through team collaboration.

**Executive branch**  Promulgates regulations and issues executive orders. At the federal level, this branch is led by the president; at the state level, by governors.

**Experience rating**  A method of predicting medical expenses based exclusively on prior medical expenses of the individual or group.

**Externalities**  Positive or negative outcomes where the market fails to produce the right quantity at the right price.

**Federalism**  A system dividing powers and responsibilities between multiple levels of government, such as federal, state, and local levels.

**Feedback loops**  Mechanisms where a system responds to changes through balancing and reinforcing loops illustrating interactions between elements.

**Financial accounting**  The recording and reporting of an organization's financial information using standardized guidelines.

**Financial management**  Short- and long-term decision-making aimed at optimizing an organization's efficiency and profitability.

**Followership**   The ability or willingness to follow a leader. Effective followership involves understanding one's interpersonal style and its impact on others.

**Fraud**   Knowingly and willfully executing or attempting to execute a scheme to defraud any healthcare benefit program or obtain money or property through false pretenses.

**Gender identity**   An individual's internal sense of their own gender, which may or may not align with the sex assigned to them at birth. Recognizing and affirming diverse gender identities is essential for creating an inclusive and respectful space for all individuals.

**Global health**   Health problems, issues, and concerns that transcend national boundaries, influenced by circumstances in other countries, and best addressed through cooperative actions.

**Health disparities**   The state where no one is denied the opportunity to be healthy due to belonging to historically disadvantaged groups.

**Health disparity**   Preventable differences in the burden of disease, injury, violence, or opportunities to achieve optimal health experienced by socially disadvantaged groups.

**Health equity**   The principle of ensuring that all individuals have equal opportunities to achieve optimal health outcomes, regardless of their social or economic background. It involves addressing underlying social determinants of health and removing barriers that lead to health disparities.

**Health ethics**   The consideration of values in prioritizing and justifying actions by health professionals, researchers, and policymakers.

**Health inequity**   Refers to disparities in health outcomes or access to healthcare services that result from systemic injustices and discriminatory practices. It disproportionately affects marginalized communities, perpetuating existing social disparities.

**Health outcomes**   Results from applying interventions, assessed through clinical measures, observations, or self-reported data.

**Health policy**   Decisions aimed at influencing the health of society, including the delivery and payment of healthcare services and addressing social determinants of health.

**Health reform**   Efforts to make healthcare more affordable, accessible, and high quality through systemic changes.

**Health status risk**   The probability that an individual or population will fall ill and seek medical care, introducing uncertainty around health.

**Healthcare access**   Timely use of personal health services to achieve optimal health outcomes.

**Healthcare organizations**   Organizations categorized by the services they predominantly provide, ranging from preventive to end-of-life care.

**Healthcare quality**   The provision of effective and safe care that meets current professional knowledge and leads to desired health outcomes.

**Healthy People 2030**   A road map setting goals to create healthy communities by addressing inequalities and raising awareness of environmental impacts on health.

**High reliability**   The ability to consistently deliver high-quality products or services without failure in complex systems.

**Implicit bias**   Unconscious attitudes or stereotypes that influence our perceptions and decisions about others based on their characteristics, such as race, gender, or age. Acknowledging and addressing implicit biases are essential for promoting fairness and inclusivity.

**Improved patient outcomes**  Refer to measurable enhancements in a patient's health status as a result of effective, inclusive, and equitable healthcare delivery. DEI practices contribute to better diagnosis, treatment adherence, and overall satisfaction.

**Inclusion**  Creating a welcoming environment where diverse perspectives are encouraged and all individuals feel valued and involved in decision-making.

**Innovation**  The process of turning ideas into products or services that address problems and create value for organizations and customers.

**Innovative technology**  Technologies that expand care, integrate experiences, and generate data to improve individual and population health.

**Institutional racism**  Refers to the policies, practices, and structures within organizations or institutions that perpetuate racial disparities and inequities, even without explicit intent. It can result in unequal access to opportunities, resources, and services for individuals from marginalized racial groups.

**Integrity**  Adherence to strong moral and ethical principles.

**Interconnectedness**  Refers to how various elements within a healthcare system are linked and impact one another in the real world.

**Interpersonal/internalized racism**  Encompasses the individual-level acts of racism, such as racial slurs, microaggressions, or discriminatory behavior, directed at someone based on their race. Internalized racism refers to the internalized belief or acceptance of racial stereotypes and prejudices by individuals from marginalized racial groups.

**Intersectionality and nationality**  Recognizes that individuals may experience multiple layers of identity-based oppression or privilege simultaneously. It highlights the interconnectedness of social categorizations, such as race, gender, and class, and the unique experiences and challenges faced by individuals based on these intersections. Nationality refers to a person's citizenship or country of origin.

**Intervention**  Actions taken to produce an effect or alter the course of a pathological process.

**Investment capital**  Funds sourced from debt or equity to support new initiatives and grow an organization.

**Job demands-resource theory**  A theory stating that motivation, well-being, and engagement thrive when individuals have the resources to meet job demands.

**Judicial branch**  The branch of government responsible for interpreting laws. At the federal level, the U.S. Supreme Court is the highest authority.

**Language services**  Refer to providing interpretation and translation assistance to individuals with limited English proficiency or other language barriers. Ensuring language access is essential for equitable access to information and services, particularly in healthcare settings.

**Leader-member exchange**  A theory predicting changes in leader-follower relationships based on organizational conditions and the perceived value of exchanges.

**Leadership development**  The process of cultivating leadership skills through training, interpersonal interaction, and job performance.

**Leadership skills (attributes)**  DEI contexts include empathy, cultural intelligence, inclusive decision-making, and advocacy for equity. Effective leaders model inclusive values, empower diverse teams, and drive systemic change.

**Leadership skills**  The knowledge and ability to drive change; foster inclusive environments; and uphold diversity, equity, and inclusion (DEI) principles.

**Lean**  A methodology focused on optimizing flow, minimizing waste, and creating value through continuous experimentation.

**Lean Six Sigma**   A strategy combining Lean and Six Sigma principles to improve processes, enhance customer satisfaction, and deliver quality outcomes.

**Legal compliance**   The process of adhering to federal and state laws, regulations, and policies in the healthcare industry.

**Legislative branch**   The branch of government that enacts and rescinds statutes, led by Congress at the federal level in the United States.

**Limited English proficient (LEP)**   Refers to individuals with limited ability to read, speak, write, or understand the English language. Ensuring language access and providing language services are vital for equitable communication and access to services for LEP individuals.

**Loading factors**   Overhead expenses and required margins necessary to maintain an organization's long-term financial viability.

**Long-term care**   Services provided to patients with chronic or degenerative conditions requiring extended care, including therapy, recreation, and case management.

**Machine learning**   A subset of artificial intelligence focused on developing algorithms that enable machines to learn from data and make predictions.

**Malpractice**   Negligence by a professional who fails to act in accordance with acceptable standards, directly causing harm.

**Managed care organization (MCO)**   Groups of providers working collaboratively to deliver care. Examples include health maintenance organizations (HMOs), preferred provider organizations (PPOs), and point-of-service (POS) plans.

**Managerial accounting**   The measurement, analysis, and interpretation of financial data to help managers make optimal decisions.

**Market failure**   When market processes fail to yield socially optimal outcomes, often due to information asymmetry.

**Market segments**   Categories of customers targeted by marketers to deliver tailored content and drive action.

**Marketing mix**   A model encompassing product, price, place, and promotion that is used to develop effective marketing strategies.

**Medicaid**   A jointly funded program by federal and state governments providing health insurance to low-income or disabled individuals.

**Medical care risk**   Uncertainty around the utilization and costs of medical treatment.

**Medicare**   A federal health insurance program for individuals aged 65 and over and those under 65 with specific disabilities or conditions.

**Mentor**   A trusted advisor who provides guidance, support, and insight that can foster personal as well as professional growth

**Microaggressions**   Subtle, everyday actions or comments that convey derogatory messages toward individuals based on their race, gender, or other identities. These seemingly harmless remarks can contribute to a hostile or unwelcoming environment and perpetuate systemic inequalities.

**Mid-career**   A growth period involving leadership, expanded responsibilities, continued leadership development and aligning work with long-term career goals.

**Mitigation**   The process of preventing harm by evaluating data, assessing risks, and providing options for handling potential threats.

**Monitoring**   Ensures a healthcare project aligns with its objectives during execution, using metrics and key performance indicators (KPIs) to assess progress.

**Moral hazard**   Occurs when consumers use more healthcare resources because costs are covered by others, such as insurance companies.

**Needs assessment**   The systematic collection, analysis, and prediction of community health data to address health issues and prevent future occurrences.

**Nonmaleficence**   The principle of "do no harm," requiring healthcare managers to weigh the benefits and burdens of actions, balancing costs, effectiveness, and quality of care.

**Normative decision-making**   A leadership model focused on applying decision-making styles based on organizational state and goals, ensuring operational success.

**Oppression/anti-oppression**   Refers to the unjust and cruel exercise of authority or power to subjugate or marginalize specific groups. Anti-oppression involves actively challenging oppressive systems and promoting equitable treatment and inclusion for all individuals, particularly those from marginalized communities.

**Organizational culture**   The shared values, norms, and practices within an organization that impact staff engagement, diversity, equity, and inclusion.

**Organizational design**   How healthcare leaders design and develop operational processes to achieve strategic goals, aligning with structure and culture.

**Organizational development**   Mechanisms to recruit, retain, and engage the best talent in an organization.

**Organizational health literacy**   Refers to the capacity of healthcare institutions to provide clear, accessible, and culturally appropriate health information and services to their patients and communities. It involves creating an environment that promotes health literacy for all individuals.

**Organizational structure**   The framework establishing the hierarchy, roles, and information-sharing protocols within a healthcare organization.

**Out-of-pocket maximum**   The maximum amount a patient pays per year for medical services, after which the insurance company covers 100% of essential care costs.

**Oversight**   Functions that ensure quality performance in health systems, maintaining public trust through transparency and assurance.

**Paid search marketing**   Paid advertisements, also known as pay-per-click (PPC), that appear ahead of organic search results based on purchased keywords.

**Pandemic**   A widespread epidemic occurring across a country, population, or the world.

**Path-goal theory**   A leadership theory focusing on setting clear paths to goal achievement, matching rewards to achievements, and removing obstacles to success.

**Patient care**   Encompasses services provided by healthcare professionals to maintain or improve a patient's health. In a DEI context, it emphasizes culturally competent, equitable, and person-centered practices tailored to diverse populations.

**Patient Protection and Affordable Care Act (ACA)**   A 2010 healthcare reform law aimed at making healthcare affordable, expanding Medicaid, and lowering costs through innovative solutions.

**Patient-centered care**   Care that is respectful of and responsive to individual patient preferences, needs, and values.

**Personal health literacy**   Refers to an individual's ability to obtain, understand, and act on health information and make informed decisions about their health. It involves critical thinking and communication skills necessary to navigate the healthcare system effectively.

**Personal selling**   A promotional tool involving direct interaction with potential buyers, often used for high-cost services or products.

**Plan-Do-Check-Act (PDCA)**   A four-step iterative technique (plan, do, check, act) to improve business processes.

**Planning**   The process of identifying stakeholders, defining project scope, conducting risk assessments, and creating resource plans and schedules.

**Policy cycle**   A cyclical process of policy development encompassing evidence collection, stakeholder engagement, drafting, implementation, and evaluation.

**Policy development**   The process of gathering evidence to inform policymakers and build partnerships to implement policies improving health and reducing harm.

**Population health**   An interdisciplinary approach connecting practice to policy, enabling health departments to drive local change.

**Post-acute care**  Medical services provided after an acute care stay, focusing on recovery, restoring functionality, and easing transitions back into the community.
**Preemption**  When higher levels of government override lower level laws. For instance, federal law supersedes conflicting state or local laws under the U.S. Constitution's Supremacy Clause.
**Premium**  The payment made to an insurance provider to ensure coverage.
**Preparedness**  The development of crisis plans and readiness activities, such as training and exercises, to respond effectively to emergencies.
**Prevention**  Efforts to prevent disease or injury in unaffected individuals through immunizations, screenings, or regular health exams.
**Preventive care**  Healthcare services aimed at preventing health issues and supporting robust primary care to identify and mitigate risks early.
**Primary care**  Healthcare services covering prevention, wellness, and treatment of common illnesses provided by doctors, nurses, and other practitioners.
**Privilege**  Refers to unearned advantages or benefits granted to individuals based on their social identities, such as race, gender, or socioeconomic status. Recognizing privilege is crucial for understanding the differential experiences of individuals and addressing systemic inequalities.
**Professional development**  Enhancing professional skills, knowledge, and competence to meet job demands and advance in a career.
**Project management**  A methodology for achieving specific objectives within set constraints, essential in healthcare for improving patient care and streamlining operations.
**Promotional mix**  The collection of marketing tools used to promote an organization's brand, products, or services, including advertising, personal selling, and digital marketing.
**Psychological safety**  A shared belief among team members that it is safe to speak up, voice concerns, and express ideas without fear of negative consequences.
**Public health**  The science of protecting and improving the health of populations through research, policy, and education.
**Publicity and Public relations**  Managing the organization's brand and relationships with media, stakeholders, and the community.
**Quality of care**  The degree to which healthcare services improve health outcomes and align with professional standards.
**Race and ethnicity**  Refer to social constructs used to categorize people based on shared physical and cultural traits. While race generally pertains to physical characteristics, ethnicity encompasses shared cultural practices, language, and history. Understanding and valuing diverse racial and ethnic backgrounds is crucial for promoting inclusivity and cultural understanding.
**Racism**  Refers to the belief in the inherent superiority or inferiority of certain racial groups, leading to discrimination and mistreatment based on race. Racism can manifest at individual, institutional, and systemic levels, perpetuating social inequities and injustices.
**Recruitment**  The process of attracting qualified individuals to apply for jobs in a timely manner to meet organizational needs.
**Regulations**  Laws or rules designed to ensure quality performance in health systems and maintain public trust.
**Reporting**  Calling out misconduct or compliance violations, empowering staff to address issues, and ensuring transparency.
**Reputation management**  A field of healthcare marketing focused on tracking patient and consumer opinions to manage the organization's public image.

**Resilience**   The ability of a system or community to adapt, recover, and transform after exposure to hazards or disruptions.
**Retain**   Refers to sustaining a diverse and inclusive workforce by fostering an organizational climate where employees feel valued, safe, and supported. This includes offering mentorship, sponsorship, equitable compensation, and benefits. Celebrating diverse contributions and ensuring career advancement opportunities are essential strategies for long-term retention.
**Risk management**   The systematic process of identifying, assessing, and mitigating threats or uncertainties that can affect an organization.
**Sales promotions**   Limited-time deals such as discounts, rebates, or coupons that encourage consumers to try new products or services.
**Scarce resources**   A limited amount of resources, such as income, wealth, and time, requiring choices to allocate them effectively.
**Search Engine Marketing (SEM)**   A strategy to connect with consumers actively seeking healthcare services through search engines, using paid ads or optimized content.
**Search engine optimization (SEO)**   The practice of optimizing website content and tagging to rank higher in search engine results, driving organic traffic.
**Self-awareness**   The ability to recognize and understand one's own emotions, motivations, and their impact on others.
**Self-management**   The ability to regulate and manage emotions, behaviors, and responses in a constructive and goal-oriented manner.
**Senior career**   The highest career stage, involving leadership of entire organizations or significant parts, with responsibilities spanning strategy, quality, safety, finance, and more.
**Sexual orientation**   Refers to a person's emotional, romantic, or sexual attraction to individuals of the same and/or different gender. Understanding and valuing diverse sexual orientations are crucial for promoting inclusivity and support for LGBTQ+ individuals.
**Sexuality**   Refers to a broad range of sexual desires, behaviors, and identities that individuals may experience. Recognizing and respecting diverse sexualities contribute to a more inclusive and supportive environment for all individuals.
**Situational leadership**   A leadership theory emphasizing adaptability by assessing followers' abilities and willingness to achieve organizational goals.
**SMART goals**   Goals that are **S**pecific, **M**easurable, **A**chievable, **R**ealistic, and **T**ime bound.
**Social determinants of health (SDoH)**   The economic, social, and environmental factors that influence an individual's health and well-being. These determinants, such as housing, education, and income, can significantly impact health outcomes and create health disparities.
**Stakeholders**   Individuals or groups interested in or affected by a project, including government agencies, medical practitioners, research institutions, and patients.
**Strategic control**   Mechanisms to ensure organizational goals are achieved, fostering innovation, learning, and development.
**Strategic direction**   Long-term goals an organization aims to achieve, guiding strategic planning.
**Strategic framework**   A framework focusing on data use, prevention, treatment access, and partnerships to ensure organizational sustainability.
**Strategic planning**   The process of making informed choices to achieve long-term goals through environmental analysis, setting objectives, and implementing strategies.
**Structural/systemic racism**   Refers to the embedded racism within societal structures, including government, education, and economic systems. It goes beyond individual

attitudes and behaviors and affects entire communities or racial groups through discriminatory policies and practices.

**Succession planning**   A strategic process to identify and develop future leaders for key organizational roles.

**Supply**   The provision of goods or services by individuals or organizations in exchange for compensation.

**Support for healthcare professionals**   Includes mentoring, professional development, inclusive work environments, employee resource groups, and mental health resources to promote retention and success.

**Systems dynamics modeling**   A method using tools to understand system behaviors over time, focusing on stocks, flows, and feedback loops to address complex problems.

**Systems engineering**   The science of developing systems that meet requirements within given constraints.

**Systems mapping**   A visual representation of system components and their interrelationships to understand system behavior.

**Systems thinking**   The ability to make reliable inferences about system behavior by understanding underlying structures and improving problem-solving skills.

**Talent management**   A strategic process for identifying, developing, and retaining high-potential employees to meet organizational needs.

**Target marketing strategy**   Focusing on specific audiences to deliver customized messages and achieve maximum impact.

**Technological progress**   Advancements in technology that drive demand, resulting in increased healthcare delivery and higher prices.

**Technology plans**   Short- and long-term plans for leveraging technology and data to drive organizational strategy and improve healthcare delivery.

**Transformational leadership**   A leadership approach rooted in inspiring change, fostering innovation, and aligning with servant leadership principles.

**Turnover**   The loss of employees, leading to financial costs, quality and safety issues, and reputational damage for organizations.

**Underrepresented minority (UDM)**   Refers to individuals from racial or ethnic groups that have lower representation in a particular setting, such as the workplace or educational institutions. This term is often used in contexts where certain groups are underrepresented and aims to address disparities and promote inclusivity.

**Vicarious liability**   A legal principle where employers can be held responsible for the actions of their employees while performing job duties.

**Waste**   The overutilization of services or practices resulting in unnecessary healthcare system costs, including Medicare and Medicaid programs.

**Workforce planning**   The process of ensuring the right people are in the right roles at the right time to meet organizational goals.

# INDEX

AAMC. *See* American Association of Medical Colleges
AAR. *See* after-action reviews
ABM. *See* agent-based modeling
academic medical centers, 23, 69, 242
access to care, 21, 107, 285, 286
accountability, 128, 195, 246, 364
Accountable Care Organizations (ACOs), 69–70, 93, 108, 161
accounting data, 257
ACHE. *See* American College of Healthcare Executives
ACOs. *See* Accountable Care Organizations
action learning, 310–312
actuarially fair premium, 159
acute care, 22–24
ADA. *See* Americans with Disabilities Act
adaptive systems theory, 7, 8
administrative service-only (ASO) contract, 163
Advanced Alternative Payment Models (APMs), 108
advanced leadership skills, 251
advanced premium tax credits (APTC), 164
advertising, 235, 237
affinity groups, 345, 348
after-action reviews (AAR), 334
agent-based modeling (ABM), 10, 11
Agile methodologies, 226
AHA. *See* American Hospital Association
AI. *See* artificial intelligence
AIDS, 78
AKS. *See* Anti-Kickback Statute
ALFs. *See* assisted living facilities
all-payor claims data, 257
alternative payment models, 107
alternative strategies, 124
ambulatory surgery centers (ASCs), 23
American Association of Medical Colleges (AAMC), 351, 353
American Cancer Society, 286
American College of Healthcare Executives (ACHE), 351, 352
American Hospital Association (AHA), 54, 351, 352
Americans with Disabilities Act (ADA), 174
Anti-Kickback Statute (AKS), 275, 324

antitrust laws, 323
APMs. *See* Advanced Alternative Payment Models
APTC. *See* advanced premium tax credits
artificial intelligence (AI), 12, 94–95, 243, 264
Asana, 227
ASCs. *See* ambulatory surgery centers
ASO contract. *See* administrative service-only contract
assisted living facilities (ALFs), 25
asymmetric information, 54–55
auditing, 274
autonomy, 320–321

BA. *See* business analytics
balance sheet, 150
balanced scorecard (BSC) approach, 137, 245
behavioral health data, 258
behavioral health hospitals, 22
belonging, 38, 345
benchmarking data, 262–263
beneficence, 320
beneficiary, 116, 158, 161
big data analytics, 12, 15, 136, 257
birth centers, 24
blockchain technology, 228, 247
Blue Cross, 162
breach of contract, 323
BSC approach. *See* balanced scorecard approach
budgeting process, 152
burnout, 32–33
  work-related causes of, 34–35
business analytics (BA), 257
buyer behavior, 233–236

CAH. *See* critical access hospital
California Consumer Privacy Act, 65
call center, 287
cancer centers, 24, 285
capital investment options, 148
CAPTE. *See* Commission on Accreditation in Physical Therapy Education
career framework, 295

career stages, healthcare leader, 295
  early career, 296
  encore career, 297–298
  mid-career, 297
  senior career, 297
CAS theory. *See* complex adaptive systems theory
case law, 320
case rate, 58
case study
  accountable care organizations, 69–70
  care for cancer patients, 284–287
  crisis management, 331–332
  data utilization, 266–267
  digital marketing, 238–239
  diversity in healthcare leadership, 353–354
  electronic health records, 70
  electronic health records implementation, 222–223
  financial health assessment, 150–151
  health economics, 58–59
  health insurance, 159
  health provider organization, 250–251
  healthcare compliance officer, 280
  healthcare law, 324–325
  healthcare leadership, 374–376
  improvement in practice, 203–204
  leadership theory, 313
  long-term capital investments, 148
  management control process, 152–153
  maternal and child health in rural America, 115–118
  multiple stakeholders, 109–110
  perception and communication, 37
  recruitment and retention strategies, 184–185
  rural emergency hospital model, 91
  solicit employee feedback, 36
  staff augmentation and virtualization, 223–224
  strategic management, 124–126
  strategic planning, 130–134
  systems thinking, 13–14
casualty, 6, 9, 128, 302, 330
causal loop diagrams (CLDs), 9, 11, 15
CBOs. *See* community-based organizations
CCH. *See* community care cub
CCRCs. *See* continuing care retirement communities
CDC. *See* Centers for Disease Control and Prevention
CDOs. *See* chief diversity officers
CEM. *See* comprehensive emergency management
Centers for Disease Control and Prevention (CDC), 74, 76, 77, 79, 101, 258, 263, 276
Centers for Medicare & Medicaid Services (CMS), 87, 192, 276

CEO. *See* chief executive officer
CFO. *See* chief financial officer
chaos theory, 7, 13–14
charismatic leader theory, 303
chief diversity officers (CDOs), 352, 354
chief equity officers, 352, 354
chief executive officer (CEO), 144, 310–311, 352–353
chief financial officer (CFO), 69, 144, 149
Children's Health Insurance Program (CHIP), 108, 158, 160
children's hospitals, 22
CHIP. *See* Children's Health Insurance Program
CHNA. *See* community health needs assessment
CIAs. *See* Corporate Integrity Agreements
civil laws, 321–323
  contract, 323
  Stark Law, 322
  tort reform, 322
  torts, 321–322
Civil Monetary Penalties Law, 276
Civil Rights Act (1964), 174, 179
CLAS. *See* culturally and linguistically appropriate services
CLDs. *See* causal loop diagrams
clinical trials, 285
clinical trials data, 257–258
CMS. *See* Centers for Medicare & Medicaid Services
coinsurance, 159
collaborative decision-making processes, 10, 11
Commission on Accreditation in Physical Therapy Education (CAPTE), 53
community-based organizations (CBOs), 109–110
community care cub (CCH), 110
community health centers, 20, 21
community health, definition of, 100
community health needs assessment (CHNA), 105–107, 116–117
community rating, 160
community stakeholders, 107
compensation strategies, 174
complementary and alternative medicine, 22
complex adaptive systems (CAS) theory, 8, 15
compliance committee, 274
compliance, definition of, 271–272
compliance officer, 274
compliance program
  areas of regulatory oversight, 275–276
  benefits of, 272
  case study, 280
  compliance committee, 274
  compliance officer, 274
  Corporate Integrity Agreements, 278
  culture and risk management, 278–280

definition of, 272
detect offenses, 275
disciplinary guidance, 274
enforcement agencies, 276
enforcement initiatives, 276–277
fraud, waste, and abuse laws, 272, 275–276
history of, 272–273
Integrity Agreements, 278
internal monitoring and auditing, 274
key elements of, 273–275
lines of communication, 274
procedures, 274
repayments, 277–278
self-disclosures, 277–278
standards of conduct, 274
training and education, 274
written policies, 274
Compliance Program Guidance for Hospitals, 273
comprehensive emergency management (CEM), 332
conceptual framework, 66–68
conflict, 38–39
    types of, 39
content marketing, 236
contingency planning, 333
contingency theory, 66, 304–305
continuing care retirement communities (CCRCs), 25–26
Continuity of Operations (COOP), 333
continuum of care, 19–21, 24, 26
contract, 323
convenient care, 21
COOP. *See* Continuity of Operations
copayment (copay), 56–57, 158–159, 284
Corporate Integrity Agreements (CIAs), 278
cost accounting, 152
cost-sharing reductions (CSR), 164
County Health Rankings & Roadmaps (CHR&R), 109
COVID-19 pandemic, 5, 7, 9, 32, 78–79, 318, 319, 330, 336–337
criminal law, 323–324
    Anti-Kickback Statute, 324
    False Claims Act, 323–324
crisis communications, 335
crisis leadership, 330
crisis management
    after-action reviews, 334
    analyze strategic failures, 334
    areas and types of, 330–334
    case study, 331–332
    communication, 334–335
    comprehensive emergency management, 332
    contingency planning, 333
    Continuity of Operations, 333
    COVID-19 pandemic, 336–337

definition of, 330
enterprise risk management, 332
hazard vulnerability analysis, 333
incident command system, 333
preparedness, 332
root cause analysis, 334
strengths and weaknesses, 335–336
critical access hospital (CAH), 23, 91
CRM. *See* customer relationship management
Cross Industry Standard Process for Data Mining (CRISP-DM), 264
CSR. *See* cost-sharing reductions
cultural competency, 346, 347, 350
culturally and linguistically appropriate services (CLAS), 348
Culture of Health, 109
customer relationship management (CRM), 244
cybersecurity threats, in healthcare, 145, 146
Cynefin Framework, 8–9, 14

data analytics
    approaches, 264
    artificial intelligence, 264–265
    benchmarking data, 262–263
    case study, 266–267
    data cleaning and preprocessing, 261–262
    data collection, 261
    data life cycle, 263–264
    data visualization, 263
    definition of, 256
    descriptive analytics, 259–260
    diagnostic analytics, 260
    operational analytics, 260
    overview of, 255–256
    personalized analytics, 260
    predictive analytics, 260
    prescriptive analytics, 260
    tools, 265
    types of, 259–260
data cleaning and preprocessing, 261–262
data collection, 261
data dictionary, 261
data-driven targeting, 238
data life cycle, 263–264
Data Management Competency Framework, 265–266
data visualization, 263
decision-making, 8–9, 11, 12, 58–59, 66, 69, 79, 82, 143–144, 147, 149, 227, 233, 256, 297, 308, 345, 348, 352, 361–363
deductible, 145, 159, 284
Defense Health Agency, 23
DEI. *See* diversity, equity, and inclusion
demand, 44–45
demographics, 117
dental clinics, 24

Department of Health and Human Services (DHHS), 76, 81, 88, 276, 319
Department of Health and Human Services Office of the Inspector General (HHS-OIG), 273, 275–278
DHHS. *See* Department of Health and Human Services
diagnostic imaging centers, 21–22
dialysis centers, 24
digital marketing, 236–237
   display advertising, 237
   paid search marketing, 237
   pay-per-click advertising, 237
   search engine marketing, 237
   social media platform advertising, 237
direct marketing, 236
disciplinary guidance, 274
discounted payback period, 147
discrimination, 179, 181
disease management data, 257–258
disease registries data, 258
display advertising, 237
diversity, equity, and inclusion (DEI), 344
   application of, 350–354
   case study, 353–354
   cultural competencies, 346–347
   definitions in healthcare, 347–348
   importance of, 344–345
   leadership skills, 346–347
   management techniques, 345–346
   organizational best practices, 345
   quantitative, 352–354
   social determinants of health, 348–350
diversity leadership CORE framework, 344–345
divided government, 88
DMAIC (Define, Measure, Analyze, Improve, and Control), 200
Doctor of Physical Therapy (DPT), 53
Donabedian's model for evaluation, 192
DPT. *See* Doctor of Physical Therapy

Ebola outbreaks, 78
EEOC. *See* Equal Opportunity Employment Commission
EFQM excellence model, 137
EHRs. *See* electronic health records
electronic health records (EHRs), 5, 70, 216, 257
Electronic Medical Record Adoption Model (EMRAM), 200
email marketing, 236
emergence, 5, 82, 89–90
Emergency Medical Treatment and Labor Act (EMTALA), 275, 318, 326
emotional intelligence, 367
employee engagement, 175
employee referral, 178

employee relations, 174
employee resource groups (ERGs), 345
employer-sponsored insurance, 160
employment contracts, 323
employment laws, 174
Employment Retirement Income Security (ERISA) Act, 163
EMRAM. *See* Electronic Medical Record Adoption Model
EMTALA. *See* Emergency Medical Treatment and Labor Act
end-of-life care services, 20, 26
End-Stage Renal Disease (ESRD) Quality Initiative Program, 107
enterprise risk management (ERM), 332
environmental data, 258
Equal Opportunity Employment Commission (EEOC), 174
equilibrium, 47–49
equity, 127
ERGs. *See* employee resource groups
ERISA Act. *See* Employment Retirement Income Security Act
ERM. *See* enterprise risk management
Ethics, 246, 264, 272, 299. *See also* law and ethics
evaluation phase, project management, 219
evidence-based practice, 5
execution phase, project management, 218
executive branch, 88, 319
executive order, 319
experience ratings, 159
external recruitment, 178

FAB. *See* features, advantages, and benefits
Facebook, 237
factory farming. *See* livestock farming
False Claims Act (FCA), 275, 323–324
Family Medical Leave Act (FMLA), 174, 184
FCA. *See* False Claims Act
FDA. *See* Food and Drug Administration
features, advantages, and benefits (FAB), 234
federal public health departments, 76
Federal Trade Commission (FTC), 276
federalism, 86–87, 318
federally qualified health centers, 21
fee-for-service (FFS), payment system, 165–166, 168
feedback loops, 5
   balancing loop, 6
   reinforcing loops, 6
FFS. *See* fee-for-service
finance/billing data, 257
financial accounting, 144, 150
financial management, 144, 147–149
   case study, 148
   definition of, 144
   long-term decision-making, 147

FMLA. *See* Family Medical Leave Act
followership, 362, 363
Food and Drug Administration (FDA), 54, 276
fraud, definition of, 272
fraud, waste, and abuse (FWA) laws, 272
freestanding emergency departments (FSEDs), 23
FSEDs. *See* freestanding emergency departments
FTC. *See* Federal Trade Commission
FWA laws. *See* fraud, waste, and abuse laws

GAAP. *See* generally accepted accounting principles
Gantt charts and timelines, 224–225
general acute care hospitals, 22, 23
generally accepted accounting principles (GAAP), 144, 150
geographic information systems (GIS), 109
GIS. *See* geographic information systems
GMC. *See* Greater Medical Center
great resignation, 32
Greater Medical Center (GMC), 285–286

HAC Program. *See* Hospital-Acquired Conditions Program
hazard vulnerability analysis (HVA), 333
HCFAC. *See* Health Care Fraud and Abuse Control Program
Health Care Fraud and Abuse Control Program (HCFAC), 277
health, definition of, 74
health disparities, 74, 104–105, 117
health economics
　asymmetric information, 54–55
　case study, 58–59
　demand, 44–45, 49–52
　externalities, 55
　health insurance, 55–58
　healthcare services, national market for, 49
　macro level, 49
　markets and prices, 44–45
　micro level, 45
　physical therapists, supply of, 45–46
　physical therapy, local market for, 45
　subsidies, 52
　supply, 44–45, 52–54
　taxes, 52
health equity, 81, 104–105
Health Information Technology for Economic and Clinical Health (HITECH) Act, 65, 220
health insurance, 55–58
　case study, 159
　co-pay, 56–57
　definition of, 158–160
　history of, 161–162
　managed care organization, 160–161
　moral hazard, 58
　national health expenditures, 165, 167
　private health insurance coverage, 160
　public health insurance coverage, 160
　regulation, 162–164
　reimbursement, 164–169
Health Insurance Portability and Accountability Act (HIPAA), 65, 220, 236, 276–277
health maintenance organization (HMO), 161
health outcomes, 77
health policy
　artificial intelligence, 94–95
　case study, 91
　defined, 85–86
　divided government, 88
　executive branch, 88
　federalism, 86–87
　healthcare reform, 91–94
　judicial branch, 89
　legislative branch, 88
　by level of government, 87
　market failure, 90–91
　Patient Protection and Affordable Care Act (PPACA), 88, 93–94
　policy cycle, 89–90
　supply and demand, 89
　telehealth, 95
　workforce development, 95
health status risk, 158
healthcare access, 76
healthcare compliance. *See also* compliance program
　definition of, 271–272
　importance of, 272
healthcare data
　accounting data, 257
　administrative data, 257
　all-payor claims data, 257
　behavioral health data, 258
　characteristics, 259
　clinical trials data, 257–258
　disease management data, 257–258
　disease registries data, 258
　electronic health records data, 257
　environmental data, 258
　finance/billing data, 257
　longitudinal claims data, 257
　market data, 257
　patient self-reported data, 258
　pharmacy data, 258
　social determinants of health data, 258
healthcare data breaches, 146
healthcare ethics, 320–321

healthcare finance
  access to care, 286
  case study, 284–287
  challenges and dilemma, 284–285
  closing the gap on access to care, 286–287
  organizational overview, 285–286
healthcare financial management
  case study, 150–153
  chief financial officer (CFO), 144
  definition of, 144
  financial accounting, 144, 150
  financial issues in health industry, 144–146
  financial management, 147–149
  managerial accounting, 144, 151–152
Healthcare Fraud Prevention and Action Team (HEAT), 277
healthcare information technology
  administrative functions, 247
  case study, 250–251
  customer relationship management, 244
  leadership considerations, 247–249
  leadership opportunities, 244
  market, 247–249
  modular stages, 245–247, 249
  stages of technology evolution, 248
  stakeholder, 247–249
  technology, 247–249
  technology plans, 245
healthcare infrastructure, 76–77
healthcare leaders
  career stages and competencies, 295–298
  early career, 296
  encore career, 297–298
  enhancing effectiveness, 293–294
  mid-career, 297
  opportunities, roadblocks, and potential pitfalls, 298–299
  past and future, 292–293
  senior career, 297
healthcare marketing
  advertising, 235
  buyer behavior, 233–236
  case study, 238–239
  data-driven targeting, 238
  in digital age, 238
  digital marketing, 236–237
  direct marketing, 236
  email marketing, 236
  market and competitor analysis, 232–233
  market segments, 233
  marketing leadership, 232
  marketing mix, 234–236
  marketing strategy, 232
  personal selling, 235–236
  promotional mix, 235
  public relations, 236
  sales promotions, 236
  target marketing strategy, 233
healthcare organizations, 20
  acute care, 22–24
  employee turnover, 31
  end-of-life care services, 26
  long-term care, 24–26
  post-acute care, 24–26
  preventive care, 20–22
  primary care, 20–22
healthcare providers, 63
healthcare quality, 4
healthcare reform, 91–94
healthcare vendor contract, 323
healthcare workforce management
  aging population, 32
  belonging, 38
  burnout, 32–35
  case study, 36
  changing work expectations and priorities, 34
  collective action and unionization, 31
  conflict, 38–39
  COVID-19 pandemic, 32
  financial cost of turnover, 30–31
  great resignation, 32
  harm to reputation, 31
  job demands-resources theory, 35–36
  manager, 38
  perception and communication, 36–37
  psychological safety, 38
  psychological strain, 32–33
  Quintuple Aim, 30
  reimbursement, 33–34
  threat to quality and safety, 31
Healthy People 2030 Initiative (HP2030), 81–82
HEAT. *See* Healthcare Fraud Prevention and Action Team
HHVBP Model. *See* Home Health Value-Based Purchasing Model
high reliability, 195
high-reliability organizations (HROs), 195, 196
HIPAA. *See* Health Insurance Portability and Accountability Act
HITECH Act. *See* Health Information Technology for Economic and Clinical Health Act
HIV, 78
HMO. *See* health maintenance organization
home health, 25
Home Health Value-Based Purchasing (HHVBP) Model, 107
hospice, 26
hospital, 63, 64. *See also specific types*
Hospital-Acquired Conditions (HAC) Program, 107

Hospital Readmission Reduction (HRR) Program, 107
Hospital Value-Based Purchasing (HVBP) Program, 107
HRIS. *See* human resource information system
HROs. *See* high-reliability organizations
HRR Program. *See* Hospital Readmission Reduction Program
human capital, 174
human resource (HR) management
   case study, 184–185
   employee and labor relations, 178–181
   employee recruitment and retention, 177–178
   enforcement and litigation statistics, 181
   metrics and organizational outcomes, 176–177
   organizational development, 182–183
   recent worker strikes and protests, 182
   workforce design, 175–176
human resource information system (HRIS), 247
HVA. *See* Hazard vulnerability analysis
HVBP Program. *See* Hospital Value-Based Purchasing Program

IAs. *See* Integrity Agreements
ICD-10-CM codes, 103
ICS. *See* incident command system
ICT. *See* Information and Communication Technologies
incident command system (ICS), 333–334
income statement, 150, 151
Information and Communication Technologies (ICT), 65
initiation phase, project management, 216
innovative technology, 244
   administrative functions, 247
   modular stages, 245–247
   technology plans, 245
   transformative change, 244–247
inpatient rehabilitation facilities (IRFs), 24–25
Instagram, 237
Institute of Medicine (IOM), 193
Integrity Agreements (IAs), 278
intentional tort, 321–322
interconnectedness, 4–5
internal rate of return (IRR), 147
internal recruitment, 177–178
Internal Revenue Service (IRS), 106
investment capital, 147
IOM. *See* Institute of Medicine
IRFs. *See* inpatient rehabilitation facilities
IRR. *See* internal rate of return
IRS. *See* Internal Revenue Service

job demands-resources theory, 35
   physical resources, 35
   reducing demands, 36
   social resources, 36
   structural resources, 36
judicial branch, 89, 320
jurisdiction, overlapping levels of, 87
just culture, 279
justice, 321

KDD. *See* knowledge discovery in databases
Key performance indicators (KPIs), 138
knowledge discovery in databases (KDD), 264
KPIs. *See* Key performance indicators

Labor Management Relations Act (LMRA), 179
Labor-Management Reporting and Disclosure Act (LMRDA), 181
Landrum-Griffin Act. *See* Labor-Management Reporting and Disclosure Act (LMRDA)
Large language models (LLMs), 265
law and ethics
   Anti-Kickback Statute, 324
   case law, 320
   case study, 324–325
   civil laws, 321–323
   contract, 323
   criminal law, 323–324
   executive order, 319
   False Claims Act, 323–324
   healthcare pillars, 320–321
   regulations, 319
   Stark Law, 322
   statutes, 319
   tort reform, 322
   torts, 321–322
leader-member exchange theory, 306–307
leadership, 66, 174, 244
   average of five, 364
   care in healthcare, 363–364
   case study, 374–376
   challenges/dilemma, 374
   competencies, 366–368
   dyad, 365–366
   leading others, 362–366
   leading self, 360–362
   organizational overview, 375
   positive in mistakes, 363
   self-awareness, 361–362
   snake wrangling, 364
   strengths versus weaknesses, 365
leadership skills, 346

leadership theories
  ancient, early, and niche, 302–303
  case study, 313
  contingency theory, 304–305
  leader-member exchange theory, 306–307
  leadership development, 310–312
  multidimensional model of leadership development, 312–313
  normative decision-making model of leadership, 308–309
  path-goal theory, 303–304
  situational leadership theory, 305–306
  transformational leadership theory, 309–310
Lean, 200
legal compliance, 174
legislative branch, 88, 319
livestock farming, 55
LLMs. *See* Large language models
LMRA. *See* Labor Management Relations Act
LMRDA. *See* Labor-Management Reporting and Disclosure Act
loading factors, 159
local public health departments, 77
long-term acute care hospitals (LTACs), 25
long-term capital investments, 148
long-term care, 24–26
long-term decision-making, 147
long-term goals, 124
longitudinal claims data, 257
LTACs. *See* long-term acute care hospitals

machine learning, 12, 13, 228, 260, 264
MACRA. *See* Medicare Access and CHIP Reauthorization Act of 2015
malpractice, 89, 322, 323
managed care organization (MCO), 160–161
managerial accounting, 144, 151–152
market data, 257
market failure, 55, 90
  asymmetric information, 54–55
  cause of, 91
  externalities, 55
  health insurance, 55–58
market segments, 233
marketing leadership, 232
marketing mix, 234–236
marketing strategy, 232
McCarran-Ferguson Act, 162–163
MCO. *See* managed care organization
Medicaid, 92, 93, 149, 158, 160
Medicaid Fraud Control Units (MFCUs), 276
Medical Assistance (MA) program. *See* Medicaid
medical care risk, 158, 169
medically based fitness and wellness centers, 22

Medicare, 92, 93, 108, 149, 158, 160
Medicare Access and CHIP Reauthorization Act of 2015 (MACRA), 108
Medicare Electronic Health Record Incentive Program, 108
mental health, 5, 36, 76, 79, 82, 109, 127, 235, 258
mentor, 183, 294, 298, 299, 311–313
Merit-Based Incentive Payment System (MIPS), 108
MFCUs. *See* Medicaid program, Medicaid Fraud Control Units
MHS. *See* Military Health System
Microsoft Excel, 265
Microsoft Projects, 227
Military Health System (MHS), 22–23
MIPS. *See* Merit-Based Incentive Payment System
MIRR. *See* modified internal rate of return
mitigation, 279
mobile clinics, 21
modified internal rate of return (MIRR), 147
modular stages, 245–247, 249
  Stage 1, 246
  Stage 2, 246
  Stage 3, 246–247
monitoring phase, project management, 218
moral hazard, 58
multidimensional feedback, 311
multidimensional model of leadership development, 312–313
multiple stakeholders, 109–110
multiservice outpatient centers, 23

NALHE. *See* National Association of Latino Healthcare Executives
National Association of Latino Healthcare Executives (NALHE), 351–352
National Cancer Institute (NCI), 285
National Health Expenditures Account (NHE), 92
National Institute of Safety and Health (NIOSH), 77
National Institutes of Health (NIH), 104
National Labor Relations Act (NLRA), 179
natural disasters, 330, 337
NCI. *See* National Cancer Institute
needs assessments, 105
negative externality, 55
negligence, 321
NEO PI-R™ (NEO Personality Inventory-Revised™), 365
net present value (NPV), 147
network theory, 7–8
NHE. *See* National Health Expenditures Account
NIH. *See* National Institutes of Health

NIOSH. *See* National Institute of Safety and Health
NLRA. *See* National Labor Relations Act
nonmaleficence, 320
normative decision-making model of leadership, 308–309
NoSQL. *See* Not only SQL
Not only SQL (NoSQL), 265
NPV. *See* net present value

Occupational Safety and Health Administration (OSHA), 77
OCR. *See* Office for Civil Rights
Office for Civil Rights (OCR), 276
opioid crisis, 79
organizational crisis, 330
organizational culture, 66, 344
organizational design
    antecedents and consequences of, 67
    case study, 69–70
    conceptual framework, 66–68
    contingency theory, 66
    definition of, 63–64
    infrastructure development, 64–65
    inventory management, 64
    operational elements of, 64
    organizational structure, 68–69
    outcomes of efficient, 68
    patient-centered care, 65
    quality and safety, 65
    resource allocation, 64
    resource-based view, 66
    structural contingency theory, 66
    technology integration, 65–66
organizational development, 182–183
organizational structure, 68–69
OSHA. *See* Occupational Safety and Health Administration
out-of-pocket maximum, 159
outpatient rehabilitation clinics/centers, 25

paid search marketing, 237
palliative care, 26
pandemics, 78, 330. *See also specific types*
path-goal theory, 303–304
patient-centered approach, 65, 221, 350
patient contracts, 323
patient experience, 284
Patient Protection and Affordable Care Act (PPACA), 88, 93–94, 162–164
patient self-reported data, 258
pay-per-click (PPC) advertising, 237
payback period, 147
PCC. *See* person-centered care

PDCA. *See* Plan-Do-Check-Act
performance prism model, 137
person-centered care (PCC), 117–118
personal protective equipment (PPE), 336–337
personal selling, 235–236
Peter principle, 178, 367
pharmacy data, 258
physical therapists (PTs), 45
    demand for, 46–47
    equilibrium price for visits, 47–49
    supply of, 45–46
Physician Quality Reporting System, 108
Physician Self-Referral Law, 276
Plan-Do-Check-Act (PDCA), 190
    Deming's method, 191
planning phase, project management, 216–218
PMIS. *See* project management information systems
point of service (POS) plans, 161
policy development, 75
policymakers, 103
population/community health
    case study, 109–110, 115–118
    challenges and dilemma, 116
    community health needs assessment (CHNA), 105–107
    Culture of Health, 109
    definition of, 100–101
    emerging technologies, 109
    health disparities, 104–105
    health equity, 104–105
    organizational overview, 116–117
    payment models, 107–108
    person-centered care, 117–118
    Robert Wood Johnson Foundation (RWJF), 109
    social determinants of health, 101–104
POS plans. *See* point of service plans
positive externality, 55
positive leadership, attributes and behaviors, 347
post-acute care, 24–26
Power BI, 265
PPACA. *See* Patient Protection and Affordable Care Act
PPC advertising. *See* pay-per-click advertising
PPE. *See* personal protective equipment
PPO. *See* preferred provider organization
PPS. *See* prospective payment system
predictive modeling, 12
preemption, 318
preferred provider organization (PPO), 161
premium, 158
preparedness, 332
preponderance of evidence, 321
prevention, public health, 74

preventive care, 20–22
primary care, 20–22
private health insurance coverage, 160
procedures, 274
process mapping, 9, 10
professional development, 360
profitability index, 147
project management
　Agile methodologies, 226
　case study, 222–224
　evaluation phase, 219
　execution phase, 218
　Gantt charts and timelines, 224–225
　initiation phase, 216
　interdisciplinary collaboration, 220
　monitoring phase, 218
　overview of, 215–216
　patient-centered approach, 221
　planning phase, 216–218
　project management information systems, 227
　project plan, 227
　regulatory and compliance, 219–220
　resource constraints, 220–221
　risk assessment and management, 225–226
　sample issue register, 217
　sample risk register, 217
project management information systems (PMIS), 227
project plan, 225, 227
promotional mix, 235, 236
prospective payment system (PPS), 166
psychological safety, 38
PTs. *See* physical therapists
public goods, 91
public health
　core functions, 74–76
　definition of, 74
　emerging challenges, 79
　federal public health departments, 76
　health determinants, 79–81
　Healthy People 2030 Initiative, 81–82
　infrastructure, 76–77
　local public health departments, 77
　practitioners, 77–78
　purpose of, 74–76
　response in past century, 78–79
　social determinants of health, 80–81
　stakeholders, 76–77
　state and territorial public health departments, 76–77
public health insurance coverage, 160
public hospitals, 22
public policy, 85
public relations, 236
Python, 265

QPP. *See* Quality Payment Program
quality and performance improvement
　business strategy, 197–198
　case study, 203–204
　Change Acceleration Process (CAP) model, 201
　culture and high reliability, 194–196
　Lean, 200
　measurement as impetus to improvement, 192–193
　ripple effect, 196–197
　robust process improvement (RPI), 198–199
　Six Sigma technique, 199–201
　tools for data analysis and presentation, 207–209
　tools for problem identification, improvement, and analysis, 205–206
　traits of success, 202–203
　voice of patient, 193–194
quality of care, 74, 192
Quality Payment Program (QPP), 108
quality trilogy, 190

R, programming language, 265
RADAR, 137
ransomware attacks, 146
RBV. *See* resource-based view
RCMC. *See* Reynolds County Medical Center
recruitment, 177
　external, 178
　internal, 177–178
regulations, 319
REH model. *See* rural emergency hospital model
Reimbursement, 23, 30, 33–34, 136, 145, 146, 164–169
repayments, 277–278
resource allocation, 64
resource-based view (RBV), 66
retention, 34, 177–178
return on investment (ROI), 110
revenue cycle management, 149
Reynolds County Medical Center (RCMC), 116–117
risk management, 225, 226, 228, 273, 278–280
roadmap, 218, 224, 294
Robert Wood Johnson Foundation (RWJF), 108, 109
robust process improvement (RPI), 198–199, 204
ROI. *See* return on investment
root cause analysis, 303, 334
RPI. *See* robust process improvement
Rule of Five, 364
rural emergency hospital (REH) model, 91
rural hospitals, 23, 51, 335
RWJF. *See* Robert Wood Johnson Foundation

sales promotions, 236
SAS/Minitab/QI Macros, 265
scarce resource allocation, 336
scarce resources, 44, 220
scenario planning, 10, 11
school-based health centers, 21
SCT. *See* structural contingency theory
SDM. *See* systems dynamics modeling
SDOH. *See* social determinants of health
search engine marketing, 237
search engine optimization (SEO), 237
self-awareness, 361–362
self-disclosures, 277–278
SEMMA process, for data analytics, 264
SEO. *See* search engine optimization
short-term decision-making, 149
situational leadership theory, 305–306
skilled nursing facilities (SNFs), 25
Skilled Nursing Facility Value-Based Purchasing (SNF VBP) Program, 107
SMART goals, 232
Smartsheet, 227
SNAP. *See* Supplemental Nutrition Assistance Program
SNF VBP Program. *See* Skilled Nursing Facility Value-Based Purchasing Program
SNFs. *See* skilled nursing facilities
social determinants of health (SDOH), 80–81, 101–104, 128, 348–350
social determinants of health data, 258
SOPs. *See* Standard operating procedures
Spanish flu, 78
specialty hospitals, 22
SQL. *See* Structured query language
stakeholders, 375–376
Standard operating procedures (SOPs), 65
standards of conduct, 274
Stark Law, 322
state and territorial public health departments, 76–77
statutes, 319
stock and flow diagrams, 9, 10
strategic control, 124
strategic direction, 124
strategic framework, 128
strategic management, 124–126
strategic planning
 application of, 130–136
 benefits of, 138
 case study, 124–126, 130–134
 chronic conditions, 130
 definition of, 124
 direct interactions with patients, 128
 elements of, 126–128
 equity, 136
 focused action, 135
 framework for, 126–127, 135
 healthcare, 136–137
 interventions for impact, 135
 pitfalls, 138
 research, 136
 social determinants of health (SDOH), 129
 sustainability, 136
 tools, 137
Strengths, Weaknesses, Opportunities, and Threats (SWOT) analysis, 137
structural contingency theory (SCT), 66
Structured query language (SQL), 265
subsidies, 52
succession planning, 174
Supplemental Nutrition Assistance Program (SNAP), 52
supply, 44–45
supply chain management, 149
surgicenters, 23
SWOT analysis. *See* Strengths, Weaknesses, Opportunities, and Threats analysis
Synthesis, 4, 5
systems dynamics modeling (SDM), 10–11
systems mapping, 6–7
systems thinking
 adaptive systems theory, 8
 agent-based modeling, 10, 11
 artificial intelligence, 12
 big data analytics, 12
 case study, 13–14
 causal loop diagrams, 9
 challenges and limitations in healthcare, 11–12
 chaos theory, 7
 collaborative decision-making processes, 10, 11
 Cynefin Framework, 8–9
 definition of, 4
 emerging research areas, 13
 examples of, 4
 foundations of, 4–7
 in healthcare education, 13
 machine learning, 12
 network theory, 7–8
 predictive modeling, 12
 process mapping, 9, 10
 scenario planning, 10, 11
 stock and flow diagrams, 9, 10
 tools, 9–10

Tableau, data visualization tool, 265
Taft-Hartley Act, 179
talent management, 174
Tallahassee Memorial Healthcare (TMH), 201

target marketing strategy, 233
taxes, 52
teaching hospitals, 23
technological progress, 51–52
technology plans, 245
telehealth, 95, 336
telemedicine, 287
TikTok, 237
tort, 321–322
tort reform, 322
training and development, 175, 182
training and education, 274
transformational leadership theory, 309–310
turnover, 30–31
21st Century Cures Act, 258

underrepresented minorities (URMs), 352
URMs. *See* Underrepresented minorities
U.S. Department of Labor (USDOL), 77
U.S. Department of Veterans Affairs, 22
U. S. House of Representatives, 319
U.S. Public Health Service (USPHS), 76
U. S. Senate, 319
U.S. uninsured population, 94
USDOL. *See* U.S. Department of Labor
USPHS. *See* U.S. Public Health Service

VA. *See* Veterans Affairs
value-based care, 93, 145, 168–169, 292, 322
Value Modifier (VM) Program, 107, 108

Veterans Affairs (VA), 22, 276, 331
vicarious liability, 322
vision centers, 24
VM Program. *See* Value Modifier Program

WhatsApp, 236
WHO. *See* World Health Organization
workforce. *See* healthcare workforce management
workforce design, in healthcare, 175
    best practices, 176
    challenges, 175
    key elements, 175
workforce development, 95
World Health Organization (WHO), 74
    data competencies description, 265
    health definition, 74, 85
    health ethics definition, 320
    health policy definition, 86
wound care centers, 24
written policies, 274

X (formerly Twitter), 237

YouTube, 236, 237, 266

Z codes, 103